Clinical Updates in Physiotherapy for Musculoskeletal Disorders

Clinical Updates in Physiotherapy for Musculoskeletal Disorders

Guest Editor

Santiago Navarro Ledesma

MDPI

Basel • Beijing • Wuhan • Barcelona • Belgrade • Novi Sad • Cluj • Manchester

Guest Editor
Santiago Navarro Ledesma
Department of Physical
Therapy
University of Granada
Melilla
Spain

Editorial Office
MDPI AG
Grosspeteranlage 5
4052 Basel, Switzerland

This is a reprint of the Special Issue, published open access by the journal *Journal of Clinical Medicine* (ISSN 2077-0383), freely accessible at: https://www.mdpi.com/journal/jcm/special_issues/294K1H451Q.

For citation purposes, cite each article independently as indicated on the article page online and as indicated below:

Lastname, A.A.; Lastname, B.B. Article Title. *Journal Name* **Year**, *Volume Number*, Page Range.

ISBN 978-3-7258-7318-0 (Hbk)
ISBN 978-3-7258-7319-7 (PDF)
https://doi.org/10.3390/books978-3-7258-7319-7

Contents

About the Editor

Santiago Navarro Ledesma

Santiago Navarro Ledesma is an Associate Professor for the Department of Physiotherapy and Director of the Chair of Clinical Psychoneuroimmunology at the University of Granada. His teaching, research, and clinical work focus on musculoskeletal physiotherapy, clinical psychoneuroimmunology, and lifestyle as a therapeutic cornerstone, integrating exercise, sleep, stress, nutrition, and inflammation into the management of pain and disability. He holds two doctoral degrees from the University of Málaga, where he received the Extraordinary Doctorate Award, and a PhD in Medical Sciences from the University of Antwerp (Belgium), with international distinction. His expertise is centered on the study and treatment of musculoskeletal disorders from a biopsychosocial and immunometabolic perspective, with a particular interest in translating scientific evidence into clinical physiotherapy practice. He maintains an active academic and scientific profile through the publication of scientific papers, the supervision and co-supervision of doctoral theses, the leadership of a research group and research projects, and active participation in numerous national and international conferences.

Journal of
Clinical Medicine

MDPI

Article

Multidimensional Recovery Trajectories Following Physiotherapy with or Without Pain Education in People with Chronic Low Back Pain

Ahmed Alalawi

Department of Medical Rehabilitation Sciences, Faculty of Applied Medical Sciences, Umm Al-Qura University, Makkah 24382, Saudi Arabia; amalawi@uqu.edu.sa

Abstract

Background/Objective: To investigate short-term multidimensional recovery trajectories after physiotherapy with or without adjunctive pain education in individuals with Chronic low back pain (CLBP). **Methods:** This was a secondary analysis of a randomized controlled trial (RCT) of 92 participants (46 participants per group) comparing physiotherapy alone with physiotherapy plus pain education. Changes from baseline values over six weeks were calculated for pain intensity, disability, psychological well-being, and self-efficacy to define short-term recovery trajectories across domains, and were standardized prior to analysis. Descriptive characterization of recovery dimensions by principal component analysis and identification of different recovery trajectory clusters by k-means clustering were performed. Sensitivity analyses with multinomial logistic regression were performed to determine robustness after adjustment for baseline characteristics. **Results:** Three recovery trajectories were found: minimal recovery (n = 40), psychosocial-dominant recovery (n = 26), and global recovery (n = 26). In the physiotherapy-only group, participants were classified as minimal recovery (61%) or psychosocial-dominant recovery (39%), with no cases of global recovery. In contradistinction, 57% of participants receiving physiotherapy with pain education were classified as within the global recovery trajectory, with fewer classified as minimal recovery (26%) or psychosocial-dominant recovery (17%). Psychosocial-dominant recovery occurred in both groups, and was characterized by large improvements in psychological well-being and self-efficacy with more modest changes in pain and disability. The distribution of recovery trajectories between treatment groups was large ($\chi^2(2) = 36.25$, $p < 0.001$; Cramer's V = 0.63). **Conclusions:** Distinct short-term recovery trajectories were found after physiotherapy with or without pain education in individuals with CLBP, reflecting heterogeneity in multidimensional recovery that is not reflected in mean-based outcome analyses.

Keywords: chronic low back pain; recovery trajectories; pain education; physiotherapy; multidimensional outcomes

1. Introduction

Low back pain (LBP) represents a major cause of disability worldwide and remains a major challenge for healthcare systems, despite extensive research and development of clinical guidelines [1–3]. In addition to the severity of pain, people with chronic low back pain (CLBP) often experience ongoing disability, low psychological well-being, and low confidence in their ability to cope with symptoms, which reflects the multidimensional nature of the condition [4,5]. Although physiotherapy-based interventions are widely recommended and routinely implemented, the effects of these treatments tend to be small, and large variability in individual responses is consistently observed [6,7].

CLBP is largely conceptualized within a biopsychosocial model. According to this model, biological factors interact with psychological and social factors to influence pain and disability [5,8,9]. The purpose of pain education is to change maladaptive beliefs about pain and reduce perceived threat [10]. It also promotes an adaptive understanding of central sensitization and pain mechanisms [10–12]. These interventions can affect multiple domains simultaneously by modifying the cognitive appraisal of pain. These domains include psychological well-being, self-efficacy, and functional engagement [13]. Improvements in psychological well-being may enhance motivation and resilience [14]. Increased confidence in symptom management may support activity despite pain [14–16]. Recovery may therefore occur as coordinated change across pain and disability and psychological outcomes rather than single measure improvement. Multivariate trajectory approaches may be appropriate to capture these multidimensional patterns of recovery that mean-based analyses may miss.

Despite the multidimensional and heterogeneous nature of LBP, most randomized controlled trials continue to measure treatment effectiveness by mean changes in isolated outcomes (mainly pain intensity or disability). This can be seen in many RCTs where pooled treatment effects are primarily reported as average between-group differences in pain and functional limitation [17–19]. While this approach is appropriate for estimating the average treatment effect, it has limited consideration of normal individual variability [20–22]. Consequently, it offers limited information on how patients recover individually in several domains of outcomes. Clinically meaningful patterns of improvement, for example, changes that do not occur simultaneously between symptoms and psychological outcomes, may therefore be masked when recovery is summarized with aggregate statistics only [23,24]. This limitation is especially relevant in LBP, in which improvements in coping, self-efficacy, or well-being may be independent of, or precede, improvements in pain and disability [4].

In response to these limitations, an emerging interest has emerged in approaches that characterize recovery as a multidimensional and heterogeneous process rather than a uniform change in a single outcome. Several studies have found subgroups of patients with different recovery profiles, highlighting that individuals may follow different courses despite receiving similar interventions [24–27]. However, much of this literature has focused on long-term trajectories or single outcome domains, most commonly pain or disability. Recovery trajectories incorporating both clinical and psychosocial outcomes after intervention remain relatively understudied, leaving the immediate post-treatment recovery of patients across multiple domains incompletely understood.

In a recent study, improvements in psychological well-being partially mediated reductions in disability following a program of pain education combined with physiotherapy, whereas self-efficacy did not [28]. Although the study provided insight into possible pathways of change, it did not examine whether patients demonstrated distinct multidimensional recovery trajectories over time. Exploring how outcomes change in parallel across domains may therefore provide insight beyond mediation models that focus on isolated causal pathways.

Therefore, the aim of this study was to identify short-term multidimensional recovery trajectories following physiotherapy with or without pain education in individuals with CLBP. It was hypothesized that different recovery trajectories would be identified across pain, disability, psychological well-being, and self-efficacy, and that the distribution of these patterns would differ between treatment groups.

https://doi.org/10.3390/jcm15062320

2. Materials and Methods

2.1. Study Design

This study is a secondary analysis of a previously published randomized controlled trial (RCT) [13]. The study examined the effect of adding a structured pain education program to physiotherapy in individuals with CLBP [13]. The primary trial was a two-arm, parallel-group trial with random assignment of participants to standard physiotherapy or physiotherapy combined with pain education.

Block randomization (block size = 4) was used. The sequences of allocations were pre-generated and hidden in sealed, opaque envelopes, which were opened sequentially once participants were enrolled. The allocation of treatment was not disclosed to the participants, and the assessments of outcomes were performed by physiotherapists who were blinded to group assignment. Additional details about the study methodology have been reported elsewhere [13].

The trial was conducted in accordance with the Declaration of Helsinki. The study was approved by the Institutional Ethics Committee (RP/114/2021) and registered in advance on the Clinical Trial Registry (CTRI/2021/08/035963). The current study is based on the initial trial [13], with an emphasis on short-term follow-up changes and multivariate analysis of recovery trajectories at the 6-week follow-up.

2.2. Participants

Participants were recruited for the original RCT until the target sample size was reached. Adults aged 18 to 60 years with a clinical diagnosis of non-specific low back pain persisting for more than three months were eligible for inclusion. Diagnosis was established by a qualified medical professional based on clinical assessment. Participants were excluded if they failed to attend more than two scheduled intervention sessions or chose to withdraw from the study. Written informed consent was obtained from all participants prior to enrollment. A total of 92 participants were available for analysis, with 46 allocated to the physiotherapy-only (control) group and 46 to the physiotherapy with pain education group.

2.3. Interventions

2.3.1. Physiotherapy (Control Group)

Participants in both groups received a standardized physiotherapy intervention for LBP, consistent with current clinical practice guidelines [7,29]. The program included recommendations to stay active, superficial heat application, lumbar stretching, aerobic conditioning via stationary cycling, and core stabilization with a focus on trunk strength and endurance. The sessions were about 40 min long and provided based on a pre-established protocol [13].

2.3.2. Pain Education (Intervention Group)

In addition to the physiotherapy program, participants assigned to the intervention group received a structured pain education program. The program covered the main concepts regarding chronic pain, pain neurophysiology, central sensitization, fear-avoidance, and the role of psychological and social factors in pain perception. Presentation, visual aids, and interactive discussion were used to deliver the educational program.

The intervention included two pain education sessions per week for the first three weeks, with reflective question-and-answer discussions in weeks four and five. A printed pain education handbook was designed specifically for the trial and distributed to participants at the end of the intervention period [10–12].

https://doi.org/10.3390/jcm15062320

2.4. Outcome Measures

Clinical and psychosocial outcomes were measured at baseline and post-intervention (6 weeks). The present analysis focuses on change over this interval in pain intensity, disability, psychological well-being, and self-efficacy. All outcomes were collected by assessors who were trained and blinded to the group allocation.

Pain intensity was measured using a 10-point Visual Analog Scale (VAS), with 0 representing no pain and 10 representing the worst imaginable pain. The VAS is a valid and reliable tool for measuring pain intensity [30]. Disability was measured using the Roland–Morris Disability Questionnaire (RMDQ), which has 24 items with a range of 0 to 24; the higher the score, the greater the disability [31]. The validity and reliability of the RMDQ have been established [31].

The psychological well-being was measured using the World Health Organization Five-Item Well-Being Index (WHO-5) [32]. The instrument comprises five items that measure participants' current emotional well-being. Item responses are summed to give a raw score between 0 and 25; the lower the score, the poorer the well-being. For interpretability, raw scores were standardized to a 0–100 scale by multiplying the total score by 4, with higher values indicating better psychological well-being. The WHO-5 has good validity, reliability, and responsiveness in both clinical and general populations [32].

The General Self-Efficacy Scale (GSE) was used to measure self-efficacy [33]. GSE is a 10-item self-report instrument that assesses a person's perceived ability to cope with difficult situations. The range is 10–40, with higher scores indicating greater perceived self-efficacy. The scale has a high construct validity and internal consistency between different populations [33].

2.5. Baseline and Clinical Covariates

In addition to the primary outcomes, a set of demographic and clinical variables was collected at baseline to support adjusted and sensitivity analyses. These variables were selected a priori based on their established associations with pain severity, disability, and recovery trajectories in individuals with CLBP [2,4,34].

Age and sex were used as demographic variables. Clinical and lifestyle-related variables included body mass index (BMI), smoking (yes/no), the duration of LBP (in months), and self-reported sleep duration. These variables were not treated as outcomes in the present analysis. Rather, they were applied to (i) determine baseline comparability between treatment groups and (ii) adjust multivariable models in sensitivity analysis of the robustness of recovery trajectory classification and group differences.

2.6. Statistical Analysis

Baseline characteristics were summarized by treatment group using means and standard deviations for continuous variables and frequencies with percentages for categorical variables. For each participant, within-participant change scores were calculated as the difference between post-intervention and baseline values for all outcomes: VAS, RMDQ, WHO-5, and GSE. These changes represented the treatment effect over the 6-week intervention period. In the present study, recovery trajectories were defined as short-term change between baseline and post-intervention across multiple outcome domains. For multivariate analyses, the within-participant change scores were standardized to z-scores to ensure comparable scaling across outcomes [35], before dimension reduction and clustering.

2.6.1. Principal Component Analysis

Principal component analysis (PCA) [36] was applied to the standardized within-participant change values of VAS, RMDQ, WHO-5, and GSE to explore underlying dimen-

https://doi.org/10.3390/jcm15062320

sions of short-term recovery trajectories across all outcomes. Components were retained based on eigenvalues > 1, the amount of variance explained, or considering the elbow criterion in the scree plot [35–37]. Variable loadings were examined to characterize the contribution of each outcome to the derived components [38].

2.6.2. Recovery Trajectory Identification

Recovery trajectory clusters were identified using k-means clustering [39] applied to the standardized multidimensional change-score space. Solutions with two to four clusters were evaluated. The optimal number of clusters was determined based on a combination of within-cluster sum of squares, mean silhouette width, and clinical interpretability of cluster profiles [40].

A three-cluster solution was selected as the final model. Clusters were labeled post hoc according to their mean change profiles across pain, disability, psychological well-being, and self-efficacy, resulting in the following recovery trajectories: minimal recovery, psychosocial-dominant recovery, and global recovery. Each recovery trajectory was summarized using the mean of within-participant change scores, standard deviations, and 95% confidence intervals for all outcomes. These summaries were used to describe the clinical and psychosocial profiles of each trajectory.

2.6.3. Group Comparisons of Recovery Trajectories

Differences in the distribution of recovery trajectories between treatment groups were assessed using a chi-square test of independence. Effect size was quantified using Cramer's V. For comparisons involving sparse cells, particularly when examining the presence versus absence of global recovery, Fisher's exact test was used in place of the chi-square test.

2.6.4. Sensitivity Analyses

Additional sensitivity analyses using multinomial logistic regression [41] were undertaken to assess the robustness of recovery trajectory cluster classification after adjustment for baseline characteristics (e.g., age, sex, duration of LBP, baseline pain and disability, and smoking status). Detailed results are provided in the Supplementary Materials. Analyses were performed in R software (version 4.5.2) and conducted using complete-case data.

3. Results

3.1. Participants and Baseline Characteristics

Ninety-two participants were included in the analyses, with 46 allocated to the control group and 46 to the pain education group. Baseline data were complete for all reported variables (Table 1). Groups were broadly comparable at baseline: age, pain intensity, well-being, self-efficacy, body mass index, and hours of sleep all showed small standardized mean differences (SMDs $\leq$ 0.27). More substantial imbalances were observed for the duration of LBP (35.85 [50.37] vs. 20.93 [34.33] months; SMD = −0.35), with longer symptom duration in the control group. The pain education group also included a higher proportion of smokers (26.1% vs. 8.7%).

Table 1. Baseline characteristics of participants by treatment group.

Variable	Level	Control (n = 46)	Pain Education (n = 46)
Age (years)		42.52 (13.32)	42.02 (8.24)
Sex	Female	35 (76.1)	25 (54.3)
	Male	11 (23.9)	21 (45.7)
Duration of low back pain (months)		35.85 (50.37)	20.93 (34.33)

https://doi.org/10.3390/jcm15062320

Table 1. *Cont.*

Variable	Level	Control (n = 46)	Pain Education (n = 46)
VAS (0–10)		5.98 (1.71)	5.70 (1.66)
RMDQ (0–24)		15.02 (4.78)	12.65 (4.71)
WHO-5 (0–100)		54.41 (18.56)	53.48 (17.53)
GSE (10–40)		25.78 (6.40)	25.83 (5.61)
BMI (kg/m^2)		26.96 (4.08)	27.76 (4.28)
Hours of sleep (per night)		6.33 (1.73)	6.74 (1.32)
Smoker	No	42 (91.3)	34 (73.9)
	Yes	4 (8.7)	12 (26.1)
Level of activity	Light	14 (30.4)	17 (37.0)
	Moderate	23 (50.0)	20 (43.5)
	Very active	9 (19.6)	9 (19.6)

Values are mean (SD) unless otherwise stated; categorical variables are presented as n (%). GSE = General Self-Efficacy Scale; WHO-5 = World Health Organization-5 Well-Being Index; RMDQ = Roland–Morris Disability Questionnaire; VAS = Visual Analogue Scale for pain; BMI = body mass index.

3.2. Recovery Dimensions and Trajectory Cluster Identification

Clustering of multidimensional change scores identified three distinct recovery trajectories. The three recovery trajectories are summarized in Table 2. The minimal recovery trajectory (n = 40) was characterized by small average improvements across all outcomes: pain intensity decreased by −0.83 (SD 1.77; 95% CI: [−1.39]–[−0.26]), disability decreased by −1.58 (SD 3.20; 95% CI [−2.60]–[−0.55]), and gains in well-being and self-efficacy were modest (WHO-5 2.50 [SD: 7.62]; 95% CI 0.06–4.94; GSE 0.75 [SD: 2.22]; 95% CI 0.04–1.46).

Table 2. Recovery trajectory clusters by outcome (mean change [SD] and 95% confidence intervals.

Outcomes	Minimal Recovery (n = 40)		Psychosocial-Dominant Recovery (n = 26)		Global Recovery (n = 26)	
	Mean (SD)	95% CI	Mean (SD)	95% CI	Mean (SD)	95% CI
VAS (0–10)	−0.83 (1.77)	−1.39, −0.26	−1.54 (1.58)	−2.18, −0.9	−4.00 (1.30)	−4.52, −3.48
RMDQ (0–24)	−1.58 (3.20)	−2.6, −0.55	−1.73 (2.16)	−2.6, −0.86	−9.77 (3.44)	−11.16, −8.38
WHO-5 (0–100)	2.50 (7.62)	0.06, 4.94	4.92 (7.03)	2.09, 7.76	24.19 (12.28)	19.23, 29.15
GSE 10–40)	0.75 (2.22)	0.04, 1.46	9.46 (2.75)	8.35, 10.57	2.69 (4.36)	0.93, 4.45

Values are mean change (SD) from baseline to post-intervention. Negative values for pain intensity and disability represent improvement; positive values for well-being and self-efficacy represent improvement. 95% CI = 95% confidence interval. GSE = General Self-Efficacy Scale; WHO-5 = World Health Organization-5 Well-Being Index; RMDQ = Roland–Morris Disability Questionnaire; VAS = Visual Analogue Scale for pain.

The psychosocial-dominant recovery trajectory (n = 26) showed a different profile: pain and disability improved only modestly (VAS −1.54 [SD: 1.58]; 95% CI [−2.18]–[−0.90]; RMDQ −1.73 [SD: 2.16], 95% CI [−2.60]–[−0.86]), whereas self-efficacy and well-being increased substantially (GSE 9.46 [SD: 2.75], 95% CI 8.35–10.57) and well-being (WHO-5 4.92 [SD: 7.03], 95% CI 2.09–7.76).

The global recovery trajectory (n = 26) showed large and coherent improvements across domains, with substantial reductions in pain (VAS −4.00 [SD: 1.30], 95% CI [−4.52]–[−3.48]) and disability (RMDQ −9.77 [SD: 3.44], 95% CI [−11.16]–[−8.38]), accompanied by marked increases in well-being (WHO-5 24.19 [SD: 12.28], 95% CI 19.23–29.15) and moderate gains in self-efficacy (GSE 2.69 [SD: 4.36], 95% CI 0.93–4.45).

Together, these trajectories represent distinct magnitudes and combinations of short-term change across clinical and psychological outcomes.

https://doi.org/10.3390/jcm15062320

3.3. Distribution of Recovery Trajectories by Treatment Group

The distribution of recovery patterns differed between groups (Table 3, Figure 1). In the control group, participants were classified exclusively into the minimal recovery (28/46; 61%) and psychosocial-dominant recovery trajectories (18/46; 39%), with no participants achieving global recovery. In contrast, in the pain education group, more than half of the participants were classified as global recovery (26/46; 57%), while substantially fewer were classified as minimal recovery (12/46; 26%) or psychosocial-dominant recovery (8/46; 17%).

Table 3. Distribution of recovery trajectory by treatment group (n and %).

Trajectory	Control n (%)	Pain Education n (%)
Minimal recovery	28 (61)	12 (26)
Psychosocial-dominant recovery	18 (39)	8 (17)
Global recovery	0 (0.0)	26 (57)

Values are n (% of group). Percentages are calculated within the treatment group (columns sum to 100%). Minimal recovery = minimal change in pain, disability, well-being, and self-efficacy; Psychosocial-dominant recovery = modest symptom changes with large gains in self-efficacy and well-being; Global recovery = large, coherent improvements across all outcomes.

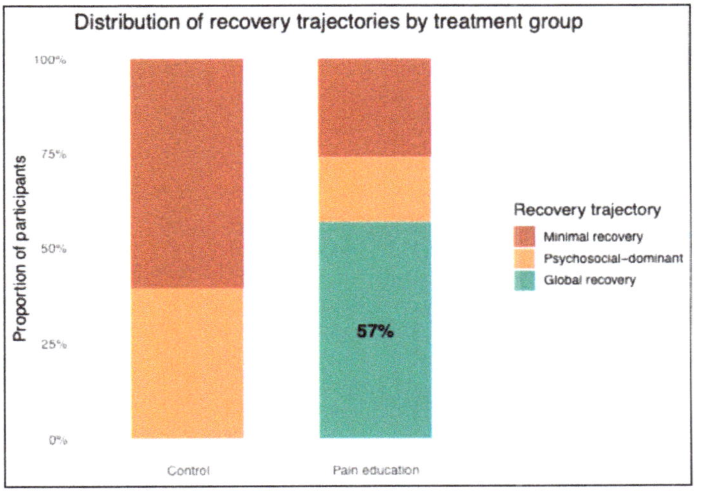

Figure 1. Distribution of short-term recovery trajectories by treatment group. Participants in the control group were exclusively classified within the minimal recovery and psychosocial-dominant recovery trajectories, with none achieving global recovery. In contrast, a higher proportion of participants in the pain education group were classified as being in the global recovery trajectory.

The association between treatment allocation and recovery trajectory was statistically large and highly significant ($\chi^2(2) = 36.25$, $p < 0.001$; Cramer's V = 0.63). When recovery trajectories were dichotomized into global recovery versus all other patterns, global recovery occurred in 26 of 46 participants (57%) in the pain education group and none of the 46 participants in the control group (Fisher's exact $p < 0.001$). Together, these findings indicate that pain education was associated with a marked redistribution of recovery trajectories toward the global recovery trajectory.

3.4. Sensitivity Analyses

Sensitivity analyses using multinomial logistic regression, adjusting for baseline pain, disability, age, sex, smoking status, and symptom duration, yielded results consistent with the primary analyses. The association between pain education and psychosocial-dominant

https://doi.org/10.3390/jcm15062320

recovery trajectory was not statistically significant (adjusted OR 1.61, 95% CI 0.41–6.29; $p = 0.49$). Estimation of the global recovery trajectory was limited by the absence of global recovery cases in the control group (Table S1).

4. Discussion

4.1. Summary of Findings

This secondary analysis identified three distinct short-term recovery trajectories following physiotherapy alone or physiotherapy combined with pain education in people with CLBP. These trajectories reflected different multidimensional changes across pain, disability, psychological well-being, and self-efficacy, rather than differences in a single outcome. The trajectories were labeled minimal recovery, Psychosocial-dominant recovery, and global recovery.

The distribution of recovery trajectories differed between treatment groups. More than half of the participants who received physiotherapy with pain education were classified within the global recovery trajectory, showing large and consistent improvements across all measured outcomes. In contrast, no participants in the physiotherapy-only group were classified within the global recovery trajectory. Participants in this group were classified only as minimal recovery or psychosocial-dominant trajectory.

A psychosocial-dominant recovery trajectory was observed in both groups, characterized by improvements in well-being and self-efficacy alongside relatively modest changes in pain and disability. After adjustment for baseline factors, this pattern was not clearly associated with treatment allocation. Overall, the findings suggest that adding pain education to the physiotherapy program was associated with a marked redistribution of short-term recovery patterns, particularly an increased representation of the global recovery trajectory.

4.2. Global Recovery Pattern

The global recovery trajectory was characterized by large improvements in multiple outcomes that occurred simultaneously (e.g., pain intensity, disability, psychological well-being, and self-efficacy), indicating coherent change across multiple outcome domains rather than isolated improvement in symptoms. This trajectory resulted from an exploratory and data-driven clustering approach. Thus, it describes an observed recovery pattern rather than a discrete, mechanistically defined recovery state. Global recovery was only observed in participants who received the pain education plus physiotherapy group, indicating a significant redistribution of recovery trajectories between treatment groups and movement towards broad and multidimensional improvement.

However, this observed difference in recovery distribution should not be interpreted as evidence that pain education alone fully accounts for the observed global recovery pattern. Although baseline characteristics were broadly comparable between groups, moderate imbalances were observed in symptom duration and smoking status. Sensitivity analyses adjusting for baseline pain, disability, age, sex, smoking status, and symptom duration yielded findings consistent with the primary analyses (Table S1). Nevertheless, the absence of global recovery cases in the control group limited the precision of adjusted effect estimates. Accordingly, these findings indicate an association between treatment allocation and recovery trajectory classification and should not be interpreted as evidence of a definitive causal effect.

The pattern of global recovery seen in this study is consistent with the current models of LBP that highlight the interdependence of pain, psychological processes, and coping capacity [2,4]. The simultaneous improvements in these outcomes could be explained by alterations in pain-related understandings and threat appraisals that may influence multiple domains of outcome at the same time, not just pain alone. In support of this interpretation,

https://doi.org/10.3390/jcm15062320

recent syntheses of pain neuroscience education report modest average effects on pain and disability but more consistent effects on psychosocial outcomes, and with substantial heterogeneity across individuals [1,17]. Taken together, this body of evidence suggests that there may be broad, multidimensional recovery in a subset of patients and that mean-based analyses may not adequately capture this recovery.

The physiotherapy intervention assigned to the control group was delivered in accordance with current clinical practice guidelines and reflects standard evidence-based care [1–3]. Although no participants in the physiotherapy-only group were classified within the global recovery trajectory, this finding should be interpreted with caution. It should not be interpreted as suggesting that physiotherapy alone is incapable of producing global recovery. Rather, within this sample and the six-week follow-up period, global recovery was observed only among participants who received additional pain education. Several methodological considerations may help explain this pattern. The sample size in this secondary analysis was modest and not specifically powered to detect differences in trajectory distribution, and the clustering approach was exploratory and data-driven. Moderate baseline imbalances were also observed, and although adjusted sensitivity analyses yielded consistent findings, residual confounding cannot be excluded. In addition, the follow-up period reflects short-term recovery only, and broader multidimensional improvements following physiotherapy alone may emerge over longer time horizons.

4.3. Psychosocial Recovery Pattern

The pattern of recovery in the psychosocial-dominant trajectory was characterized by large improvements in psychological well-being and self-efficacy with modest improvements in pain intensity and disability. This profile suggests a type of recovery where psychosocial adaptation improves more quickly than physical symptoms, rather than a partial or incomplete response to treatment. Importantly, this trajectory was found in both treatment groups, indicating that it is not specific to the addition of pain education.

After controlling for baseline characteristics, the analyses showed no clear association between allocation to the treatment arm and classification within the psychosocial-dominant recovery trajectory (see Supplementary Table S1). Consequently, the observed improvements in well-being and self-efficacy cannot be attributed solely to the pain education component of the intervention. More likely, these improvements reflect participants' responsiveness to the physiotherapy intervention provided to both groups. All participants undertook a standardized physiotherapy regimen that adhered to guidelines and included advice to remain active, supervised exercise sessions, and repeated therapist–patient interactions. The structured nature of this rehabilitation program may have facilitated improvements in psychological well-being and self-efficacy, independent of the additional pain education material. Indeed, similar psychosocial-dominant response patterns have been observed in previous trajectory and subgroup studies, in which psychological improvements occurred despite relatively modest reductions in pain intensity or functional disability [24,26].

Clinically, this trajectory should not be interpreted as treatment failure. Rather, it may represent an intermediate or alternative form of recovery in which psychological adaptation precedes, or occurs independently of, symptomatic improvement. However, given the short follow-up period, it remains unclear whether psychosocial-dominant recovery is a stable trajectory, a transient response, or a precursor to later improvements in pain and disability. Longer-term follow-up is required to determine whether this trajectory translates into sustained functional recovery or reduced healthcare use over time.

https://doi.org/10.3390/jcm15062320

4.4. Clinical Implications

The findings of this study indicate that short-term recovery following treatment for CLBP is heterogeneous, with patients exhibiting different recovery trajectories over the same intervention period. These differences are not apparent when outcomes are summarized using single outcomes or mean changes alone [23,24], which may obscure clinically meaningful variation in how patients respond to treatment.

The high proportion of participants classified within the global recovery trajectory in the pain education group should not be interpreted as evidence that pain education reliably produces comprehensive recovery at the individual level. Rather, the results suggest that some patients experience broad improvements across pain, disability, and psychosocial domains, while others demonstrate predominantly psychological improvements, with more modest changes in symptoms.

Importantly, improvements in psychological well-being and self-efficacy may represent meaningful clinical progress, even in the absence of large reductions in pain or disability. However, the present findings do not support changes in treatment selection, stratification, or clinical decision-making based on recovery trajectory membership. Instead, these results support a broader, multidimensional view of recovery and suggest that trajectory-based interpretation of outcomes may improve understanding of heterogeneous short-term responses to treatment in individuals with LBP.

4.5. Strengths and Limitations

One of the strengths of this study is that a multivariate, trajectory-based analytic approach was used to investigate the short-term recovery after intervention for people with CLBP. By incorporating changes across pain, disability, psychological well-being, and self-efficacy, this approach goes beyond single-outcome or mean-based summaries and offers a more comprehensive perspective on heterogeneous responses to recovery, a perspective increasingly advocated [42]. The use of data from an RCT provides additional internal validity, enhancing the interpretation of observed recovery trajectories as reflecting differences in response rather than systematic variation in intervention delivery. In addition, sensitivity analyses based on adjusted multinomial models were performed to assess the robustness of trajectory-group associations, accounting for statistical uncertainty.

However, several limitations should also be noted. Recovery trajectories in this study were determined using an exploratory, data-driven clustering approach and, as such, should be interpreted as descriptive rather than definitive classifications. The sample size was based on the primary RCT and was not specifically calculated for the exploratory clustering analyses performed in this secondary study. An additional limitation relates to the duration of follow-up. The identified recovery trajectories reflect patterns observed over a six-week period only. It remains unclear whether these trajectories represent sustained recovery states or short-term treatment responses, and their prognostic significance over longer follow-up is unknown. Future studies incorporating extended follow-up are required to evaluate the stability of multidimensional recovery patterns. Furthermore, the absence of global recovery cases in the control group led to quasi-complete separation in the adjusted multinomial models, limiting the precision and reliability of independent effect estimates for this trajectory.

5. Conclusions

This secondary analysis identified three different short-term recovery trajectories after physiotherapy with or without pain education for people with CLBP. Rather than reflecting change in a single outcome, these trajectories described parallel changes in pain intensity, disability, psychological well-being, and self-efficacy over the six weeks of intervention. Most of the participants who received physiotherapy with pain education were classified within a global recovery trajectory. In contrast, those who were assigned to physiotherapy alone were represented only within the minimal recovery and psychosocial-dominant trajectories. The psychosocial-dominant trajectory was observed in both groups and characterized improvements in psychological outcomes, with relatively small changes in pain and disability.

Supplementary Materials: The following supporting information can be downloaded at https://www.mdpi.com/article/10.3390/jcm15062320/s1. Table S1: Multinomial logistic regression for recovery trajectories (reference: Minimal recovery trajectory).

Funding: This research received no external funding.

Institutional Review Board Statement: The original randomized controlled trial from which the dataset was derived received approval from the Institutional Ethics Committee of SKIMS (reference RP/114/2021) and was registered with the Clinical Trial Registry (CTRI/2021/08/035963). The ethical approval refers to the original randomized controlled trial from which the dataset was derived. The present study is a secondary analysis of that trial and did not involve new participant recruitment or data collection.

Informed Consent Statement: The ethical approval refers to the original randomized controlled trial from which the dataset was derived. The present study is a secondary analysis of that trial and did not involve new participant recruitment or data collection.

Data Availability Statement: This is a secondary analysis of a published randomized controlled trial. The data is available publicly. The R code used to perform the analyses was implemented in R software (version 4.5.2) and is available from the author upon reasonable request.

Acknowledgments: The author acknowledges the investigators of the original randomized controlled trial for conducting the study and making the dataset available for secondary analysis.

Conflicts of Interest: The author declares no conflicts of interest.

References

1. Foster, N.E.; Anema, J.R.; Cherkin, D.; Chou, R.; Cohen, S.P.; Gross, D.P.; Ferreira, P.H.; Fritz, J.M.; Koes, B.W.; Peul, W.; et al. Prevention and treatment of low back pain: Evidence, challenges, and promising directions. *Lancet* **2018**, *391*, 2368–2383. [CrossRef]
2. Hartvigsen, J.; Hancock, M.J.; Kongsted, A.; Louw, Q.; Ferreira, M.L.; Genevay, S.; Hoy, D.; Karppinen, J.; Pransky, G.; Sieper, J.; et al. What low back pain is and why we need to pay attention. *Lancet* **2018**, *391*, 2356–2367. [CrossRef]
3. Aldera, M.; Alturkistany, A.; Al Rayes, H.; Rada, G.; Alsulaimany, H.H.; Alsobayel, H.I.; Alghamdi, K.; Awwad, W.; Alyamani, O.A.; Bedaiwi, M.; et al. Saudi Clinical Practice Guideline for the Assessment and Management of Low Back Pain and Sciatica in Adults. *J. Clin. Med.* **2026**, *15*, 528. [CrossRef] [PubMed]
4. Lee, H.; Hübscher, M.; Moseley, G.L.; Kamper, S.J.; Traeger, A.C.; Mansell, G.; McAuley, J.H. How does pain lead to disability? A systematic review and meta-analysis of mediation studies in people with back and neck pain. *Pain* **2015**, *156*, 988–997. [CrossRef] [PubMed]
5. Vlaeyen, J.W.; Linton, S.J. Fear-avoidance model of chronic musculoskeletal pain: 12 years on. *Pain* **2012**, *153*, 1144–1147. [CrossRef] [PubMed]
6. Costa, L.d.C.M.; Maher, C.G.; Hancock, M.J.; McAuley, J.H.; Herbert, R.D.; Costa, L.O. The prognosis of acute and persistent low-back pain: A meta-analysis. *CMAJ* **2012**, *184*, E613–E624. [CrossRef]
7. Qaseem, A.; Wilt, T.J.; McLean, R.M.; Forciea, M.A.; Clinical Guidelines Committee of the American College of Physicians; Denberg, T.D.; Barry, M.J.; Boyd, C.; Chow, R.D.; Fitterman, N.; et al. Noninvasive treatments for acute, subacute, and chronic low back pain: A clinical practice guideline from the American College of Physicians. *Ann. Intern. Med.* **2017**, *166*, 514–530. [CrossRef]
8. Gatchel, R.J.; Peng, Y.B.; Peters, M.L.; Fuchs, P.N.; Turk, D.C. The biopsychosocial approach to chronic pain: Scientific advances and future directions. *Psychol. Bull.* **2007**, *133*, 581. [CrossRef]
9. McCracken, L.M.; Morley, S. The psychological flexibility model: A basis for integration and progress in psychological approaches to chronic pain management. *J. Pain* **2014**, *15*, 221–234. [CrossRef]
10. Moseley, G.L.; Butler, D.S. *The Explain Pain Handbook: Protectometer*; Noigroup: Adelaide, Australia, 2015.

https://doi.org/10.3390/jcm15062320

11. Moseley, G.L.; Butler, D.S. *Explain Pain Supercharged*; Noigroup: Adelaide, Australia, 2017.
12. Sharma, S.; Jensen, M.P.; Moseley, G.L.; Abbott, J.H. Pain education for patients with non-specific low back pain in Nepal: Protocol of a feasibility randomised clinical trial (PEN-LBP Trial). *BMJ Open* **2018**, *8*, e022423. [CrossRef]
13. Sidiq, M.; Muzaffar, T.; Janakiraman, B.; Masoodi, S.; Vasanthi, R.K.; Ramachandran, A.; Bansal, N.; Chahal, A.; Kashoo, F.Z.; Rizvi, M.R.; et al. Effects of pain education on disability, pain, quality of life, and self-efficacy in chronic low back pain: A randomized controlled trial. *PLoS ONE* **2024**, *19*, e0294302. [CrossRef] [PubMed]
14. Ryum, T.; Stiles, T.C. Changes in pain catastrophizing, fear-avoidance beliefs, and pain self-efficacy mediate changes in pain intensity on disability in the treatment of chronic low back pain. *Pain Rep.* **2023**, *8*, e1092. [CrossRef] [PubMed]
15. Jackson, T.; Wang, Y.; Wang, Y.; Fan, H. Self-efficacy and chronic pain outcomes: A meta-analytic review. *J. Pain* **2014**, *15*, 800–814. [CrossRef]
16. Linton, S.J.; Shaw, W.S. Impact of psychological factors in the experience of pain. *Phys. Ther.* **2011**, *91*, 700–711. [CrossRef]
17. Cancela, J.G.; Vázquez, O.C.; Ledesma, S.N.; Pruimboom, L. The effectiveness of pain neuroscience education in people with chronic non-specific low back pain: An umbrella review with meta-analysis. *Ann. Phys. Rehabil. Med.* **2025**, *68*, 102020. [CrossRef]
18. Fleckenstein, J.; Floessel, P.; Engel, T.; Krempel, L.; Stoll, J.; Behrens, M.; Niederer, D. Individualized exercise in chronic non-specific low back pain: A systematic review with meta-analysis on the effects of exercise alone or in combination with psychological interventions on pain and disability. *J. Pain* **2022**, *23*, 1856–1873. [CrossRef]
19. Hayden, J.A.; Ellis, J.; Ogilvie, R.; Malmivaara, A.; van Tulder, M.W. Exercise therapy for chronic low back pain. *Cochrane Database Syst. Rev.* **2021**, CD009790. [CrossRef]
20. Kent, D.M.; Rothwell, P.M.; Ioannidis, J.P.; Altman, D.G.; Hayward, R.A. Assessing and reporting heterogeneity in treatment effects in clinical trials: A proposal. *Trials* **2010**, *11*, 85. [CrossRef]
21. Lesko, C.R.; Henderson, N.C.; Varadhan, R. Considerations when assessing heterogeneity of treatment effect in patient-centered outcomes research. *J. Clin. Epidemiol.* **2018**, *100*, 22–31. [CrossRef]
22. Varadhan, R.; Seeger, J.D. Estimation and reporting of heterogeneity of treatment effects. In *Developing a Protocol for Observational Comparative Effectiveness Research: A User's Guide*; Agency for Healthcare Research and Quality (US): Rockville, MD, USA, 2013.
23. Kent, P.; Keating, J.L.; Leboeuf-Yde, C. Research methods for subgrouping low back pain. *BMC Med. Res. Methodol.* **2010**, *10*, 62. [CrossRef] [PubMed]
24. Kongsted, A.; Kent, P.; Axen, I.; Downie, A.S.; Dunn, K.M. What have we learned from ten years of trajectory research in low back pain? *BMC Musculoskelet. Disord.* **2016**, *17*, 220. [CrossRef] [PubMed]
25. Ailix K.; Campbell, P.; Michaleff, Z.A.; Strauss, V.Y.; Jordan, K.P.; Bremander, A.; Croft, P.; Bergman, S. Long-term trajectories of chronic musculoskeletal pain: A 21-year prospective cohort latent class analysis. *Pain* **2021**, *162*, 1511–1520. [CrossRef]
26. Dunn, K.M.; Campbell, P.; Jordan, K.P. Long-term trajectories of back pain: Cohort study with 7-year follow-up. *BMJ Open* **2013**, *3*, e003838. [CrossRef]
27. Kongsted, A.; Andersen, C.H.; Hansen, M.M.; Hestbaek, L. Prediction of outcome in patients with low back pain–a prospective cohort study comparing clinicians' predictions with those of the start back tool. *Man. Ther.* **2016**, *21*, 120–127. [CrossRef]
28. Aladawi, A. Causal Mediation Analysis of the Effects of Pain Education on Disability and Pain Intensity in Individuals with Chronic Low Back Pain. *J. Clin. Med.* **2026**, *15*, 348. [CrossRef] [PubMed]
29. National Guideline Centre (UK). *Low Back Pain and Sciatica in over 16s: Assessment and Management*; National Institute for Health and Care Excellence (NICE): London, UK, 2016.
30. Hawker, G.A.; Mian, S.; Kendzerska, T.; French, M. Measures of adult pain: Visual analog scale for pain (vas pain), numeric rating scale for pain (nrs pain), mcgill pain questionnaire (mpq), short-form mcgill pain questionnaire (sf-mpq), chronic pain grade scale (cpgs), short form-36 bodily pain scale (sf-36 bps), and measure of intermittent and constant osteoarthritis pain (icoap). *Arthritis Care Res.* **2011**, *63*, S240–S252.
31. Roland, M.; Fairbank, J. The Roland–Morris disability questionnaire and the Oswestry disability questionnaire. *Spine* **2000**, *25*, 3115–3124. [CrossRef]
32. Topp, C.W.; Østergaard, S.D.; Søndergaard, S.; Bech, P. The WHO-5 Well-Being Index: A systematic review of the literature. *Psychother. Psychosom.* **2015**, *84*, 167–176. [CrossRef]
33. Luszczynska, A.; Scholz, U.; Schwarzer, R. The general self-efficacy scale: Multicultural validation studies. *J. Psychol.* **2005**, *139*, 439–457. [CrossRef]
34. Vlaeyen, J.W.; Linton, S.J. Fear-avoidance and its consequences in chronic musculoskeletal pain: A state of the art. *Pain* **2000**, *85*, 317–332. [CrossRef] [PubMed]
35. Jolliffe, I.T.; Cadima, J. Principal component analysis: A review and recent developments. *Philos. Trans. R. Soc. A Math. Phys. Eng. Sci.* **2016**, *374*, 20150202. [CrossRef]
36. Ringnér, M. What is principal component analysis? *Nat. Biotechnol.* **2008**, *26*, 303–304. [CrossRef]
37. Costello, A.B.; Osborne, J. Best practices in exploratory factor analysis: Four recommendations for getting the most from your analysis. *Pract. Assess. Res. Eval.* **2005**, *10*, 7.

https://doi.org/10.3390/jcm15062320

38. Jolliffe, I. Principal component analysis. In *Encyclopedia of Statistics in Behavioral Science*; Wiley Online Library: Hoboken, NJ, USA, 2005.
39. Hastie, T.; Tibshirani, R.; Friedman, J.; Franklin, J. The elements of statistical learning: Data mining, inference and prediction. *Math. Intell.* **2005**, *27*, 83–85. [CrossRef]
40. Kaufman, L.; Rousseeuw, P.J. *Finding Groups in Data: An Introduction to Cluster Analysis*; John Wiley & Sons: Hoboken, NJ, USA, 2009.
41. Bilder, C.R.; Loughin, T.M. *Analysis of Categorical Data with R*; Chapman and Hall/CRC: Boca Raton, FL, USA, 2024.
42. Kent, D.M.; Paulus, J.K.; Van Klaveren, D.; D'Agostino, R.; Goodman, S.; Hayward, R.; Ioannidis, J.P.; Patrick-Lake, B.; Morton, S.; Pencina, M.; et al. The predictive approaches to treatment effect heterogeneity (PATH) statement. *Ann. Intern. Med.* **2020**, *172*, 35–45. [CrossRef] [PubMed]

https://doi.org/10.3390/jcm15062320

Journal of
Clinical Medicine

MDPI

Article

Causal Mediation Analysis of the Effects of Pain Education on Disability and Pain Intensity in Individuals with Chronic Low Back Pain

Ahmed Alalawi

Department of Medical Rehabilitation Sciences, Faculty of Applied Medical Sciences, Umm Al-Qura University, Makkah 24382, Saudi Arabia; amalawi@uqu.edu.sa

Abstract

Background/Objective: The purpose of this study was to determine whether the effects of pain education combined with physiotherapy could be explained by changes in psychological well-being and self-efficacy in individuals with chronic low back pain (LBP). **Methods:** This study includes a secondary analysis (mediation analysis) of a randomized controlled trial (RCT) that compares the effect of physiotherapy and pain education with physiotherapy alone. The Roland-Morris Disability Questionnaire, assessed at six weeks, was used as a primary outcome in this study, with pain intensity as a secondary outcome. The World Health Organization Five Well-Being Index (WHO-5) and the General Self-Efficacy Scale were evaluated as potential mediators. Causal mediation analysis based on a counterfactual framework was employed to estimate both direct and indirect effects. **Results:** The analyses comprised 46 participants (mean age = 42.2 years; 54.3% female) who received pain education along with physiotherapy. In the mediation models, improvements in emotional well-being (assessed by WHO-5) explained approximately one quarter of the effect of the intervention on disability (average causal mediation effect = −1.66, 95% CI [−2.8, −0.72], $p < 0.001$). By contrast, self-efficacy did not significantly mediate disability, and neither factor accounted for changes in pain intensity. Sensitivity analyses suggested that the indirect effect on psychological well-being was reasonably robust against potential unmeasured confounding factors. **Conclusions:** Enhancements in psychological well-being were associated with reductions in disability following pain education, whereas self-efficacy did not emerge as a significant mediator. These findings may support the value of incorporating mental well-being strategies within rehabilitation programs for chronic LBP.

Keywords: chronic low back pain; pain education; psychological well-being; self-efficacy; mediation analysis

1. Introduction

One of the leading causes of disability worldwide and a significant public health concern is chronic low back pain (LBP). According to estimates from around the world, LBP is the leading cause of years spent disabled in many different areas and demographic groups. Over the coming decades, it is anticipated that the number of people who suffer from LBP will keep rising [1]. High healthcare expenses, lost productivity, and a reduced quality of life are just a few of the significant personal, social, and financial costs associated with LBP [2].

According to current treatment guidelines, the first-line treatment for LBP should involve non-invasive techniques such as physiotherapy, exercise therapy, and patient education [3]. These interventions result in modest improvements in pain and function, but recurrence rates are still high, and many patients experience long-term disability [4]. This highlights how important it is to fully understand how rehabilitation interventions work in order to improve outcomes.

A biopsychosocial model recognizes that physical impairments, in addition to psychological and social factors, have an impact on pain and disability [5]. There is a consistent correlation between outcomes in chronic LBP and psychological measures such as self-efficacy, catastrophizing, and fear-avoidance [6]. Specifically, self-efficacy has been demonstrated to predict disability levels and quality of life in musculoskeletal pain conditions [7,8]. More general signs of mental health, mood, and resilience have also been linked to pain-related outcomes, and they often have a stronger link to disability than to pain severity itself [9]. Within biopsychosocial frameworks such as the fear-avoidance model [10] and the psychological flexibility model [11], cognitive and emotional processes play a central role in shaping pain-related disability. Both self-efficacy and psychological well-being are conceptually aligned with these frameworks, making them theoretically relevant mediators of rehabilitation outcomes. Unlike constructs such as catastrophizing or affective distress, psychological well-being reflects positive mental health and resilience rather than negative symptom burden [12] and has been relatively understudied as a mediator in LBP rehabilitation. Psychological responses to pain, including factors such as well-being and self-efficacy, can vary across age groups [13]. A recent umbrella review in individuals with chronic LBP reported that pain neuroscience education, when combined with exercise or physiotherapy, leads to improvements in pain and disability. However, the review also highlighted substantial heterogeneity and noted that the mechanisms underlying these benefits remain preliminary and require further research [14].

Despite this evidence, there exist relatively few randomized controlled trials (RCTs) that have systematically investigated the psychological mechanisms by which rehabilitation interventions confer their benefits. Numerous secondary analyses and mediation studies indicate that psychosocial alterations could explain a portion of the effects of interventions such as cognitive behavioral therapy (CBT), cognitive functional therapy (CFT), and exposure-based methodologies [15–18]. The Back Skills Training trial illustrated that modifications in cognitive and affective processes partially mediated enhancements in disability [18]. Concurrently, mediation analyses in exposure-based treatments identified significant pathways of change, including reductions in catastrophizing and fear-avoidance, alongside increases in self-efficacy [15]. Mindfulness-based stress reduction (MBSR) and CBT have demonstrated efficacy in alleviating pain and enhancing psychological and functional outcomes, partially through the enhancement of mindfulness, acceptance, and self-efficacy [19,20]. Recent mediation studies on physiotherapy, yoga, and chiropractic care have yielded inconclusive results, indicating that certain psychological factors, such as stress and self-efficacy, serve as partial mediators, whereas others, such as catastrophizing or sleep disturbances, do not [16,17,21,22].

This expanding body of literature highlights the necessity to identify the psychological mechanisms that most significantly impact clinical outcomes and to determine whether these mechanisms differ by intervention type. Nevertheless, significant gaps persist, as the majority of trials conducted thus far have excluded psychological well-being as a mediator, despite evidence correlating it with pain-related disability. Despite extensive mediation research in chronic LBP, the role of psychological well-being in pain education interventions remains largely unexamined, creating a conceptual gap that this study addresses. We hypothesized that improvements in psychological well-being would partially mediate the

https://doi.org/10.3390/jcm15010348

effect of pain education on disability. This study aimed to assess whether the impact of a pain education intervention on disability and pain intensity in individuals with chronic LBP was mediated by changes in self-efficacy, psychological well-being, and pain intensity itself. In line with this aim, the present work focuses on the effects of this intervention by applying a counterfactual causal mediation framework.

2. Materials and Methods

2.1. Study Design

The data from a previously published RCT that evaluated the effects of a structured pain education and physiotherapy program on people with chronic LBP were secondary analyzed in this study. Details about the study methodology, participants' details, recruitment, and key findings are published elsewhere [23]. Briefly, a two-arm parallel-group design was used in the trial, and participants were randomized 1:1 to receive either standard physiotherapy or physiotherapy plus a pain education intervention. Randomization was performed using block randomization (block size = 4), with allocation sequences concealed in sealed, opaque envelopes to ensure allocation concealment. Participants were blinded to their group assignment, as were the physiotherapists who conducted the clinical outcome examinations. This study was conducted in accordance with the Declaration of Helsinki and reported in accordance with the Guidelines for Reporting Mediation Analysis [24]. Ethical approval was granted by the Institutional Ethics Committee (RP/114/2021), and the trial was registered with the Clinical Trial Registry (CTRI/2021/08/035963).

2.2. Participants

Until a sufficient sample size of 92 was reached, participants were recruited on a rolling basis [23]. Adults of either sex, ages 18 to 60, who had been diagnosed with nonspecific chronic LBP that had persisted for longer than three months were eligible. A medical professional used appropriate diagnostic investigations and clinical assessment to establish the diagnosis. Participants who missed more than two scheduled sessions or voluntarily withdrew were excluded from the study. Group assignment was concealed from both participants and outcome assessors. Prior to enrollment, all participants provided written informed consent.

2.3. Interventions

2.3.1. Physiotherapy

A standardized physiotherapy program for chronic LBP was provided to both groups, based on international clinical practice guidelines [3,25]. The program included advice to avoid prolonged bed rest, application of superficial heat for 10 min, and stretching of the lumbar musculature for 10 min. It also comprised static cycling for 10 min and core stabilization exercises aimed at enhancing strength and endurance for 10–15 min. A study calendar was used to monitor adherence during the roughly 40 min sessions.

2.3.2. Pain Education

Participants in the intervention group received a structured pain education program in addition to a regular physiotherapy program. The education intervention session covered topics like the nature of chronic pain, how pain affects the brain, how central sensitization works, what fear-avoidance beliefs are, and how social and psychological factors affect how pain is perceived. For individual education sessions, PowerPoint presentations, pictures, lectures, and interactive discussions were used. There were two sessions per week for the first three weeks. Reflective Q&A sessions took place in weeks four and five. Participants were given a printed pain education handbook at the end of the six-week program.

https://doi.org/10.3390/jcm15010348

Following Butler and Moseley's methodological framework, a culturally specific pain education handbook was developed specifically for this study [26–28]. Relevant clinical guidelines for LBP and the body of existing literature on pain education were used as the basis for the content. Additionally, the Explain Pain handbook [28] was used. The drafts of the education handbook were reviewed by several co-authors to ensure clarity, and final proofreading was performed by a physiotherapist, a clinical psychologist, a rehabilitation doctor, and a native speaker.

2.4. Measurement

2.4.1. Outcome Measures

The disability and pain intensity were the primary outcomes of this mediation analysis. Disability was assessed using the Roland-Morris Disability Questionnaire (RMDQ), which consists of 24 items with a score range of 0 to 24 [29]. Higher disability is indicated by higher scores. The reliability and validity of the RMDQ have been demonstrated [29]. Pain intensity during routine tasks was measured using a 10-point Visual Analog Scale (VAS; 0 = no pain, 10 = worst imaginable pain). In clinical and research settings, the VAS is a valid and reliable measure for assessing pain intensity [30]. Scores of both measures were collected at baseline and at the end of the 6-week intervention [23].

2.4.2. Mediators

Self-efficacy and psychological well-being were used as mediators in this study. Self-efficacy was assessed using the General Self-Efficacy Scale (GSE) [31]. This 10-item self-report test assesses a person's level of confidence in their capacity to manage and succeed in challenging circumstances. Higher GSE scores indicate that people believe they are more self-sufficient. The scores range from 10 to 40. The construct validity and internal consistency have been demonstrated in a range of populations [31].

Psychological well-being was assessed using the World Health Organization Five Well-Being Index (WHO-5) [32]. It is composed of five questions that evaluate the current emotional state of participants. A raw score ranging from 0 (the lowest level of well-being) to 25 (the highest level). Additionally, a percentage score between 0 and 100 is calculated by multiplying the raw scores by 4, where higher values indicate greater well-being. In both clinical and non-clinical populations, the WHO-5 is known to have robust psychometric characteristics, including validity, reliability, and sensitivity to change [12]. Since psychological well-being and self-efficacy are key elements in biopsychosocial models of chronic pain and have both been shown to have an effect on pain-related outcomes and disability in people with chronic LBP, these mediators were chosen [33]. Pain intensity was included as a potential mediator because prior mediation research shows that pain contributes to disability indirectly by influencing cognitive and emotional processes such as fear of movement, catastrophizing, and self-efficacy [34].

2.5. Analysis

The proposed causal framework was designed to divide the total effect of the intervention into direct and indirect components, as previously employed [16]. A causal mediation analysis was conducted utilizing a counterfactual-based methodology to estimate the natural direct effect (NDE) and the average causal mediation effect (ACME), or natural indirect effect [35]. Within this framework, the NDE signifies the impact of the intervention on the outcome that remains unexplained by the mediator, whereas the ACME quantifies the degree to which the intervention affects the outcome via alterations in the mediator. The proportion mediated was determined by the ratio of the ACME to the total effect, indicating the extent to which the mediator pathway accounts for the intervention's effect [16].

https://doi.org/10.3390/jcm15010348

The analyses relied on the assumption of sequential ignorability: namely, no unmeasured confounding between intervention and mediator, between mediator and outcome, and no mediator–outcome confounders affected by the intervention [16]. Given the randomized design, confounding between intervention and mediator was not expected. Potential mediator–outcome confounders considered in the models included baseline age, sex, pain intensity, disability, and baseline values of the mediator.

To further assess robustness, additional sensitivity mediation models were estimated that included baseline smoking status, BMI, and duration of low back pain as covariates in both the mediator and outcome equations. These extended models yielded ACME, average direct effect (ADE), and total effect estimates that were nearly identical to the primary models, indicating that these baseline variables did not confound the mediation pathway.

The original RCT reported three missing baseline item responses (two items from the GSE and one item from the WHO-5), which were addressed using mean substitution at the item level, as described elsewhere [23]. Following this minimal item-level imputation conducted in the primary trial, the dataset used for the present secondary analysis contained no missing mediator, outcome, or covariate values at either baseline or follow-up. Therefore, no additional imputation procedures were performed, and the current mediation analysis was conducted on a complete-case dataset.

Although baseline mediator and outcome values were included as covariates, the mediator and outcome values used in the mediation pathway were both assessed at the 6-week follow-up. Baseline adjustment reduces confounding but does not establish temporal ordering. Consequently, the mediation findings should be interpreted as exploratory. To address assumptions underlying causal mediation, particularly the sequential ignorability assumption, we conducted a sensitivity analysis following the recommendations of Imai et al. (2010), quantifying the degree of unmeasured mediator–outcome confounding required to nullify the ACME [35].

Although baseline mediator and outcome values were collected and statistically adjusted for, mediator and outcome assessments were obtained at the same 6-week follow-up.

Separate models were estimated for each hypothesized mediator (self-efficacy, psychological well-being, pain intensity, and disability) and each outcome (pain intensity and disability). Following the approach of Imai et al. (2010), counterfactual mediator and outcome values were simulated based on fitted regression models: the mediator model regressed the mediator on intervention and covariates, while the outcome model regressed the outcome on the mediator, intervention, and covariates [35]. All confidence intervals (CIs) were derived from 2000 parametric bootstrap replications [35]. All analyses were performed in R software (version 4.5.2) using the 'mediation' package.

Sensitivity Analyses

To examine robustness, we conducted a sensitivity analysis to assess the degree to which the estimated ACME would be affected by potential unmeasured confounding in the mediator–outcome relationship, as proposed by Imai et al. (2010) [35]. For the linear regression models underlying the mediation analyses, model adequacy was assessed using standard diagnostics (residual-versus-fitted and normal Q-Q plots, scale–location plots, and Cook's distance), and model fit was summarized using R^2, adjusted R^2, and the residual standard error [36]. In exploratory analyses, we also examined the association between change in self-efficacy and change in disability and tested whether the relationship between change in self-efficacy and change in disability differed by treatment group in a linear regression model predicting change in RMDQ [36].

https://doi.org/10.3390/jcm15010348

3. Results

3.1. Participant Characteristics

Table 1 presents the baseline characteristics and post-intervention outcomes for participants in the control and pain education groups (n = 46 each). Both groups were generally comparable at baseline in terms of age, gender distribution, BMI, smoking status, physical activity level, sleep duration, and baseline clinical measures. The mean age was similar (42.52 ± 13.32 years in the control group vs. 42.02 ± 8.24 in the pain education group), and most participants were female. Sleep duration was comparable at baseline (6.33 ± 1.73 h vs. 6.74 ± 1.32), and smoking prevalence was higher in the intervention group (26.1%) compared to the control group (8.7%).

Table 1. Baseline and Post-Intervention Characteristics of Participants in the Pain Education and Control Groups of 92 participants.

Variable	Level	Control (n = 46)	Pain Education (n = 46)	Control (6 Weeks Post-Intervention) (n = 46)	Pain Education (6 Weeks Post-Intervention) (n = 46)
Age (years)		42.52 (13.32)	42.02 (8.24)		
Gender	Female	35 (76.1)	25 (54.3)		
	Male	11 (23.9)	21 (45.7)		
BMI (kg/m^2)		26.96 (4.08)	27.76 (4.28)		
Duration of LBP (months)		35.85 (50.37)	20.93 (34.33)		
Level of activity	Light	14 (30.4)	17 (37.0)		
	Moderate	23 (50.0)	20 (43.5)		
	Very active	9 (19.6)	9 (19.6)		
Smoker	No	42 (91.3)	34 (73.9)		
	Yes	4 (8.7)	12 (26.1)		
Hours of sleep		6.33 (1.73)	6.74 (1.32)		
VAS (0–10)		5.98 (1.71)	5.70 (1.66)	5.57 (1.15)	2.26 (0.88)
RMDQ (0–24)		15.02 (4.78)	12.65 (4.71)	14.00 (4.74)	5.80 (2.49)
WHO-5 (0–100)		54.41 (18.56)	53.48 (17.53)	56.39 (16.34)	70.13 (14.42)
GSE (10–40)		25.78 (6.40)	25.83 (5.61)	30.28 (5.84)	28.85 (5.54)

Values are presented as mean (SD) or frequency (%), as appropriate. Abbreviations: BMI = Body Mass Index; LBP = Low Back Pain; VAS = Visual Analog Scale for pain intensity; RMDQ = Roland-Morris Disability Questionnaire; WHO-5 = World Health Organization-5 Well-Being Index; GSE = General self-efficacy scale.

At baseline, pain intensity scores were 5.98 ± 1.71 for the control group and 5.70 ± 1.66 for the pain education group. Following the intervention, the control group exhibited minimal change in pain intensity (5.57 ± 1.15), whereas the intervention group demonstrated a significant reduction (2.26 ± 0.88). In the control group, disability scores (RMDQ) exhibited a minor decrease (from 15.02 ± 4.78 to 14.00 ± 4.74), while the intervention group demonstrated a significant reduction (from 12.65 ± 4.71 to 5.80 ± 2.49).

Improvements were also observed in the emotional well-being assessed by WHO-5, increasing from 53.48 ± 17.53 to 70.13 ± 14.42 in the intervention group, while the control group changed only modestly (54.41 ± 18.56 to 56.39 ± 16.34). GSE followed a similar pattern, with greater post-intervention improvement in the pain education group (from 25.83 ± 5.61 to 28.85 ± 5.54) compared to the control group (from 25.78 ± 6.40 to 30.28 ± 5.84).

3.2. Mediation Analysis

3.2.1. Causal Mediation Effects on Disability (RMDQ)

As shown in Table 2, causal mediation analysis revealed that the WHO-5 significantly mediated the effect of pain education on disability scores (ACME = −1.66, 95% CI [−2.8, −0.72], $p < 0.001$), accounting for approximately 23.6% of the total effect. Neither self-efficacy (ACME = 0.10, 95% CI [−0.15, 0.37], $p = 0.41$) nor pain intensity (ACME = −0.69, 95% CI [−2.67, 1.40], $p = 0.51$) showed significant indirect effects. The mediation model, including multiple mediators, did not yield significant indirect effects on disability for the

https://doi.org/10.3390/jcm15010348

physiotherapy versus physiotherapy and education model (Table S1). The ADE and total effect estimates corresponding to these mediation results are also reported in Table 2 to provide a complete decomposition of effects. In exploratory stratified mediation analyses, the indirect effect of pain education versus control on disability at 6 weeks via WHO-5 was consistently negative across sex, smoking status, and duration of LBP subgroups, with broadly overlapping 95% confidence intervals (Table S2).

Table 2. Estimated total, direct (ADE), and indirect (ACME) effects of pain education versus control on Roland-Morris Disability Questionnaire scores at 6 weeks, with effect estimates and 95% confidence intervals for each potential mediator.

Mediator	Path a [1]	Path b [2]	Total Effect [3] [95% CI]	Direct Effect (ADE) [95% CI]	Indirect Effect (ACME) [95% CI]	ACME p-Value	% Mediated
GSE	−1.66 [−3.48, 0.16]	−0.06 [−0.21, 0.09]	−7.02 [−8.37, −5.66]	−7.11 [−8.5, −5.68]	0.1 [−0.15, 0.38]	0.410	−1.4
WHO-5	14.49 [10.53, 18.45]	−0.11 [−0.18, −0.05]	−7.02 [−8.37, −5.69]	−5.37 [−7.13, −3.67]	−1.66 [−2.8, −0.72]	0.001	23.6
VAS	−3.23 [−3.6, −2.86]	0.21 [−0.51, 0.94]	−7.01 [−8.4, −5.68]	−6.32 [−8.67, −4.09]	−0.69 [−2.56, 1.39]	0.508	9.9

Abbreviations: WHO-5 = World Health Organization-5 Well-Being Index; ADE = Average Direct Effect; ACME = Average Causal Mediation Effect; CI = Confidence Interval; VAS = Visual Analog Scale for pain intensity. [1] Path a is intervention–mediator estimates in units of the mediator scale. [2] Path b is mediator–outcome estimates in units of the outcome scale. [3] Total effect estimates are presented in terms of back-related disability on the RMDQ scale. All estimates are presented as mean differences between pain education and the control group and their 95% confidence interval. All estimates are presented as mean differences between pain education and the control group, with 95% confidence intervals.

The mediator and outcome regression models showed good fit, explaining 70.7% and 76.5% of the variance in WHO-5 and RMDQ scores at 6 weeks, respectively (adjusted R^2 = 0.697 and 0.754), and diagnostic plots did not indicate major violations of linear regression assumptions or any highly influential observations (Table S3, Figure S1). Exploratory analyses examining the association between change in self-efficacy and change in disability, and testing whether this relationship differed between groups, did not provide evidence of a meaningful relationship or differential effect between groups. Full results are presented in Table S4.

3.2.2. Causal Mediation Effects on Pain Intensity (VAS)

As shown in Table 3, none of the tested mediators significantly mediated the effect of pain education on post-intervention pain intensity. The indirect effects (ACME) through the General Self-Efficacy Scale, WHO-5 Well-being Index, and Roland-Morris Disability Questionnaire were all non-significant (ACME = 0.05, 95% CI [−0.02, 0.16], p = 0.254; ACME = −0.18, 95% CI [−0.47, 0.1], p = 0.226; and ACME = −0.13, 95% CI [−0.54, 0.29], p = 0.580, respectively). The proportion of the total effect mediated ranged from −1.4% to 5.7%. The mediation model, including multiple mediators, did not yield significant indirect effects on pain intensity for the physiotherapy versus physiotherapy and education model (Table S5).

Table 3. Estimated total, direct (ADE), and indirect (ACME) effects of pain education versus control on pain intensity at 6 weeks, with effect estimates and 95% confidence intervals for each potential mediator.

Mediator	Path a [1]	Path b [2]	Total Effect [3] [95% CI]	Direct Effect (ADE) [95% CI]	Indirect Effect (ACME) [95% CI]	ACME p-Value	% Mediated
GSE	−1.35 [−3.11, 0.4]	−0.03 [−0.08, 0.01]	−3.21 [−3.57, −2.86]	−3.26 [−3.61, −2.92]	0.05 [−0.02, 0.16]	0.254	−1.4
WHO-5	14.32 [10.47, 18.17]	−0.01 [−0.03, 0.01]	−3.21 [−3.57, −2.85]	−3.02 [−3.47, −2.58]	−0.18 [−0.47, 0.1]	0.226	5.7
RMDQ	−7.01 [−8.27, −5.74]	0.02 [−0.04, 0.08]	−3.23 [−3.59, −2.88]	−3.1 [−3.59, −2.58]	−0.13 [−0.54, 0.29]	0.580	4.0

Abbreviations: WHO-5 = World Health Organization-5 Well-Being Index; ADE = Average Direct Effect; ACME = Average Causal Mediation Effect; CI = Confidence Interval; RMDQ = Roland-Morris Disability Questionnaire. [1] Path a is intervention–mediator estimates in units of the mediator scale. [2] Path b is mediator–outcome estimates in units of the outcome scale. [3] Total effect estimates are presented in terms of pain intensity on the VAS scale. All estimates are presented as mean differences between the pain education and control group and their 95% confidence interval.

https://doi.org/10.3390/jcm15010348

3.3. Sensitivity Analyses

Sensitivity analysis indicated that the mediating effect of psychological well-being (WHO-5) on disability was robust to a meaningful degree of unmeasured mediator–outcome confounding. Although psychological variables such as depression, catastrophizing, or fear-avoidance were not measured in the original trial, the sensitivity curve demonstrates that the ACME would remain statistically significant unless the residual correlation (ρ) between the mediator and outcome models exceeded approximately −0.40 (equivalent to a shared variance of 16%). Confidence intervals for the ACME remained above zero across most of the plausible range of ρ values, suggesting that unmeasured psychological confounders would need to exert a strong and unlikely degree of correlated influence to fully explain away the mediation effect. The sensitivity curve illustrating this robustness is presented in Figure 1, with detailed numerical estimates included in Table S6.

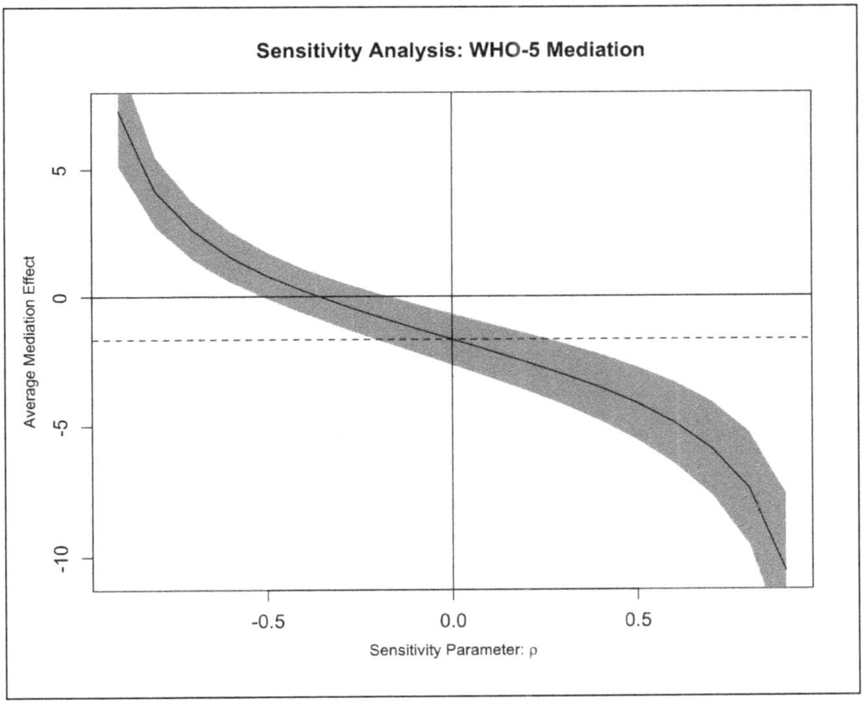

Figure 1. Sensitivity analysis for the confounding assumption in the mediation model for WHO-5. The solid curve represents the estimated average causal mediation effect (ACME) of the WHO-5 Well-being Index on disability (RMDQ) as a function of the sensitivity parameter (ρ). The shaded area indicates the 95% confidence interval, the horizontal dotted line denotes the null indirect effect (ACME = 0), and the vertical line at ρ = 0 represents the assumption of no residual correlation between the mediator and outcome models.

4. Discussion

4.1. Summary of Findings

This secondary analysis of an RCT investigated whether the impacts of a pain education program on pain and disability were facilitated by self-efficacy and psychological well-being. The findings offer partial support for the proposed hypothesis of the mediation pathways. Pain education, when provided together with physiotherapy, substantially

https://doi.org/10.3390/jcm15010348

reduced pain and disability in comparison to physiotherapy alone, as evidenced in the initial RCT [23]. Mediation analyses indicated that improvements in emotional well-being were associated with approximately 24% of the overall difference in disability between groups. On the other hand, self-efficacy did not have a significant effect on disability, and neither self-efficacy nor psychological well-being had an effect on the intervention's effect on pain intensity. Because the mediator and outcome were measured concurrently at the 6-week follow-up, the temporal ordering required for definitive causal mediation cannot be confirmed.

4.2. The Mediating Role of Psychological Well-Being in the Effect of Pain Education on Disability

Our results indicate that improvements in emotional well-being were associated with lower disability scores and partially explained the differences observed between groups. This suggests that improvements in the general quality of life could be partly responsible for the reduction in disability observed in the intervention group. On the other hand, the observed treatment effect was not significantly explained by other mediators that were assessed in this study, such as pain intensity and pain self-efficacy.

These results are consistent with a growing body of research highlighting the importance of psychological health in musculoskeletal rehabilitation. Psychological interventions improve physical function and quality of life for people with chronic LBP, particularly when paired with physiotherapy [37]. CBT and mindfulness-based stress reduction (MBSR) have also shown promise in improving psychological and functional outcomes and reducing pain in this population [19,20]. Additionally, a comprehensive analysis by O'Keeffe et al. [38] emphasized that pain-related disability can be considerably reduced by addressing maladaptive pain-related thoughts, feelings, and behavioral tendencies.

The study's findings regarding the mediating role of psychological well-being align with the biopsychosocial model of chronic pain. This model recognizes that social and psychological factors, in addition to biological influences, have a substantial impact on disability [5]. The WHO-5 is an internationally recognized tool for assessing well-being and has been validated among clinical groups, including those with chronic pain [12]. It might also cover broader aspects of mental health that are not just connected to pain. In line with evidence showing that psychosocial constructs often show a stronger correlation with disability than with pain severity, this could help explain why well-being mediated disability but not pain intensity [9]. These findings suggest that interventions that support psychological well-being may enhance functional outcomes and could serve as a valuable addition to traditional rehabilitation approaches. Integrating mental health components into pain education and rehabilitation programs may be a vital approach to improve long-term outcomes for those with LBP. The absence of mediation through pain intensity further suggests that psychological well-being may influence disability via affective-motivational or attentional pathways, rather than through direct modulation of nociceptive processing [39]. However, because well-being and disability were measured at the same time point in this study, alternative temporal sequences cannot be excluded, and the proposed pathway should be regarded as preliminary.

4.3. Self-Efficacy as a Non-Significant Mediator

Although self-efficacy is widely acknowledged as a key predictor of outcomes in chronic LBP, our mediation analysis did not support its role in explaining the benefits of pain education on either pain or disability. These null mediation findings are consistent with exploratory analyses in the present dataset, which showed only a very weak, non-significant association between change in self-efficacy and change in disability and no evidence that this association differed between intervention and control groups (Table S4).

This contrasts with prior evidence. For example, van Hooff et al. demonstrated that post-treatment self-efficacy was a stronger predictor of functional improvements than traditional constructs such as fear-avoidance or catastrophizing [40]. Similarly, Ryum and Stiles reported that increases in self-efficacy significantly mediated the relationship between changes in pain intensity and disability in the treatment of LBP [15]. Meta-analyses also highlight self-efficacy as a robust determinant of pain-related disability across musculoskeletal conditions [7].

Several explanations may account for the absence of mediation effects in the present study. First, the short intervention duration (six weeks) may not have been sufficient to produce measurable improvements in self-efficacy. A recent meta-analysis indicated that exercise or combined physiotherapy programs typically yield only small improvements in self-efficacy over longer periods of 4–6 months [7]. Second, the content of the pain education program primarily focused on neurophysiological understanding and promoting psychological well-being, rather than mastery-based or behavioral strategies such as graded exposure, goal setting, or cognitive-behavioral therapy techniques that directly enhance self-efficacy. Finally, although baseline self-efficacy scores were in the moderate range, suggesting scope for improvement, the intervention may not have sufficiently targeted the mechanisms necessary to shift this construct, thereby limiting its potential role as a mediator. It is also possible that the content of the pain education intervention targeted emotional appraisal more directly than behavioral confidence, and that the use of a global (non-pain-specific) self-efficacy measure may have reduced sensitivity to detect change in this context.

4.4. Implications and Future Directions

The findings from this study have both clinical and research implications. Clinically, the results highlight the importance of addressing psychological well-being in rehabilitation programs for individuals with chronic LBP. The observation that improvements in well-being, but not self-efficacy, mediated reductions in disability suggests that interventions that foster positive mental health and resilience may be particularly effective in improving functional outcomes. Routine use of brief, validated tools such as the WHO-5 could help clinicians identify patients with low emotional well-being who may benefit most from pain education and complementary psychosocial support [12]. Integrating strategies that actively target mental well-being, such as mindfulness-based interventions, positive psychology techniques, and stress management, in physiotherapy and pain education programs may therefore optimize long-term outcomes [41,42]. These implications should therefore be interpreted cautiously and primarily as guidance for future mechanistic and clinical trials, rather than as definitive evidence. These exploratory findings are consistent with a recent umbrella review showing that pain neuroscience education combined with exercise or physiotherapy yields small-to-moderate improvements in pain and disability in chronic LBP, while the mechanisms underlying these benefits still require further clarification [14].

An alternative explanation for the observed pattern is moderation rather than mediation, for example, that individuals with higher baseline well-being or self-efficacy may derive greater benefit from pain education. Although exploratory analyses did not reveal significant interaction effects, this remains a plausible conceptual model and warrants examination in future trials with repeated mediator assessments.

From a research perspective, the findings underscore the need to broaden the scope of mediation analyses in chronic LBP. While this study focused on psychological well-being and self-efficacy, other psychosocial mechanisms, including fear-avoidance, catastrophizing, stress, and mood disturbance, may also contribute significantly to the effects of education

https://doi.org/10.3390/jcm15010348

and rehabilitation programs [10,34]. In addition, future studies should investigate physiological and behavioral pathways, such as nociceptive modulation and physical activity, to capture a more comprehensive understanding of treatment mechanisms [43]. Longer follow-up periods are also essential to determine whether improvements in psychological well-being translate into sustained functional benefits and whether self-efficacy requires greater time and targeted intervention strategies to emerge as a significant mediator [44,45].

4.5. Strengths and Limitations

This study has several notable strengths. First, it was based on a rigorously conducted RCT, which enhances internal validity by minimizing selection bias and treatment–mediator confounding. The use of a counterfactual causal mediation framework allowed for the decomposition of total effects into direct and indirect components, providing a nuanced understanding of how pain education exerts its influence on clinical outcomes. To further ensure robustness, confidence intervals were generated using bootstrap resampling, and sensitivity analyses were conducted, demonstrating that the mediating role of psychological well-being was relatively stable even under moderate levels of unmeasured confounding. In addition, supplementary sensitivity models that included baseline smoking status, BMI, and duration of low back pain yielded ACME estimates nearly identical to the primary model, further supporting the robustness of the mediating effect of psychological well-being. These methodological features strengthen confidence in the validity of the observed findings.

Despite the strengths of this study, several limitations should be noted. First, because this was a secondary analysis, the original trial was not specifically powered to detect mediation effects, which may have limited our ability to identify smaller indirect pathways. This limitation is even more pronounced for the exploratory subgroup mediation analyses (Table S2), which were based on smaller strata and multiple comparisons. Accordingly, these subgroup results were presented primarily to assess consistency of the mediation pattern across key clinical characteristics, rather than to support formal hypothesis testing, and the associated p-values should be regarded as descriptive. Second, the follow-up period was relatively short (six weeks), making it difficult to draw conclusions about the durability of the intervention's effects and potentially explaining why self-efficacy did not emerge as a mediator. Third, this study focused on only two mediators (psychological well-being and self-efficacy) while other psychosocial factors, such as fear-avoidance, catastrophizing, stress, or anxiety, were not measured and may also play important roles in treatment mechanisms. Fourth, mediators and outcomes were collected at the same post-intervention time point. Although this study adjusted for baseline levels, this limits the ability to establish temporal ordering, and the mediation findings should be interpreted with caution. Finally, as with any causal mediation analysis, the sequential ignorability assumption cannot be fully verified, even though the sensitivity analyses suggest that a substantial degree of unmeasured confounding would be required to eliminate the observed mediation effect.

5. Conclusions

This secondary analysis found that improvements in psychological well-being were associated with reductions in disability following pain education, whereas self-efficacy did not appear to explain treatment effects. These mediation findings should be interpreted cautiously, as mediators and outcomes were assessed concurrently, and the short intervention period limits conclusions about temporal ordering or durability. Nonetheless, the results suggest that psychological well-being may play a meaningful role in functional

https://doi.org/10.3390/jcm15010348

improvement and highlight the value of incorporating well-being-oriented content into rehabilitation programs.

Supplementary Materials: The following supporting information can be downloaded at https://www.mdpi.com/article/10.3390/jcm15010348/s1. Table S1: Decomposition of the total effect of physical therapy versus physical therapy and education on disability score assessd by RMDQ using combined multiple mediator model; Table S2: Stratified causal mediation analyses of the effect of pain education plus physiotherapy versus physiotherapy alone on disability (RMDQ) at 6 weeks via WHO-5, by sex, smoking status, and duration of low back pain; Table S3: Model fit indices for the mediator and outcome regression models used in the primary causal mediation analysis; Table S4: Exploratory analyses of the association between self-efficacy and disability; Table S5: Decomposition of the total effect of physical therapy versus physical therapy and education on disability score assessd by RMDQ using combined multiple mediator model; Table S6: Sensitivity Analysis of the Average Causal Mediation Effect (ACME) for the WHO-5 Mediator on Disability Outcomes; Figure S1: Diagnostic plots for the linear regression models underlying the primary mediation analysis. The top row shows the mediator model (WHO-5 at 6 weeks); the bottom row shows the outcome model (RMDQ at 6 weeks). Residual-versus-fitted, normal Q-Q, scale-location, and Cook's distance plots did not indicate major violations of linear regression assumptions or any highly influential observations.

Funding: This research received no external funding.

Institutional Review Board Statement: The trial received approval from the Institutional Ethics Committee of SKIMS under reference RP/114/2021 and was registered with the Clinical Trial Registry of India (CTRI/2021/08/035963).

Informed Consent Statement: Informed consent was obtained from all subjects involved in the study. Written informed consent has been obtained from the patient(s) to publish this paper.

Data Availability Statement: This is a secondary analysis of a published randomized control trial. The data is available publicly. The R code used to perform the mediation analyses is available from the author upon reasonable request.

Acknowledgments: The author reviewed and edited the output and takes full responsibility for the content of this publication.

Conflicts of Interest: The author declares no conflicts of interest. The funders had no role in the design of the study; in the collection, analyses, or interpretation of data; in the writing of the manuscript; or in the decision to publish the results.

References

1. Ferreira, M.L.; De Luca, K.; Haile, L.M.; Steinmetz, J.D.; Culbreth, G.T.; Cross, M.; Kopec, J.A.; Ferreira, P.H.; Blyth, F.M.; Buchbinder, R. Global, regional, and national burden of low back pain, 1990–2020, its attributable risk factors, and projections to 2050: A systematic analysis of the Global Burden of Disease Study 2021. *Lancet Rheumatol.* **2023**, *5*, e316–e329. [CrossRef] [PubMed]
2. Hartvigsen, J.; Hancock, M.J.; Kongsted, A.; Louw, Q.; Ferreira, M.L.; Genevay, S.; Hoy, D.; Karppinen, J.; Pransky, G.; Sieper, J. What low back pain is and why we need to pay attention. *Lancet* **2018**, *391*, 2356–2367. [CrossRef] [PubMed]
3. Qaseem, A.; Wilt, T.J.; McLean, R.M.; Forciea, M.A.; Clinical Guidelines Committee of the American College of Physicians. Noninvasive treatments for acute, subacute, and chronic low back pain: A clinical practice guideline from the American College of Physicians. *Ann. Intern. Med.* **2017**, *166*, 514–530. [CrossRef] [PubMed]
4. Hayden, J.A.; Ellis, J.; Ogilvie, R.; Malmivaara, A.; van Tulder, M.W. Exercise therapy for chronic low back pain. *Cochrane Database Syst. Rev.* **2021**, *9*, CD009790. [CrossRef]
5. Gatchel, R.J.; Peng, Y.B.; Peters, M.L.; Fuchs, P.N.; Turk, D.C. The biopsychosocial approach to chronic pain: Scientific advances and future directions. *Psychol. Bull.* **2007**, *133*, 581. [CrossRef]
6. Vlaeyen, J.W.; Linton, S.J. Fear-avoidance model of chronic musculoskeletal pain: 12 years on. *Pain* **2012**, *153*, 1144–1147. [CrossRef]
7. Jackson, T.; Wang, Y.; Wang, Y.; Fan, H. Self-efficacy and chronic pain outcomes: A meta-analytic review. *J. Pain* **2014**, *15*, 800–814. [CrossRef]

8. Denison, E.; Åsenlöf, P.L. Self-efficacy, fear avoidance, and pain intensity as predictors of disability in subacute and chronic musculoskeletal pain patients in primary care health. *Pain* **2004**, *111*, 245–252. [CrossRef]
9. Linton, S.J.; Shaw, W.S. Impact of psychological factors in the experience of pain. *Phys. Ther.* **2011**, *91*, 700–711. [CrossRef]
10. Vlaeyen, J.W.; Linton, S.J. Fear-avoidance and its consequences in chronic musculoskeletal pain: A state of the art. *Pain* **2000**, *85*, 317–332. [CrossRef]
11. McCracken, L.M.; Morley, S. The psychological flexibility model: A basis for integration and progress in psychological approaches to chronic pain management. *J. Pain* **2014**, *15*, 221–234. [CrossRef] [PubMed]
12. Topp, C.W.; Østergaard, S.D.; Søndergaard, S.; Bech, P. The WHO-5 Well-Being Index: A systematic review of the literature. *Psychother. Psychosom.* **2015**, *84*, 167–176. [CrossRef] [PubMed]
13. Murray, C.B.; Patel, K.V.; Twiddy, H.; Sturgeon, J.A.; Palermo, T.M. Age differences in cognitive–affective processes in adults with chronic pain. *Eur. J. Pain* **2021**, *25*, 1041–1052. [CrossRef] [PubMed]
14. García Cancela, J.; Conde Vázquez, O.; Navarro Ledesma, S.; Pruimboom, L. The effectiveness of pain neuroscience education in people with chronic nonspecific low back pain: An umbrella review with meta-analysis. *Ann. Phys. Rehabil. Med.* **2025**, *68*, 102020. [CrossRef]
15. Ryum, T.; Stiles, T.C. Changes in pain catastrophizing, fear-avoidance beliefs, and pain self-efficacy mediate changes in pain intensity on disability in the treatment of chronic low back pain. *Pain Rep.* **2023**, *8*, e1092. [CrossRef]
16. Joyce, C.T.; Chernofsky, A.; Lodi, S.; Sherman, K.J.; Saper, R.B.; Roseen, E.J. Do physical therapy and yoga improve pain and disability through psychological mechanisms? A causal mediation analysis of adults with chronic low back pain. *J. Orthop. Sports Phys. Ther.* **2022**, *52*, 470–483. [CrossRef]
17. O'Neill, A.; O'Sullivan, K.; O'Sullivan, P.; Purtill, H.; O'Keeffe, M. Examining what factors mediate treatment effect in chronic low back pain: A mediation analysis of a Cognitive Functional Therapy clinical trial. *Eur. J. Pain* **2020**, *24*, 1765–1774. [CrossRef]
18. Fordham, B.; Ji, C.; Hansen, Z.; Lall, R.; Lamb, S.E. Explaining how cognitive behavioral approaches work for low back pain: Mediation analysis of the back skills training trial. *Spine* **2017**, *42*, E1031–E1039. [CrossRef]
19. Turner, J.A.; Anderson, M.L.; Balderson, B.H.; Cook, A.J.; Sherman, K.J.; Cherkin, D.C. Mindfulness-based stress reduction and cognitive behavioral therapy for chronic low back pain: Similar effects on mindfulness, catastrophizing, self-efficacy, and acceptance in a randomized controlled trial. *Pain* **2016**, *157*, 2434–2444. [CrossRef]
20. Cherkin, D.C.; Sherman, K.J.; Balderson, B.H.; Cook, A.J.; Anderson, M.L.; Hawkes, R.J.; Hansen, K.E.; Turner, J.A. Effect of mindfulness-based stress reduction vs cognitive behavioral therapy or usual care on back pain and functional limitations in adults with chronic low back pain: A randomized clinical trial. *JAMA* **2016**, *315*, 1240–1249. [CrossRef]
21. Shannon, Z.K.; Long, C.R.; Chrischilles, E.; Goertz, C.; Wallace, R.; Casteel, C.; Carnahan, R.M. Secondary causal mediation analysis of a pragmatic clinical trial to evaluate the effect of chiropractic care for US active-duty military on biopsychosocial outcomes occurring through effects on low back pain interference and intensity. *BMJ Open* **2024**, *14*, e083509. [CrossRef] [PubMed]
22. Mansell, G.; Hill, J.C.; Main, C.J.; Von Korff, M.; Van Der Windt, D. Mediators of treatment effect in the back in action trial: Using latent growth modeling to take change over time into account. *Clin. J. Pain* **2017**, *33*, 811–819. [CrossRef] [PubMed]
23. Sidiq, M.; Muzaffar, T.; Janakiraman, B.; Masoodi, S.; Vasanthi, R.K.; Ramachandran, A.; Bansal, N.; Chahal, A.; Kashoo, F.Z.; Rizvi, M.R. Effects of pain education on disability, pain, quality of life, and self-efficacy in chronic low back pain: A randomized controlled trial. *PLoS ONE* **2024**, *19*, e0294302. [CrossRef] [PubMed]
24. Cashin, A.G.; McAuley, J.H.; Lamb, S.E.; Hopewell, S.; Kamper, S.J.; Williams, C.M.; Henschke, N.; Lee, H. Development of a guideline for reporting mediation analyses (AGReMA). *BMC Med. Res. Methodol.* **2020**, *20*, 19. [CrossRef]
25. National Guideline Centre (UK). *Low Back Pain and Sciatica in Over 16s: Assessment and Management*; National Institute for Health and Care Excellence: London, UK, 2016.
26. Sharma, S.; Jensen, M.P.; Moseley, G.L.; Abbott, J.H. Pain education for patients with non-specific low back pain in Nepal: Protocol of a feasibility randomised clinical trial (PEN-LBP Trial). *BMJ Open* **2018**, *8*, e022423. [CrossRef]
27. Butler, D.; Moseley, G. *Explain Pain Supercharged*; NOI Group Publishers: Adelaide, Australia, 2017.
28. Moseley, G.L.; Butler, D.S. *The Explain Pain Handbook: Protectometer*; NOI Group Publishers: Adelaide, Australia, 2015.
29. Roland, M.; Fairbank, J. The Roland–Morris disability questionnaire and the Oswestry disability questionnaire. *Spine* **2000**, *25*, 3115–3124. [CrossRef]
30. Hawker, G.A.; Mian, S.; Kendzerska, T.; French, M. Measures of adult pain: Visual analog scale for pain (vas pain), numeric rating scale for pain (nrs pain), mcgill pain questionnaire (mpq), short-form mcgill pain questionnaire (sf-mpq), chronic pain grade scale (cpgs), short form-36 bodily pain scale (sf-36 bps), and measure of intermittent and constant osteoarthritis pain (icoap). *Arthritis Care Res.* **2011**, *63*, S240–S252.
31. Schwarzer, R.; Jerusalem, M. Generalized self-efficacy scale. In *Measures in Health Psychology: A User's Portfolio*; Weinman, J., Wright, S., Johnston, M., Eds.; Causal and control belief; NFER-Nelson: Windsor, UK, 1995; Volume 35, p. 82-003.
32. Luszczynska, A.; Scholz, U.; Schwarzer, R. The general self-efficacy scale: Multicultural validation studies. *J. Psychol.* **2005**, *139*, 439–457. [CrossRef]

33. Nicholas, M.K. The pain self-efficacy questionnaire: Taking pain into account. *Eur. J. Pain* **2007**, *11*, 153–163. [CrossRef]
34. Lee, H.; Hübscher, M.; Moseley, G.L.; Kamper, S.J.; Traeger, A.C.; Mansell, G.; McAuley, J.H. How does pain lead to disability? A systematic review and meta-analysis of mediation studies in people with back and neck pain. *Pain* **2015**, *156*, 988–997. [CrossRef]
35. Imai, K.; Keele, L.; Tingley, D. A general approach to causal mediation analysis. *Psychol. Methods* **2010**, *15*, 309. [CrossRef] [PubMed]
36. Fox, J. *Applied Regression Analysis and Generalized Linear Models*; Sage publications: Thousand Oaks, CA, USA, 2015.
37. Williams, A.C.C.; Fisher, E.; Hearn, L.; Eccleston, C. Psychological therapies for the management of chronic pain (excluding headache) in adults. *Cochrane Database Syst. Rev.* **2020**, *8*, CD007407. [CrossRef] [PubMed]
38. O'Keeffe, M.; O'Sullivan, P.; Purtill, H.; Bargary, N.; O'Sullivan, K. Cognitive functional therapy compared with a group-based exercise and education intervention for chronic low back pain: A multicentre randomised controlled trial (RCT). *Br. J. Sports Med.* **2020**, *54*, 782–789. [CrossRef]
39. Wiech, K. Deconstructing the sensation of pain: The influence of cognitive processes on pain perception. *Science* **2016**, *354*, 584–587. [CrossRef] [PubMed]
40. van Hooff, M.L.; Vriezekolk, J.E.; Kroeze, R.J.; O'Dowd, J.K.; van Limbeek, J.; Spruit, M. Targeting self-efficacy more important than dysfunctional behavioral cognitions in patients with longstanding chronic low back pain; a longitudinal study. *BMC Musculoskelet. Disord.* **2021**, *22*, 824. [CrossRef]
41. Hofmann, S.G.; Gómez, A.F. Mindfulness-based interventions for anxiety and depression. *Psychiatr. Clin. North Am.* **2017**, *40*, 739. [CrossRef]
42. Seligman, M.E.; Steen, T.A.; Park, N.; Peterson, C. Positive psychology progress: Empirical validation of interventions. *Am. Psychol.* **2005**, *60*, 410. [CrossRef]
43. Mühlhauser, Y.; Vogt, L.; Niederer, D. How and how fast does pain lead to disability? A multilevel mediation analysis on structural, temporal and biopsychosocial pathways in patients with chronic nonspecific low back pain. *Musculoskelet. Sci. Pract.* **2020**, *49*, 102199. [CrossRef]
44. Broderick, J.E.; Keefe, F.J.; Schneider, S.; Junghaenel, D.U.; Bruckenthal, P.; Schwartz, J.E.; Kaell, A.T.; Caldwell, D.S.; McKee, D.; Gould, E. Cognitive behavioral therapy for chronic pain is effective, but for whom? *Pain* **2016**, *157*, 2115–2123. [CrossRef]
45. Turner, J.A.; Holtzman, S.; Mancl, L. Mediators, moderators, and predictors of therapeutic change in cognitive–behavioral therapy for chronic pain. *Pain* **2007**, *127*, 276–286. [CrossRef]

https://doi.org/10.3390/jcm15010348

Journal of
Clinical Medicine

MDPI

Article

Association Between Systemic Symptoms and Recovery in Acute Low Back Pain: A Retrospective Cross-Sectional Study

Ji-Ho Lee [1], Si-Hyun Han [2], Min-Su Kim [2], Dong-Ho Keum [2] and Seo-Hyun Park [3,*]

[1] College of Korean Medicine, Dongguk University Graduate School, Seoul 04620, Republic of Korea; wigh1996@naver.com
[2] Department of Rehabilitation Medicine of Korean Medicine, Dongguk University Bundang Oriental Hospital, Seongnam-si 13601, Republic of Korea; h4692@naver.com (S.-H.H.); alstn7180@naver.com (M.-S.K.); keumdh660@naver.com (D.-H.K.)
[3] College of Korean Medicine, Dongguk University Graduate School, Gyeongju 38066, Republic of Korea
* Correspondence: barksh84@naver.com; Tel.: +82-317103744

Abstract: Background: Several prognostic factors, including the early recovery pattern of acute low back pain (ALBP), are related to the chronicity of LBP. However, the association between systemic symptoms and ALBP remains underexplored from a holistic perspective. Hence, this study aimed to investigate this relationship and identify novel clinical prognostic predictors for LBP. **Methods**: This retrospective cross-sectional study included patients with ALBP admitted to the Department of Korean Medicine Rehabilitation at the Dongguk University Bundang Hospital between 1 January 2021 and 30 April 2025. Data extracted from medical records included demographics, treatment-related information, pain characteristics, past medical history, and systemic symptoms. Statistical analyses included independent *t*-tests, Mann–Whitney U tests, chi-squared tests, Fisher's exact tests, correlation analysis, and multiple linear regression models. **Results**: A total of 194 patients with ALBP were included in the analysis. Among systemic symptoms, dyspepsia was significantly associated with higher pain at discharge and smaller absolute and relative pain changes. Although sleep disturbance and constipation showed associations with higher pain at discharge in univariate analyses, these associations were not statistically significant in regression models. Beyond systemic symptoms, alcohol consumption was significantly associated with lower pain at discharge and greater relative pain change, while hospitalization and symptom duration exhibited non-linear relationships. These findings remained robust in sensitivity and subgroup analyses. **Conclusions**: Systemic symptoms, especially dyspepsia, may serve as prognostic factors impeding ALBP recovery, representing potential early markers for identifying patients at risk of chronicity. The findings highlight the prospect of multidimensional strategies in reducing pain and enhancing patients' quality of life in clinical practice.

Keywords: low back pain; prognosis; chronicity; systemic symptom; dyspepsia

1. Introduction

Low back pain (LBP) is defined as pain or discomfort localized below the costal margin and above the inferior gluteal folds, which can radiate to the lower extremities. LBP is a commonly encountered musculoskeletal symptom in primary care, with a reported lifetime prevalence of 49–70% [1]. Among various LBP classification systems, the etiological classification distinguishes mechanical from non-mechanical causes. Mechanical LBP, accounting for approximately 97% of cases, arises from structural or functional abnormalities of the spine and surrounding tissues, whereas non-mechanical LBP, comprising the remaining 3% of cases, is caused by extrinsic pathologies such as infections, malignancies, or visceral disorders [2]. LBP can also be classified according to symptom duration. Although somewhat controversial, acute LBP is generally defined as pain lasting <4–6 weeks, while subacute and chronic phases are subsequently delineated using a 12-week threshold [1,3]. Over 90% of patients with acute LBP (ALBP) recover fully within days to weeks, whereas approximately 5% progress to chronic LBP (CLBP) via the subacute phase [4].

CLBP impairs not only the patient's physical health but also psychological well-being and socioeconomic functioning. Studies showed that CLBP is frequently accompanied by sleep disturbances, depression, and anxiety [5–7]. Additionally, productivity loss imposes a substantial societal LBP-related burden [8]. Moreover, despite the availability of various treatment modalities reflecting the multifactorial nature of CLBP, treatment efficacy remains inconsistent, and the factors influencing the therapeutic response are not yet fully understood [9]. Consequently, a small subset of patients with CLBP accounts for nearly 80% of the total healthcare costs for LBP [9].

Given the considerable socioeconomic burden imposed by CLBP, early identification of patients at risk for chronicity is of utmost clinical importance. Studies demonstrated that CLBP is more strongly related to demographic, psychosocial, and occupational factors than with musculoskeletal pathology alone [10]. These findings prompted a shift toward the biopsychosocial model, which integrates biological, psychological, and social dimensions in the understanding of pain perception [11]. Several prognostic factors for chronicity, including sex, age, obesity, physical workload and awkward posture, social isolation, depression, diabetes, and smoking, have been proposed [12].

Furthermore, the short-term progression of ALBP is recognized as an indicator of chronicity risk. Recovery patterns within the first week of onset predict the LBP course at 1 and 3 months with significant accuracy [13]. Moreover, most patients with LBP who continued to experience activity limitations for 3 months from the onset had already exhibited signs of delayed recovery within the first week [14]. Therefore, early recovery patterns may serve as valuable prognostic indicators of long-term outcomes in ALBP.

Beyond the biopsychosocial model, a holistic approach has recently gained attention, seeking to investigate the relationship between LBP and systemic symptoms. Systemic symptoms, identified through comprehensive history-taking, refer to symptoms arising from other organ systems unrelated to the patient's chief complaint [15]. These symptoms are utilized to assess the overall health status, aid in differential diagnosis, and evaluate the systemic impact of diseases [15]. Studies reported a higher risk of LBP in women with frequent gastrointestinal (GI) symptoms, as well as increased rates of urinary incontinence or GI symptoms among women with LBP [16,17]. Furthermore, women with LBP who experience constipation exhibit higher pain sensitivity [18]. However, these studies did not examine the impact of systemic symptoms on the clinical LBP course. Sleep disturbances also demonstrated a bidirectional association between pain intensity, which may contribute to delayed recovery [19].

Traditional Korean Medicine (TKM) adopts a holistic diagnostic and therapeutic approach, encompassing physiological characteristics, lifestyle factors, and systemic symptoms. The *Donguibogam*, a foundational text in TKM, reflects a longstanding recognition of the association between LBP and systemic symptoms, classifying LBP into subtypes based on accompanying symptoms: urinary dysfunction (kidney deficiency type), GI symptoms (food accumulation type), and psychological symptoms (Qi stagnation type) [20]. Accordingly, TKM practitioners comprehensively assess systemic symptoms (i.e., sleep patterns, dietary habits, digestive function, bowel and urinary symptoms, and thirst) in conjunction with pain intensity, duration, and location [20]. This multidimensional information determines the underlying pathophysiology of pain and supports pattern identification and treatment planning. From this holistic perspective, systemic symptoms may plausibly influence LBP prognosis. Indeed, the prognostic value of systemic symptoms for neck pain was reported [21]. However, no studies have examined the prognostic value of systemic symptoms in ALBP.

This study retrospectively analyzed systemic symptoms in inpatients with ALBP, aiming to identify potential novel factors that may significantly influence early recovery patterns. Specifically, we aimed to evaluate the prognostic value of systemic symptoms commonly used in TKM and explore the clinical relevance of a holistic approach through univariate and multivariate statistical analyses. Given that short-term progression can predict long-term outcomes of LBP, this study is expected to provide early indicators for identifying the risk of chronicity.

2. Materials and Methods

2.1. Study Design and Eligibility Criteria

This retrospective cross-sectional study aimed to investigate potential factors influencing recovery from ALBP by analyzing the correlation between ALBP and systemic symptoms. The Institutional Review Board (IRB) of Dongguk University Bundang Oriental Hospital approved this study (IRB no. 2025-0005). All procedures adhered to the Strengthening the Reporting of Observational Studies in Epidemiology (STROBE) guidelines [22]. Patients who were admitted to the Department of Korean Rehabilitation Medicine for acute mechanical LBP between 1 January 2021 and 30 April 2025, were included in the study. LBP diagnoses were identified using the Korean Standard Classification of Diseases (KCD) diagnostic codes recorded at initial admission, specifically S30–S39 (injury to the abdomen, lower back, lumbar spine, and pelvis) and M50–M54 (other dorsopathies).

The following eligibility criteria were applied to ensure data reliability and sample consistency (Table 1). First, patients with non-mechanical LBP (such as spinal tumor, spinal infection, or ankylosing spondylitis) were excluded to focus exclusively on mechanical LBP. Mechanical LBP is generally defined as pain arising from structural or functional abnormalities of the spine and its surrounding tissues. However, this study also classified cases involving radicular pain as mechanical LBP when nerve root compression could be clearly attributable to structural lesions, such as disc herniation or spinal stenosis [2].

Furthermore, to minimize potential confounding, patients aged > 65 years, presenting with red flag signs, or with concussion at LBP onset were excluded. Older patients are subject to various confounders (including age-related degenerative changes, comorbidities, and psychosocial issues such as anxiety or cognitive impairment), which may substantially influence the prognosis of LBP [23,24]. Red flag signs indicate potential serious underlying conditions such as compression fractures, cauda equina syndrome, progressive neurological deficits, infection, or malignancy [25]. Among these, compression fractures and cauda equina syndrome, although structural in nature, were excluded due to their distinct clinical course and specific management strategies (i.e., urgent surgical intervention in cauda equina syndrome), which differ significantly from those for typical mechanical LBP [26–28]. Lastly, concussion was excluded as it may alter pain perception through central sensitization, compromising the reliability of self-reported pain measures [29,30].

Moreover, patients who received no treatment during hospitalization or were admitted for ≤3 days were excluded due to insufficient therapeutic exposure to ensure homogeneity of therapeutic outcomes. Furthermore, although ALBP is typically defined as <4–6 weeks, a more conservative cutoff of 4 weeks was adopted to avoid the inclusion of cases possibly transitioning into the subacute phase by the final assessment [2].

Table 1. Inclusion and exclusion criteria of the study.

Definition of LBP	KCD Codes S30–S39 (Injuries to the Abdomen, Lower Back, Lumbar Spine and Pelvis) or M50–M54 (Other Dorsopathies) Related to LBP
Inclusion Criteria	Age $\leq$ 65 years old Duration of LBP $\leq$ 4 weeks Hospitalization period $\geq$ 3 days
Exclusion Criteria	Age > 65 years old Duration of LBP > 4 weeks Hospitalization period < 3 days Non-mechanical LBP Red flags (Cauda equina, Compression fracture, etc.) Loss of conscious at onset Lack of sufficient information regarding systemic symptoms

Abbreviation: LBP, Low Back Pain; KCD, Korean Standard Classification of Diseases.

2.2. Data Extraction

Patient's medical records were reviewed to obtain comprehensive data. A third-party independent of the study extracted the data and removed personal identifiers to ensure patient anonymity and data protection. The processed data were subsequently provided to two independent researchers for verification and organization. Any disagreements between the researchers were resolved through discussion. Then, the finalized data set was transferred to another researcher for statistical analysis.

Demographic data were retrieved from the admission records, including sex, age, symptom duration, hospitalization length, diagnosis, smoking and alcohol history, and past medical history. The latter encompassed a history of hypertension (HTN), dyslipidemia, diabetes mellitus (DM), cardiovascular disease, gynecological disease, upper and lower GI disease, respiratory disease, musculoskeletal diseases (thoracolumbar, cervical, or other regions), and psychological history (PSY). The classification of upper and lower GI disorders was based on the anatomical landmark known as the ligament of Treitz, with disorders from the esophagus to the duodenum categorized as upper GI, whereas those from the jejunum to the anus were categorized as lower GI [31]. Only conditions with confirmed diagnoses in the hospital were included.

Details about LBP were collected from admission and discharge records, including pain intensity, pain difference, pain distribution, and range of motion (ROM). Pain intensity was examined using the Numeric Rating Scale (NRS) both at admission (NRS AD) and discharge (NRS DC). Pain difference was calculated as both an absolute change ($\triangle$NRS = NRS DC − NRS AD) and a relative change ($\triangle$NRS[%] = (NRS DC − NRS AD)/NRS AD × 100).

Systemic symptoms were identified from the admission and progress records as patient-reported symptoms based on patient interviews conducted by Korean medicine doctors with at least one year of clinical experience. This study focused on six systemic symptoms listed in the hospital records: sleep disturbance, anorexia, dyspepsia, constipation, nocturia, and thirst. Given their subjective nature, relevant diagnostic criteria and literature were referenced, if applicable, to enhance the objectivity and clinical relevance of their interpretation [32–35]. Table 2 presents the detailed definitions.

Table 2. Adapted inclusion criteria for systemic symptoms based on subjective complaints in traditional Korean medicine.

Systemic Symptoms	Referenced Diagnostic Criteria	Adapted Inclusion Criteria
Sleep disturbance	DSM-5 - Difficulty initiating or maintaining sleep, or early-morning awakening, occurring ≥3 nights per week for ≥3 months - Symptoms not attributable to mental disorder, substance use, or medical condition	- Frequency of DSM-5-defined sleep disturbance symptoms ≥3 nights per week during hospitalization - Excludes cases attributable to mental disorder, medical condition (ex. nocturia) or substance use (caffeine intake)
Anorexia	None	- Patient's dietary intake decreased to ≤50% of baseline during hospitalization
Dyspepsia	Rome IV Criteria - Presence of at least one of the following: postprandial fullness, early satiation, epigastric pain, or epigastric burning - Symptom presentation for the last 3 months, with onset ≥6 months before diagnosis - No evidence of structural disease or identifiable gastrointestinal disorder	- Occurrence of at least one Rome IV-defined symptom during hospitalization - No evidence of structural disease or identifiable gastrointestinal disorder based on past history
Constipation	Rome IV Criteria - Presence of at least two of the following: bowel movements ≤ 3 times per week, straining, hard stools, sensation of incomplete evacuation, anorectal obstruction, or manual maneuvers - Symptom presentation for the last 3 months, with onset ≥6 months before diagnosis	- Occurrence of at least two Rome IV-defined symptoms during hospitalization
Nocturia	ICS - At least one episode of awakening during the night to void Article - Clinically significant, occurring at least twice per night - Regardless of voiding frequency, clinical significance could be determined by the degree of sleep disruption	- Occurrence of voiding at least twice per night during hospitalization or - Frequency of sleep disturbance due to nocturia ≥3 times per week during hospitalization
Thirst	None	- Patient-reported thirst or increased water intake during hospitalization

Abbreviation: DSM-5, Diagnostic and Statistical Manual of Mental Disorders, Fifth Edition; ICS, International Continence Society.

2.3. Statistical Analysis

All statistical analyses were primarily conducted using IBM SPSS Statistics for Windows, Version 21 (IBM Corp., Armonk, NY, USA). Regression analyses were performed using R Studio Version 4.2.0. Continuous variables were presented as means and standard deviations, while categorical data were presented as frequencies and percentages. Binary variables included sex, smoking history, alcohol consumption, presence of past medical history, pain distribution, and presence of each systemic symptom. ROM was also classified as a binary variable (normal and abnormal) based on the hospital medical record system, with 'normal' defined as no limitation in any lumbar ROM.

The dependent variable was the pain score measured by the NRS, a continuous variable ranging from 0 to 10, with higher scores indicating greater pain severity [36]. Four subscales were analyzed: NRS AD, NRS DC, absolute pain change (ΔNRS), and relative pain change (ΔNRS [%]). Improvement was indicated by a lower NRS DC compared to NRS AD. Accordingly, negative values in both absolute and relative changes reflected pain relief, while positive values indicated worsening of pain.

Univariate analyses were conducted using the independent *t*-test or Mann–Whitney U test, depending on the normality of each independent variable. Normality was assessed through the Kolmogorov–Smirnov or Shapiro–Wilk test, depending on the sample size. Spearman or Pearson correlation coefficients were computed to examine the correlations between continuous variables, as appropriate. Chi-square or Fisher's exact tests were employed to evaluate the associations between binary variables. A p-value < 0.05 with a 95% confidence interval indicated statistical significance.

Multiple linear regression analyses were conducted to identify the independent effects of each variable on the LBP progression. Variables with statistical significance ($p < 0.05$) or suggestive trends ($p < 0.1$) in univariate analyses were included in the model. Model assumptions of linearity, normality of residuals, homoscedasticity, and multicollinearity were assessed to ensure validity. Generalized additive models (GAMs) were applied to account for potential non-linear relationships for continuous variables violating the linearity assumption. Subsequently, bootstrapping was employed to estimate confidence intervals for the regression coefficients for any remaining violations of normality and homoscedasticity. Further sensitivity and subgroup analyses were conducted to assess the robustness of the findings. Sensitivity analyses used two alternative models: (1) one including all variables and (2) one incorporating only known predictors of LBP chronicity. The same procedures were followed without bootstrapping, focusing on consistency in coefficient direction and significance. Subgroup analyses were conducted based on patients' diagnoses.

3. Results

3.1. General Characteristics of Participants

A total of 655 patients were admitted to the clinic between 1 January 2021 and 30 April 2025. Among them, 343 patients met the study criteria for LBP, whereas 194 eligible patients with ALBP were included in the statistical analysis (Figure 1). Within this cohort, 79 patients were male, and 115 patients were female, with a mean age of 47.06 ± 12.11 years. The average complaint duration was 2.65 ± 4.18 days, and the mean hospitalization length was 6.57 ± 3.84 days. Regarding diagnoses, the majority of patients were classified under "sprain and strain of lumbar spine" (n = 181), followed by "other and unspecified sprains and strains of lumbar and pelvic region" (n = 8) and "lumbar and other intervertebral disc disorders with radiculopathy" (n = 5). The mean NRS AD was 6.09 ± 1.46, and the mean NRS DC was 4.77 ± 2.01. The average absolute pain change (ΔNRS) was –1.32 ± 1.75, and the average relative change (ΔNRS [%]) was –21.61 ± 27.93% (Table 3).

Table 3. General characteristics of included patients.

Total number of cohorts	194
Gender (Male/Female)	79/115
Age (Year)	47.06 ± 12.11
Complaint duration (Day)	2.65 ± 4.18
Hospitalization period (Day)	6.57 ± 3.84

Table 3. *Cont.*

Diagnosis	Sprain and strain of lumbar spine	181 (93.3%)
	Sprain and strain of other and unspecified parts of lumbar spine and pelvis	8 (4.1%)
	Lumbar and other intervertebral disc disorders with radiculopathy	5 (2.6%)
	Spinal stenosis, lumbar region	2 (1.0%)
	Other spondylosis, lumbar region	1 (0.5%)
	Low back pain, lumbar region	1 (0.5%)
	Lumbago due to displacement of intervertebral disc	1 (0.5%)
	Spondylolysis, lumbar region	1 (0.5%)
NRS AD	6.09 ± 1.46	
NRS DC	4.77 ± 2.01	
ΔNRS	-1.32 ± 1.75	
ΔNRS (%)	-21.61 ± 27.93	

Abbreviation: NRS, Numeric rating scale; NRS AD, NRS at admission; NRS DC, NRS at discharge; ΔNRS, absolute pain change = NRS DC − NRS AD; ΔNRS (%), relative pain change = ((NRS DC − NRS AD)/NRS AD) × 100.

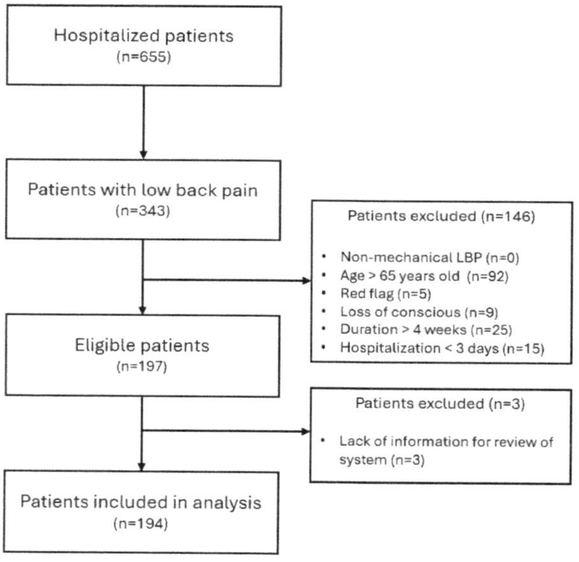

Figure 1. Flow chart of patient selection. Abbreviation: LBP, Low back pain.

3.2. Association Between Demographic Characteristics and Pain Intensity

Given the violation of normality, the Mann–Whitney U test and Spearman's rank correlation were applied to binary variables (gender, smoking, and alcohol) and continuous variables (age), respectively. Among the four variables, only smoking and alcohol consumption demonstrated a significant association with pain intensity at discharge and pain reduction ($p < 0.05$ or $p < 0.01$). None of the variables showed significant associations with initial pain intensity (Table 4A).

Table 4. Univariate associations with low back pain intensity.

Variables			NRS AD	NRS DC	ΔNRS	ΔNRS (%)
(A) Demographic characteristics	Gender	Male (79)	6.03 ± 1.41	4.71 ± 2.02	−1.32 ± 1.82	−21.08 ± 28.87
		Female (115)	6.14 ± 1.49	4.82 ± 2.02	−1.32 ± 1.70	−21.96 ± 27.39
		p-value	0.801	0.693	0.819	0.759
	Age	Correlation coefficient	0.013	0.050	0.035	0.041
		p-value	0.858	0.491	0.630	0.634
	Smoking	Yes (28)	5.96 ± 1.53	3.93 ± 1.90	−2.04 ± 2.13	−31.99 ± 32.05
		No (166)	6.11 ± 1.45	4.92 ± 2.00	−1.20 ± 1.65	−19.86 ± 26.89
		p-value	0.546	0.017 *	0.051 †	0.047 *
	Alcohol	Yes (57)	6.04 ± 1.49	4.25 ± 2.17	−1.79 ± 1.81	−30.00 ± 27.78
		No (137)	6.12 ± 1.45	4.99 ± 1.91	−1.12 ± 1.69	−18.11 ± 27.34
		p-value	0.549	0.007 **	0.018 *	0.009 **
(B) Pain characteristics	NRS AD	Correlation coefficient	-	0.506	−0.145	−0.012
		p-value	-	0.000 ***	0.044 *	0.863
	Symptom duration	Correlation coefficient	−0.072	−0.266	−0.280	−0.302
		p-value	0.320	0.000 ***	0.000 ***	0.000 ***
	Hospitalization length	Correlation coefficient	0.022	−0.181	−0.215	−0.199
		p-value	0.761	0.011 *	0.003 **	0.005 **
	Distribution of LBP	Widespread (131)	6.24 ± 1.46	4.80 ± 1.97	−1.44 ± 1.73	−22.91 ± 26.36
		Localized (63)	5.79 ± 1.43	4.71 ± 2.11	−1.08 ± 1.76	−18.90 ± 31.00
		p-value	0.067 †	0.725	0.156	0.255
	ROM	Normal (81)	5.72 ± 1.39	4.48 ± 2.09	−1.23 ± 1.62	−22.85 ± 29.34
		Abnormal (113)	6.36 ± 1.45	4.98 ± 1.94	−1.38 ± 1.83	−20.71 ± 26.97
		p-value	0.007 **	0.089 †	0.781	0.660
(C) Systemic symptoms	Sleep disturbance	Yes (114)	6.20 ± 1.42	5.01 ± 2.09	−1.19 ± 1.68	−19.78 ± 26.91
		No (80)	5.94 ± 1.51	4.44 ± 1.86	−1.50 ± 1.83	−24.21 ± 29.30
		p-value	0.262	0.049 *	0.215	0.215
	Anorexia	Yes (47)	6.17 ± 1.36	4.96 ± 1.89	−1.21 ± 1.47	−19.95 ± 22.57
		No (147)	6.07 ± 1.49	4.71 ± 2.05	−1.35 ± 1.83	−22.13 ± 29.49
		p-value	0.942	0.592	0.848	0.813
	Constipation	Yes (8)	6.88 ± 1.46	6.13 ± 2.10	−0.75 ± 1.83	−9.97 ± 26.96
		No (186)	6.06 ± 1.45	4.72 ± 1.99	−1.34 ± 1.74	−22.11 ± 27.93
		p-value	0.133	0.076 †	0.311	0.213
	Dyspepsia	Yes (68)	6.15 ± 1.56	5.16 ± 2.06	−0.99 ± 1.52	−16.34 ± 24.81
		No (126)	6.06 ± 1.41	4.56 ± 1.97	−1.50 ± 1.84	−24.45 ± 29.18
		p-value	0.771	0.091	0.052 †	0.054 †
	Nocturia	Yes (65)	6.22 ± 1.39	4.88 ± 1.89	−1.34 ± 1.88	−20.59 ± 26.91
		No (129)	6.03 ± 1.49	4.72 ± 2.08	−1.31 ± 1.68	−22.12 ± 28.52
		p-value	0.581	0.644	0.822	0.733
	Thirst	Yes (76)	6.09 ± 1.56	4.80 ± 2.03	−1.29 ± 1.78	−21.24 ± 28.40
		No (118)	6.09 ± 1.40	4.75 ± 2.01	−1.34 ± 1.73	−21.84 ± 27.74
		p-value	0.680	0.887	0.744	0.820

Annotation: Data presented as mean ± standard deviation. *p*-values were calculated by Mann–Whitney U test, except for age, NRS AD, complaint duration and hospitalization period, which were analyzed by Spearman correlation analysis. († = $p < 0.1$, * = $p < 0.05$, ** $p < 0.01$, *** = $p < 0.001$). Abbreviation: NRS, Numeric rating scale; NRS AD, NRS at admission; NRS DC, NRS at discharge; ΔNRS, absolute pain change = NRS DC − NRS AD; ΔNRS (%), relative pain change = ((NRS DC − NRS AD)/NRS AD) × 100; LBP, Low back pain; ROM, Range of motion.

3.3. Association Between Past Medical History and Pain Intensity

Given the violation of normality, the Mann–Whitney U test was conducted. Patients with a history of thoracolumbar musculoskeletal disorders exhibited significantly higher initial pain intensity ($p < 0.05$). Additionally, those with a history of lower GI disorders showed a suggestive trend toward lower initial pain ($p < 0.1$). However, no past medical history was significantly related to pain at discharge or overall pain change (Table S1)

3.4. Association Between Low Back Pain Characteristics and Pain Intensity

Given the violation of normality, the Mann–Whitney U test and Spearman's rank correlation were applied according to variable types. Initial pain intensity (NRS AD) was positively correlated with pain at discharge ($p < 0.001$) and inversely correlated with absolute pain change ($p < 0.05$) but was not associated with relative pain change. Symptom duration and hospitalization length showed a negative correlation with pain at discharge and both absolute and relative pain change (symptom duration, $p < 0.001$; hospitalization length, $p < 0.05$ or $p < 0.01$). Pain distribution did not significantly influence pain at discharge or pain change, although cases of widespread pain demonstrated a suggestive trend toward higher initial pain ($p < 0.1$). Finally, abnormal ROM was significantly associated only with initial pain and showed a marginal trend toward the association with higher pain at discharge ($p < 0.1$) (Table 4B).

3.5. Association Between Systemic Symptoms and Pain Intensity

Given the violation of normality, the Mann–Whitney U test was conducted. Sleep disturbance was significantly associated with higher pain at discharge ($p < 0.05$) but showed no significant difference in initial pain or pain change. Constipation showed a trend toward higher pain at discharge ($p = 0.076$), while dyspepsia exhibited trends toward smaller absolute and relative pain changes ($p = 0.052$ and 0.054). However, neither significantly influenced initial pain. Other systemic symptoms showed no significant association with pain intensity or pain change (Table 4C).

3.6. Association Between Systemic Symptoms and Pain Characteristics

Chi-square tests were conducted to examine the associations between systemic symptoms and LBP characteristics. Constipation and dyspepsia showed a suggestive association with widespread pain distribution ($p < 0.1$). No other significant associations were identified (Table S2).

3.7. Multiple Regression Analysis

The independent variables of the basic regression model included hospitalization length, symptom duration, initial pain intensity (NRS AD), sleep disturbance, dyspepsia, constipation, history of lower GI disorders, history of thoracolumbar musculoskeletal disorders, pain distribution, smoking status, alcohol consumption, and ROM. The dependent variables were pain at discharge (NRS DC), absolute pain change (ΔNRS), and relative pain change (ΔNRS [%]). Table 5 presents the results of multiple regression.

Table 5. The relationship between low back pain characteristics and pain intensity.

Variables	NRS DC			ΔNRS			ΔNRS (%)		
Parametric Terms	**Estimate**	***p*-Value**	**95% CI**	**Estimate**	***p*-Value**	**95% CI**	**Estimate**	***p*-Value**	**95% CI**
NRS AD	0.71	0.000 ***	(0.56, 0.90) ‡	-	-	-	-	-	-
Sleep disturbance	0.29	0.223	(−0.18, 0.77)	0.24	0.315	(−0.20, 0.76)	2.82	0.465	(−5.18, 10.27)
Dyspepsia	0.55	0.026 *	(0.05, 1.02) ‡	0.54	0.033 *	(0.06, 1.00) ‡	8.15	0.045 *	(0.27, 16.38) ‡
Constipation	0.41	0.483	(−0.95, 1.69)	0.21	0.726	(−1.29, 1.53)	7.54	0.436	(−13.35, 26.91)
Lower GI	−0.23	0.539	(−0.92, 0.43)	−0.05	0.904	(−0.75, 0.57)	−3.07	0.609	(−14.49, 7.53)
MSTL	−0.28	0.355	(−0.95, 0.35)	−0.40	0.195	(−1.07, 0.28)	−4.86	0.321	(−15.59, 5.33)
Distribution of LBP	0.03	0.908	(−0.47, 0.56)	−0.08	0.748	(−0.60, 0.41)	−0.54	0.899	(−7.91, 8.98)
Smoking	−0.60	0.10	(−1.43, 0.11)	−0.64	0.091 †	(−1.54, 0.13)	−5.22	0.384	(−19.74, 6.67)
Alcohol	−0.58	0.037 *	(−1.06, −0.03) ‡	−0.50	0.077 †	(−1.01, 0.05)	−11.57	0.011 *	(−19.33, −2.97) ‡
ROM	0.18	0.447	(−0.31, 0.64)	0.03	0.905	(−0.46, 0.49)	4.65	0.229	(−3.67, 12.44)
Smooth terms	**edf**	**F-value**	***p*-value**	**edf**	**F-value**	***p*-value**	**edf**	**F-value**	***p*-value**
Hospitalization length	3.80	3.82	0.004 **	3.96	3.56	0.005 **	3.72	2.85	0.022 **
Symptom duration	3.35	4.24	0.003 **	3.45	3.75	0.006 **	3.00	4.98	0.001 **
Model fit summary	n = 194 R^2 (adjusted) = 0.417 Deviance explained = 46.9%			n = 194 R^2 (adjusted) = 0.176 Deviance explained = 24.6%			n = 194 R^2 (adjusted) = 0.168 Deviance explained = 23.6%		

Annotation: Results from multiple regression using a Generalized Additive Model (GAM). NRS AD was excluded from ΔNRS and ΔNRS (%) models to avoid mathematical coupling, as it is a component of both outcome definitions. Non-linearity was observed in Hospitalization length and Symptom duration, for which smooth terms with k = 7 were applied. Due to violations of residual normality and homoscedasticity, all models were bootstrapped. *p*-values were obtained from GAM outputs († = $p < 0.1$, * = $p < 0.05$; ** = $p < 0.01$; *** = $p < 0.001$). The 95% confidence intervals were estimated via non-parametric bootstrapping and considered statistically significant if excluding zero (‡ = 95% CI excludes zero). Abbreviation: NRS, Numeric rating scale; NRS AD, NRS at admission, NRS DC, NRS at discharge; ΔNRS, absolute pain change = NRS DC − NRS AD; ΔNRS (%), relative pain change = ((NRS DC − NRS AD)/NRS AD) × 100; CI, Confidence Interval; Lower GI, Past history of Lower Gastrointestinal disease; MSTL, Past history of Musculoskeletal disease–thoracic or lumbar spinal region; LBP, Lower back pain; ROM, Range of motion.

3.7.1. Pain at Discharge

Violations of the linearity, residual normality, and homoscedasticity assumptions were identified through the residuals vs. fitted plot (Figure S1a), the Shapiro–Wilk normality test ($p = 0.003$), and the Breusch-Pagan test ($p = 0.026$). However, all variance inflation factors (VIFs) were <2, indicating no multicollinearity. Partial residual plots of continuous variables revealed non-linearity in hospitalization and symptom duration, for which GAMs were subsequently applied for correction (Figure S2a). Upon re-evaluation, residual diagnostics continued to show normality and heteroscedasticity violations, as indicated by the Shapiro–Wilk test ($p = 0.004$) and the residuals vs. fitted plot. Accordingly, bootstrapping was employed to obtain robust confidence intervals.

The model included 194 patients, with an adjusted R^2 of 0.417 and deviance explained at 46.9%. Initial pain intensity ($\beta = 0.71$, 95% CI: 0.56–0.90, $p < 0.001$) and dyspepsia ($\beta = 0.55$, 95% CI: 0.05–1.02, $p < 0.05$) were significantly associated with higher pain at discharge. In contrast, alcohol consumption was significantly associated with lower pain at discharge ($\beta = -0.58$, 95% CI: −1.06–−0.03, $p < 0.05$). Furthermore, hospitalization length (EDF = 3.80) and symptom duration (EDF = 3.35) exhibited significant non-linear effects (Figure 2a). No other variables showed significant associations.

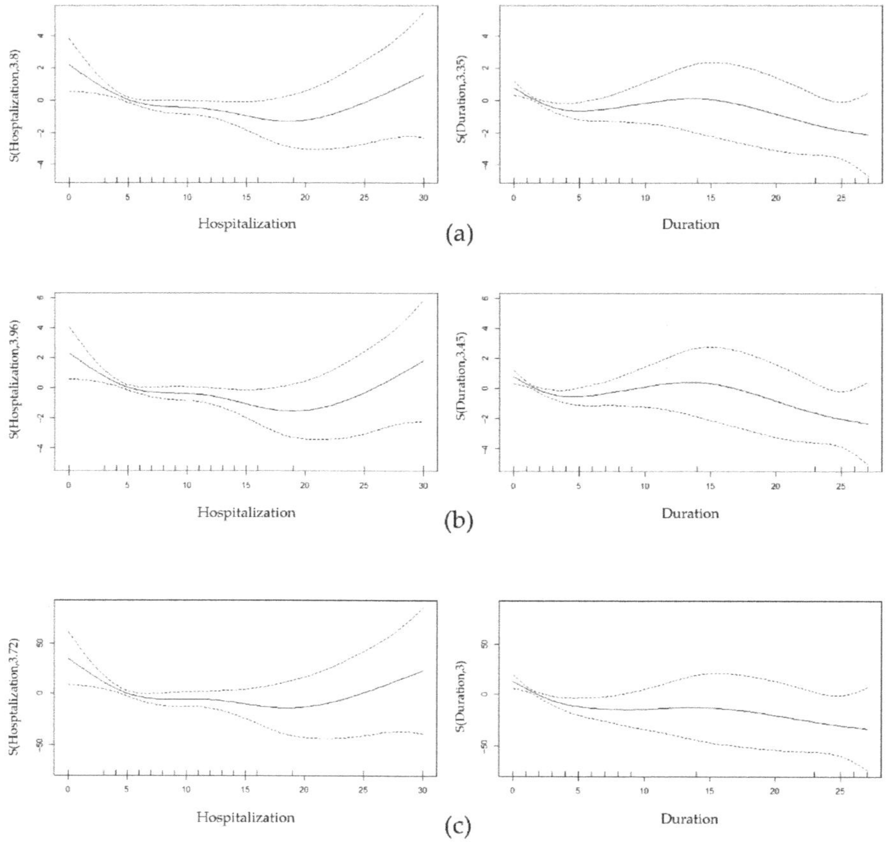

Figure 2. Graphs of estimated smooth effect of hospitalization (**left**) and duration (**right**) using GAM. (**a**) NRS DC, (**b**) ΔNRS, (**c**) ΔNRS (%). The solid line indicates the estimated smooth function, and the dashed lines represent the 95% confidence interval. The *x*-axis represents the number of days since hospitalization or symptom onset. The *y*-axis depicts the estimated smooth function, representing the non-linear effect of the predictor on the outcome while adjusting for other covariates. Deviations from zero indicate the direction and strength of this effect. The curve suggests a non-linear association between the two variables. Abbreviation: GAM, Generalized Additive Model; NRS, Numeric rating scale; NRS DC, NRS at discharge; ΔNRS, absolute pain change = NRS DC − NRS AD; ΔNRS (%), relative pain change = ((NRS DC − NRS AD)/NRS AD) × 100.

3.7.2. Absolute Pain Change

NRS AD was excluded from the model as an independent variable since the absolute change was defined as NRS DC − NRS AD, which would induce mathematical coupling. Violations of the linearity and residual normality assumptions were identified through the residuals vs. fitted plot (Figure S1b) and the Shapiro–Wilk normality test ($p = 0.000$). The Breusch-Pagan test supported homoscedasticity ($p = 0.102$); however, the residuals versus fitted values plot suggested a potential violation. VIFs were all <2, indicating no evidence of multicollinearity. Non-linearity in hospitalization and symptom duration was identified via partial residual plots, and GAMs were applied for correction (Figure S2b). Bootstrapping was employed to derive robust confidence intervals since the Shapiro–Wilk test ($p = 0.003$) and the residuals vs. fitted plot indicated persistent normality and heteroscedasticity violation.

The model included 194 patients, with an adjusted R^2 of 0.176 and deviance explained at 24.6%. Dyspepsia was significantly associated with smaller absolute pain change ($\beta = 0.54$, 95% CI: 0.06–1.00, $p < 0.05$). In contrast, alcohol consumption ($\beta = -0.50$, 95% CI: −1.01–0.05, $p < 0.1$) and smoking ($\beta = -0.64$, 95% CI: −1.54–0.13, $p < 0.1$) showed suggestive associations with greater pain change, although their bootstrapped confidence intervals included zero, indicating uncertainty in these estimates. Additionally, hospitalization length (EDF = 3.96) and symptom duration (EDF = 3.45) exhibited significant non-linear effects significant non-linear effects (Figure 2b). No other variables showed significant associations.

3.7.3. Relative Pain Change

Given that relative change was defined as (NRS DC − NRS AD)/NRS AD, NRS AD was excluded from the model as an independent variable to avoid endogeneity and potential bias in the regression estimates. Violations of the linearity and residual normality assumptions were identified by the residuals vs. fitted plot (Figure S1c) and the Shapiro–Wilk normality test ($p = 0.003$). Although the Breusch-Pagan test showed no significant heteroscedasticity ($p = 0.2825$), the residual plot suggested a potential mild dichotomous distribution. VIFs for all variables were <2, indicating no multicollinearity concerns. Partial residual plots revealed non-linearity of hospitalization and symptom duration, which was addressed using GAMs (Figure S2c). Bootstrapping was employed to adjust confidence intervals since the Shapiro–Wilk test indicated a persistent violation of normality ($p = 0.008$).

The model included 194 patients, with an adjusted R^2 of 0.168 and deviance explained at 23.6%. Dyspepsia showed a significant association with smaller relative pain change ($\beta = 8.15$, 95% CI: 0.27–16.38, $p < 0.05$). In contrast, alcohol consumption was significantly associated with a greater pain change ($\beta = -11.57$, 95% CI: −19.33–−2.97, $p < 0.05$). Furthermore, hospitalization length (EDF = 3.72) and symptom duration (EDF = 3.00) exhibited significant non-linear effects (Figure 2c). No other variables showed significant associations.

3.7.4. Sensitive and Subgroup Analysis

Table S3 presents the results of the sensitivity and subgroup analysis of multiple regression. In the full model including all covariates, the regression coefficient for dyspepsia remained consistent in both direction and magnitude across all pain outcomes (NRS DC: $\beta = 0.66$, $p < 0.05$; ΔNRS: $\beta = 0.67$, $p < 0.05$; ΔNRS [%]: $\beta = 10.21$, $p < 0.05$). Alcohol consumption also showed a consistent association with pain at discharge and relative pain change (NRS DC: $\beta = -0.66$, $p < 0.05$; ΔNRS [%]: $\beta = -13.13$, $p < 0.01$), while absolute pain change demonstrated only a suggestive association (ΔNRS: $\beta = -0.57$, $p < 0.1$). Initial pain intensity retained a significant association with pain at discharge (NRS DC: $\beta = 0.71$, $p < 0.001$). Additionally, suggestive associations were observed for smoking (NRS DC: $\beta = -0.72$, $p < 0.1$; ΔNRS: $\beta = -0.75$, $p < 0.1$), age (NRS DC: $\beta = -0.02$, $p < 0.1$, ΔNRS [%]: $\beta = -0.45$, $p < 0.1$), and ROM (ΔNRS [%]: $\beta = 6.62$, $p < 0.1$).

The regression coefficient for dyspepsia (NRS DC: $\beta = 0.69$, $p < 0.01$; ΔNRS: $\beta = 0.69$, $p < 0.01$; ΔNRS [%]: $\beta = 10.43$, $p < 0.05$) and alcohol consumption (NRS DC: $\beta = -0.70$, $p < 0.05$; ΔNRS: $\beta = -0.63$, $p < 0.05$; ΔNRS [%]: $\beta = -13.64$, $p < 0.01$) remained consistent in both direction and magnitude across all pain outcomes in the model adding known predictors of LBP chronicity (age, gender, psychological history, DM, and HTN). Initial pain intensity remained significant for pain at discharge (NRS DC: $\beta = 0.71$, $p < 0.001$). Additionally, smoking showed significant or suggestive associations (NRS DC: $\beta = -0.75$, $p < 0.05$; ΔNRS: $\beta = -0.77$, $p < 0.1$).

Subgroup analysis was performed with the basic model, including 181 patients diagnosed with lumbar sprain or strain. The regression coefficient for dyspepsia was consistently maintained across all pain outcomes, although the association reached only suggestive significance (NRS DC: $\beta = 0.49$, $p < 0.1$; ΔNRS: $\beta = 0.48$, $p < 0.1$; ΔNRS [%]: $\beta = 7.23$, $p < 0.1$). Initial pain intensity remained strongly associated with pain at discharge (NRS DC: $\beta = 0.71$, $p < 0.001$), whereas alcohol consumption showed a significant or suggestive association with pain at discharge and relative pain change (NRS DC: $\beta = -0.49$, $p < 0.1$; ΔNRS [%]: $\beta = -10.70$, $p < 0.05$).

3.7.5. Association Between Binary Variables Included in Regression

Although the absence of multicollinearity was observed in the regression analysis, a Chi-squared test was additionally conducted to examine the independence between categorical variables. Alcohol consumption and smoking demonstrated a strong association ($p < 0.001$). Furthermore, significant associations were observed between dyspepsia and constipation, dyspepsia and widespread pain, past history of lower GI disorders and thoracolumbar musculoskeletal disorders, and past history of thoracolumbar musculoskeletal disorders and widespread pain ($p < 0.05$) (Table S4).

4. Discussion

This retrospective study analyzed 194 patients hospitalized for ALBP to investigate how systemic symptoms influence the clinical course of ALBP. Progression to CLBP causes functional impairment and psychosocial issues such as sleep disturbance, anxiety, and depression while imposing a long-term socioeconomic burden through reduced productivity and increased healthcare costs [5–9]. Accordingly, numerous studies explored prognostic factors for the early prevention of LBP chronicization, emphasizing psychosocial and demographic variables, as well as the short-term recovery of ALBP [13,14]. However, to the best of our knowledge, no studies have examined systemic symptoms as prognostic factors for LBP through a holistic perspective. Recognizing that short-term recovery of ALBP may predict its chronicization, this study assessed the impact of systemic symptoms on the clinical course of ALBP, ultimately identifying long-term prognostic factors and highlighting the value of a holistic approach.

Among the systemic symptoms, dyspepsia may hinder recovery from ALBP as an independent risk factor. In univariate analysis, dyspepsia showed a suggestive association with higher pain at discharge ($p = 0.091$) and lower absolute ($p = 0.052$) and relative ($p = 0.054$) change in pain. However, dyspepsia was significantly associated with greater pain at discharge ($\beta = 0.55$, $p = 0.026$, 95% CI [0.05, 1.02]) and lower pain improvement both in absolute ($\beta = 0.54$, $p = 0.033$, 95% CI [0.06, 1.00]) and relative terms ($\beta = 8.15$, $p = 0.045$, 95% CI [0.27, 16.38]) in regression analysis. The observed discrepancy likely reflects the limitations of univariate analysis in accounting for confounding and interaction effects, whereas regression models adjust for these influences, providing a more precise estimate of the independent effect.

Dyspepsia also demonstrated a robust association in the sensitivity analyses, demonstrating consistent effects regardless of variable selection or analytic conditions. Dyspepsia consistently showed significant associations across all pain outcomes in the full model and the model with known chronicity factors, highlighting its robustness and novelty as an independent factor beyond previously identified predictors. Furthermore, dyspepsia exhibited suggestive associations across pain outcomes in subgroup analysis. Nevertheless, the directions of the coefficient remained consistent with that of the base model. Additionally, the regression coefficients for absolute pain change associated with dyspepsia were estimated at 0.48–0.69, indicating a corresponding reduction in the extent of LBP improvement. Given the average admission pain score of 6.09 ± 1.46 and the reported Minimal Clinically Important Difference (MCID) of -2 for moderate LBP (NRS 5–7), dyspepsia may meaningfully hinder the degree of pain reduction required to meet the MCID threshold [37]. Hence, the adjusted R^2, representing the explanatory power of the base regression model, ranged from 16.8% to 41.7%. Consequently, these results suggest a reasonable level of reliability since R^2 values >15% are generally considered meaningful in clinical research [38]. Taken together, these statistical and clinical interpretations suggest that dyspepsia may serve as a significant independent factor impeding the recovery of ALBP and potentially contributing to its chronicity.

No studies have yet reported an influence of dyspepsia on ALBP prognosis. Moreover, a definitive pathophysiological mechanism has yet to be established. Nevertheless, several plausible mechanisms can be proposed based on anatomical and physiological considerations. First, hyperactivation of the abdominal muscles, including the rectus abdominis, external oblique, and internal oblique, is frequently observed in LBP patients [39]. This increases intra-abdominal pressure (IAP) as a compensatory mechanism, enhancing spinal stability and reducing the mechanical load on the vertebrae [40,41]. The elevated IAP may concurrently reduce gastrointestinal blood flow, thereby contributing to dyspeptic symptoms [42]. Second, dyspepsia may impact LBP through viscerosomatic reflexes. The upper GI tract is primarily innervated by the T5–T9 spinal segments. Visceral stimuli from GI symptoms are conveyed via visceral afferent fibers to the corresponding spinal dorsal horn segments, where they may affect somatic nerves through viscerosomatic convergence [43]. Such convergence can trigger reflexive muscle tension in dorsal rami–innervated muscles at the same spinal segments [44]. These muscles, including the erector spinae, multifidus, and intertransversarii, play a critical role in segmental spinal stability and fine motor control [44]. As these muscles are anatomically integrated with the thoracolumbar fascia, sustained reflexive tension may induce fascial stress and deformation. Given previous evidence that thoracolumbar fascia deformation may contribute to the onset of ALBP, visceral stimulation associated with dyspepsia could exacerbate pain or hinder recovery [45]. Lastly, dyspepsia may induce central sensitization, leading to altered pain perception. In visceral pain disorders such as irritable bowel syndrome or functional dyspepsia, cortical reorganization has been reported in the anterior cingulate cortex (ACC) and medial prefrontal cortex [46]. These alternations affect sensory perception, pain modulation, and emotional as well as cognitive processing [46]. The ACC, in particular, is activated by acute visceral pain through glutamatergic signaling, contributing to the formation of pain memory and negative affective responses [47]. These neural changes induced by visceral pain can increase overall pain sensitivity, potentially amplifying the perception of pain arising from other regions [48]. Consequently, LBP patients with dyspepsia may experience more intense and persistent pain.

Constipation is another systemic symptom warranting attention. While univariate analysis indicated a suggestive association with higher pain at discharge ($p = 0.076$), no significant effects were observed in absolute or relative pain change across analyses. However, mean comparisons suggested a substantial negative effect of constipation on LBP recovery. Patients with constipation showed a 0.6-point smaller absolute reduction and a 12% lower relative improvement in pain compared to controls. These differences may be clinically meaningful because dyspepsia, a systemic symptom previously discussed with a suggestive association in univariate analysis, showed only a 0.5-point and 8% difference. The lack of statistical significance may reflect the limited power due to the small number of patients with constipation (8 of 194, 4.1%). Moreover, several studies reported a significant association between constipation and increased LBP intensity [18,49], attributing it to the increased mechanical load from the elevated intra-abdominal pressure during defecation and altered pain modulation due to gut microbiome dysbiosis [18,49]. Taken together, the present findings do not entirely exclude a potential association between constipation and

ALBP prognosis. Thus, further studies with larger sample sizes are recommended to clarify the clinical impact of constipation on ALBP prognosis.

Regarding sleep disturbance, a significant association with higher pain at discharge was identified only in univariate analysis ($p = 0.049$), while no significant findings emerged for absolute or relative pain change in any analyses. This finding does not fully align with prior studies indicating a bidirectional correlation between sleep disturbance and LBP, highlighting that poor sleep quality elevates next-day pain, whereas higher pain intensifies sleep disturbance, creating a vicious cycle [19]. This discrepancy may be partly attributable to the measurement of sleep disturbance. Although identified from clinical records referencing diagnostic criteria, sleep disturbances were based on subjective complaints rather than standardized tools, such as sleep diaries and the Pittsburgh Sleep Quality Index, potentially limiting diagnostic accuracy and influencing the results. Nevertheless, given that sleep disturbance exhibited consistently positive, but not significant, regression coefficients across all pain outcomes, it may interact with other clinical factors in a more complex manner. However, this finding alone cannot conclusively establish the effect due to conflicting evidence on the impact of sleep disturbances on LBP [13,19]. Therefore, further research employing rigorous and standardized sleep assessment tools is needed.

Among demographic characteristics, both smoking and alcohol consumption were significantly associated with lower pain at discharge and greater pain change in univariate analysis. However, only alcohol remained significant in multivariate regression, suggesting greater explanatory relevance. Given the strong association between the two (chi-square, $p = 0.000$), the effect of smoking may reflect the influence of alcohol consumption due to shared variance, with its independent contribution attenuated in the regression model despite the absence of multicollinearity. The observed effect of alcohol aligns with prior findings showing that moderate consumption is associated with a reduced risk of pain chronicity, lower pain intensity and extent, and enhanced physical function, especially in non-localized pain conditions [50,51]. However, the apparent analgesic effect of alcohol may reflect elevated pain thresholds rather than actual improvement in mechanical pain. Indeed, consuming 3–4 drinks at least once per month is associated with significantly higher pain thresholds compared to non-drinkers [52]. Therefore, the potential benefits of alcohol consumption for ALBP should be interpreted cautiously.

Regarding other variables, age showed only a suggestive trend in regression sensitivity analysis, with coefficients of -0.02 points and -0.45% for absolute and relative pain change, respectively, although both are clinically negligible. The impact of age on LBP recovery remains controversial, with limited clinical relevance observed in middle-aged populations but significant effects reported in those aged $\geq$65 years [53,54]. Hence, our results may reflect the age restriction to individuals aged $\leq$65 years. This restriction likely enhanced the reliability of our findings by minimizing the confounding effects of age-related degenerative changes and comorbidities observed in older adults [23,24]. However, this approach inevitably limits the external validity of our findings to relatively younger and healthier populations. Although specific evidence for ALBP is limited, advancing age is well known to be associated with higher prevalence of LBP and greater disability [55]. Consequently, generalizability of our findings may be limited, and caution is warranted when extrapolating the results to older adults in clinical settings, as advanced age may negatively impact LBP recovery.

Furthermore, past history, such as the history of DM and PSY, often linked to poor LBP recovery, showed no consistent associations in this study, nor did HTN, which had been reported to predict better prognosis [13]. This discrepancy may be partly explained by the study design focusing on the short-term prognosis of ALBP, whereas prior research examined long-term pain outcomes over months to years, which may better capture the impact of medical history. Indeed, type 2 diabetes is associated with low-grade systemic inflammation, a factor that contributes to the development of CLBP and may necessitate prolonged periods for symptom manifestation [56,57]. Furthermore, depression and CLBP share common neurotransmitters, notably serotonin, which modulate both the descending pain inhibitory pathway and emotion regulation [58]. The clinical effects of these changes often take extended periods to emerge due to neuroplasticity [59]. Therefore, the aforementioned past history may exert a progressively greater influence on LBP recovery, with PSY in particular representing a key factor [58]. These findings underscore the necessity of long-term follow-up in future studies to fully elucidate these associations.

Hospitalization length and symptom duration demonstrated strong significance across all pain outcomes in univariate analyses and exhibited non-linear relationships in regression models. Both variables showed a rapid pain improvement trend up to 5–7 days, followed by a gradual recovery until 15–20 days. However, unlike symptom duration, hospitalization length showed a potential pain rebound beyond 20 days, suggesting important clinical implications. While short-term bed rest of 2–3 days is generally considered most effective for ALBP [60], the continued improvement observed up to 20 days in this study may reflect a synergistic effect of bed rest and active therapeutic intervention during admission. Nevertheless, the negative consequences of reduced physical activity may outweigh the benefits beyond a certain point, warranting caution in considering prolonged hospitalization. Hence, results beyond 16 days for both variables should be interpreted with caution since sparse observations in this interval led to wider confidence intervals, potentially compromising the precision of the estimates.

The present findings suggest several clinical implications. Systemic symptoms in ALBP patients, particularly dyspepsia, may serve as early indicators of slower recovery, underscoring the importance of careful assessment at the initial clinical evaluation. Identifying such patients can help clinicians to prioritize early intervention and design multidimensional management strategies aimed at preventing prolonged disability. In this context, management focusing solely on pain control may result in delayed improvement for patients presenting with dyspeptic symptoms. Therefore, combining physiotherapy or acupuncture with medication for dyspepsia may offer a viable therapeutic approach, addressing both systemic and musculoskeletal components. More broadly, incorporating symptom profiling into routine assessment may enhance prognostic accuracy and facilitate tailored treatment planning. For example, considering the combined patterns of GI symptoms, PSY, and DM alongside pain intensity could enable more precise risk stratification, providing a practical foundation for more proactive and comprehensive approaches to ALBP care.

Hence, this study has some limitations. First, the results present only correlational analyses between systemic symptoms and LBP without establishing causality. Despite outlining possible mechanisms, they remain hypothetical and require further investigation to confirm causality. Second, systemic symptoms were identified based on patients' subjective reports in medical records rather than standardized assessment tools or objective diagnostic criteria. The reliance on subjective reports may have introduced measurement bias, potentially affecting patient selection and over- or underestimating associations with LBP. Future studies should employ validated tools, such as the Nepean Dyspepsia Index for dyspepsia or the Pittsburgh Sleep Quality Index for sleep disturbances, to enhance the reliability and specificity of systemic symptom assessment. Third, the generalizability of our findings may be limited. The present study focused solely on ALBP, with a mean total course of approximately 9 days (sum of symptom duration and hospitalization), thereby excluding CLBP populations. Despite the evidence that short-term recovery patterns can predict LBP chronicity, it remains unclear whether these associations extend to longer-term courses in CLBP patients, limiting the applicability of our findings. In addition, the exclusion of non-mechanical LBP patients, who often present with more severe or persistent pain and poorer overall health, may have led to an underestimation of symptom impact. Moreover, 93% of the included patients were diagnosed with lumbar sprain or strain, further limiting the generalizability of our findings to other mechanical LBP types, such as acute disc herniation. Finally, the size and gender distribution of the sample may have influenced the observed associations. With a sample size of 194 and no a priori calculation, the statistical power to detect small-to-moderate effects may have been limited given the number of covariates, particularly in subgroup analysis. The male-to-female ratio was also imbalanced at approximately 40:60. The smaller number of participants in one gender may have increased estimate variability and lowered the statistical power to detect gender-related differences or interactions. Although GAM and bootstrap methods were applied to enhance reliability, certain associations may have remained undetected, warranting caution in interpreting the results. Taken together, these limitations suggest that future research should include older adults, patients with CLBP and/or non-mechanical LBP, and a more balanced sex distribution. Studies should also employ standardized symptom assessments and longer follow-up periods, ideally in large-scale prospective longitudinal trials with diverse populations.

5. Conclusions

This retrospective cross-sectional study is the first to identify systemic symptoms, especially dyspepsia, as potential short-term prognostic factors impeding ALBP recovery. Given the influence of early recovery patterns on long-term outcomes, these findings may serve as meaningful markers for early identification of patients at risk of LBP chronicity. Furthermore, multivariable regression analysis was employed to assess the independent effects of various factors beyond systemic symptoms, acknowledging the multifactorial nature of LBP prognosis in clinical settings. This comprehensive analysis underscores the clinical relevance of a holistic approach to LBP by demonstrating the significant association between pain and dyspepsia. Despite the limitations of our study design, the obtained results suggest a novel approach for preventing chronicity and guiding proactive treatment strategies in LBP. Moreover, this study highlights the potential effectiveness of multidimensional and integrated strategies in reducing pain and enhancing patients' quality of life in clinical practice.

Supplementary Materials: The following supporting information can be downloaded at: https://www.mdpi.com/article/10.3390/jcm14196969/s1, Figure S1: Residuals Vs. Fitted plots for the initial multiple linear regression model; Figure S2: Partial residual plots of continuous variables in the initial multiple linear; Table S1: Association between Past Medical History and Pain Intensity; Table S2: Association between systemic symptoms and pain characteristics; Table S3: Sensitivity and Subgroup Analyses of between low back pain characteristics and pain intensity; Table S4: Results of association between binary indices included in the regression.

Author Contributions: Conceptualization, J.-H.L. and S.-H.P.; Methodology, S.-H.H. and D.-H.K.; Investigation, J.-H.L., S.-H.H. and M.-S.K.; Project administration, S.-H.P. and D.-H.K.; Supervision, S.-H.P.; Writing—Original draft, J.-H.L. and S.-H.P.; Writing—Review And Editing: S.-H.H., M.-S.K. and D.-H.K. All authors have read and agreed to the published version of the manuscript.

Funding: This research received no external funding.

Institutional Review Board Statement: The study protocol was approved by the Institutional Review Board of Dongguk University Bun-dang Oriental Hospital (IRB no. 2025-0005; Approval Date: 2025.07.07).

Informed Consent Statement: Informed consent was waived due to the difficulties in obtaining consent from patients who had already completed treatment. This study poses less than minimum risk, as it was conducted using data from patients who had completed treatment. Furthermore, in accordance with IRB regulations, all personal information had been removed by third party not involved in this study prior to data analysis.

Data Availability Statement: Data are not available due to ethical reasons.

Conflicts of Interest: The authors declare no conflicts of interest.

Abbreviations

The following abbreviations are used in this manuscript:

LBP	Low Back Pain
ALBP	Acute Low Back Pain
CLBP	Chronic Low Back Pain
GI	Gastrointestinal
TKM	Traditional Korean Medicine
IRB	Institutional Review Board
HTN	Hypertension
DM	Diabetes Mellitus
PSY	Psychological history
ROM	Range of Motion
NRS	Numeric Rating Scale
NRS AD	Numeric Rating Scale at Admission
NRS DC	Numeric Rating Scale at Discharge
GAM	Generalized Additive Model
VIF	Variance Inflation Factors
IAP	Intra-abdominal Pressure
ACC	Anterior Cingulate Cortex

References

1. Burton, A.K.; Balague, F.; Cardon, G.; Eriksen, H.R.; Henrotin, Y.; Lahad, A.; Leclerc, A.; Müller, G.; van der Beek, A.J. Chapter 2 European guidelines for prevention in low back pain. *Eur. Spine J.* **2006**, *15*, S136–S168. [CrossRef]
2. Chien, J.J.; Bajwa, Z.H. What is mechanical back pain and how best to treat it? *Curr. Pain Headache Rep.* **2008**, *12*, 406–411. [CrossRef] [PubMed]
3. Cooper, G. Treatment of acute lower back pain. In *Non-Operative Treatment of the Lumbar Spine*; Bono, C.M., Schoenfeld, A.J., Vaccaro, A.R., Eds.; Springer: Cham, Switzerland, 2015; pp. 15–18.
4. Apkarian, A.V.; Baliki, M.N.; Geha, P.Y. Towards a theory of chronic pain. *Prog. Neurobiol.* **2009**, *87*, 81–97. [CrossRef] [PubMed]
5. Robert, J.G.; Dana, B.; Anna, W.S.; Glenn, P. Psychosocial differences between high-risk acute vs chronic low back pain patients. *Pain Pract.* **2008**, *8*, 91–97.
6. Marin, R.; Cyhan, T.; Miklos, W. Sleep disturbance in patients with chronic low back pain. *Am. J. Phys. Med. Rehabil.* **2006**, *85*, 430–435. [CrossRef]
7. Wang, H.Y.; Fu, T.S.; Hsu, S.C.; Hung, C.I. Association of depression with sleep quality might be greater than that of pain intensity among outpatients with chronic low back pain. *Neuropsychiatr. Dis. Treat.* **2016**, *12*, 1993–1998. [CrossRef]
8. Montgomery, W.; Sato, M.; Nagasaka, Y.; Vietri, J. The economic and humanistic costs of chronic lower back pain in Japan. *Clin. Outcomes Res.* **2017**, *9*, 361–371. [CrossRef]
9. Moradi, B.; Hagmann, S.; Zahlten-Hinguranage, A.; Caldeira, F.; Putz, C.; Rosshirt, N.; Schönit, E.; Mesrian, A.; Schiltenwolf, M.; Neubauer, E. Efficacy of multidisciplinary treatment for patients with chronic low back pain: A prospective clinical study in 395 patients. *J. Clin. Rheumatol.* **2012**, *18*, 76–82. [CrossRef]
10. Valat, J.P.; Goupille, P.; Védère, V. Low back pain: Risk factors for chronicity. *Rev. Rhum. Engl. Ed.* **1997**, *64*, 189–194.
11. Waddell, G. 1987 Volvo award in clinical sciences. A new clinical model for the treatment of low-back pain. *Spine* **1987**, *12*, 632–644. [CrossRef]
12. Nieminen, L.K.; Pyysalo, L.M.; Kankaanpää, M.J. Prognostic factors for pain chronicity in low back pain: A systematic review. *Pain Rep.* **2021**, *6*, e919. [CrossRef]

13. da Silva, T.; Macaskill, P.; Mills, K.; Maher, C.; Williams, C.; Lin, C.; Hancock, M.J. Predicting recovery in patients with acute low back pain: A clinical prediction model. *Eur. J. Pain* **2017**, *21*, 716–726. [CrossRef]
14. Friedman, B.W.; O'Mahony, S.; Mulvey, L.; Davitt, M.; Choi, H.; Xia, S.; Esses, D.; Bijur, P.E.; Gallagher, E.J. One-week and 3-month outcomes after an emergency department visit for undifferentiated musculoskeletal low back pain. *Ann. Emerg. Med.* **2012**, *59*, 128–133. [CrossRef] [PubMed]
15. Schneiderman, H. The review of systems: An important part of a comprehensive examination. *Postgrad. Med.* **1982**, *71*, 151–158. [CrossRef] [PubMed]
16. Smith, M.D.; Russell, A.; Hodges, P.W. How common is back pain in women with gastrointestinal problems? *Clin. J. Pain* **2008**, *24*, 199–203. [CrossRef] [PubMed]
17. Smith, M.D.; Russell, A.; Hodges, P.W. The relationship between incontinence, breathing disorders, gastrointestinal symptoms, and back pain in women: A longitudinal cohort study. *Clin. J. Pain* **2014**, *30*, 162–167. [CrossRef]
18. Yu, H.Y.; Jeong, Y.W. Influence of constipation in women in their twenties on low back pain. *J. Korean Orthop. Manip. Phys. Ther.* **2018**, *24*, 43–49.
19. Alsaadi, S.M.; McAuley, J.H.; Hush, J.M.; Lo, S.; Bartlett, D.J.; Grunstein, R.R.; Maher, C.G. The bidirectional relationship between pain intensity and sleep disturbance/quality in patients with low back pain. *Clin. J. Pain* **2014**, *30*, 755–765. [CrossRef]
20. The Society of Korean Rehabilitation Medicine. *Korean Rehabilitation Medicine*, 5th ed.; Kunja Publisher: Seoul, Republic of Korea, 2020; pp. 6–10, 16–20, 87–88.
21. Park, S.H.; Keum, D.H. Systemic symptoms as potential predictors of chronic neck pain on initial examination: Can systemic symptoms act as a predictor of neck pain? *J. Pers. Med.* **2024**, *14*, 688. [CrossRef]
22. Cuschieri, S. The STROBE guidelines. *Saudi. J. Anaesth.* **2019**, *13*, S31–S34. [CrossRef]
23. Wong, A.Y.L.; Karppinen, J.; Samartzis, D. Low back pain in older adults: Risk factors, management options and future directions. *Scoliosis Spinal Disord.* **2017**, *12*, 14. [CrossRef] [PubMed]
24. Rundell, S.D.; Sherman, K.J.; Heagerty, P.J.; Mock, C.N.; Dettori, N.J.; Comstock, B.A.; Avins, A.L.; Nedeljkovic, S.S.; Nerenz, D.R.; Jarvik, J.G. Predictors of persistent disability and back pain in older adults with a new episode of care for back pain. *Pain Med.* **2017**, *18*, 1049–1062. [CrossRef] [PubMed]
25. Verhagen, A.P.; Downie, A.; Popal, N.; Maher, C.; Koes, B.W. Red flags presented in current low back pain guidelines: A review. *Eur. Spine J.* **2016**, *25*, 2788–2802. [CrossRef] [PubMed]
26. Kuris, E.O.; McDonald, C.L.; Palumbo, M.A.; Daniels, A.H. Evaluation and management of cauda equina syndrome. *Am. J. Med.* **2021**, *134*, 1483–1489. [CrossRef]
27. Donnally, C.J., III; Margetis, K.; Varacallo, M.A. Vertebral Compression Fractures. In *StatPearls*; StatPearls Publishing: Treasure Island, FL, USA, 2025.
28. Suzuki, N.; Ogikubo, O.; Hansson, T. The course of the acute vertebral body fragility fracture: Its effect on pain, disability and quality of life during 12 months. *Eur. Spine J.* **2008**, *17*, 1380–1390. [CrossRef]
29. Sahbaie, P.; Irvine, K.A.; Liang, D.Y.; Shi, X.; Clark, J.D. Mild traumatic brain injury causes nociceptive sensitization through spinal chemokine upregulation. *Sci. Rep.* **2019**, *9*, 19500. [CrossRef]
30. Danielli, E.; Simard, N.; DeMatteo, C.A.; Kumbhare, D.; Ulmer, S.; Noseworthy, M.D. A review of brain regions and associated post-concussion symptoms. *Front. Neurol.* **2023**, *14*, 1136367. [CrossRef]
31. Strate, L.L.; Ayanian, J.Z.; Kotler, G.; Syngal, S. Risk factors for mortality in lower intestinal bleeding. *Clin. Gastroenterol. Hepatol.* **2008**, *6*, 1004–1010. [CrossRef]
32. Center for Behavioral Health Statistics and Quality. Additional Disorders for Consideration. In *Impact of the DSM-IV to DSM-5 Changes on the National Survey on Drug Use and Health*; Substance Abuse and Mental Health Services Administration: Rockville, MD, USA, 2016; pp. 151–153.
33. Rome Foundation, Rome IV Criteria. Available online: https://theromefoundation.org/rome-iv/rome-iv-criteria/ (accessed on 4 February 2025).
34. International Continence Society Committees, Nocturia—Terminology Discussion. Available online: https://www.ics.org/committees/standardisation/terminologydiscussions/nocturia (accessed on 4 February 2025).
35. Choi, E.P.H.; Wan, E.Y.F.; Kwok, J.Y.Y.; Chin, W.Y.; Lam, C.L.K. The mediating role of sleep quality in the association between nocturia and health-related quality of life. *Health. Qual. Life Outcomes.* **2019**, *17*, 181. [CrossRef]
36. Dijkers, M. Comparing quantification of pain severity by verbal rating and numeric rating scales. *J. Spinal Cord Med.* **2010**, *33*, 232–242. [CrossRef]
37. Haase, I.; Kladny, B. Clinical relevance of changes in pain intensity in patients with specific back pain. *Z. Orthop. Unfall.* **2022**, *160*, 213–221. [CrossRef]
38. Gupta, A.; Stead, T.S.; Ganti, L. Determining a meaningful R-squared value in clinical medicine. *Acad. Med. Surg.* **2024**. [CrossRef]
39. Marras, W.S.; Davis, K.G.; Ferguson, S.A.; Lucas, B.R.; Gupta, P. Spine loading characteristics of patients with low back pain compared with asymptomatic individuals. *Spine* **2001**, *26*, 2566–2574. [CrossRef]

40. Hodges, P.W.; Eriksson, A.E.; Shirley, D.; Gandevia, S.C. Intra-abdominal pressure increases stiffness of the lumbar spine. *J. Biomech.* **2005**, *38*, 1873–1880. [CrossRef]
41. Stokes, I.A.F.; Gardner-Morse, M.G.; Henry, S.M. Intra-abdominal pressure and abdominal wall muscular function: Spinal unloading mechanism. *Clin. Biomech.* **2010**, *25*, 859–866. [CrossRef] [PubMed]
42. Gudmundsson, F.F.; Gislason, H.G.; Dicko, A.; Horn, A.; Viste, A.; Grong, K.; Svanes, K. Effects of prolonged increased intra-abdominal pressure on gastrointestinal blood flow in pigs. *Surg. Endosc.* **2001**, *15*, 854–860. [CrossRef] [PubMed]
43. Willis, W.D. Visceral inputs to sensory pathways in the spinal cord. In *Progress in Brain Research*; Cervero, F., Morrison, J.F.B., Eds.; Elsevier: Amsterdam, The Netherlands, 1986; Volume 67, pp. 207–225.
44. Beal, M.C. Viscerosomatic reflexes: A review. *J. Am. Osteopath. Assoc.* **1985**, *85*, 53–68. [CrossRef]
45. Brandl, A.; Egner, C.; Reer, R.; Schmidt, T.; Schleip, R. Associations between deformation of the thoracolumbar fascia and activation of the erector spinae and multifidus muscle in patients with acute low back pain and healthy controls: A matched pair case-control study. *Life* **2022**, *12*, 1735. [CrossRef]
46. Liu, P.; Wang, G.; Zeng, F.; Liu, Y.; Fan, Y.; Wei, Y.; Qin, W.; Calhoun, V.D. Abnormal brain structure implicated in patients with functional dyspepsia. *Brain Imaging Behav.* **2018**, *12*, 459–466. [CrossRef]
47. Yan, N.; Cao, B.; Xu, J.; Hao, C.; Zhang, X.; Li, Y. Glutamatergic activation of anterior cingulate cortex mediates the affective component of visceral pain memory in rats. *Neurobiol. Learn. Mem.* **2012**, *97*, 156–164. [CrossRef]
48. Sengupta, J.N. Visceral pain: The neurophysiological mechanism. *Handb. Exp. Pharmacol.* **2009**, *194*, 31–74.
49. Arai, Y.C.; Shiro, Y.; Funak, Y.; Kasugaii, K.; Omichi, Y.; Sakurai, H.; Matsubara, T.; Inoue, M.; Shimo, K.; Saisu, H.; et al. The association between constipation or stool consistency and pain severity in patients with chronic pain. *Anesth. Pain Med.* **2018**, *8*, e69275. [CrossRef] [PubMed]
50. Karimi, R.; Mallah, N.; Nedjat, S.; Beasley, M.J.; Takkouche, B. Association between alcohol consumption and chronic pain: A systematic review and meta-analysis. *Br. J. Anaesth.* **2022**, *129*, 355–365. [CrossRef] [PubMed]
51. Scott, J.R.; Hassett, A.L.; Schrepf, A.D.; Brummett, C.M.; Harris, R.E.; Clauw, D.J.; Harte, S.E. Moderate alcohol consumption is associated with reduced pain and fibromyalgia symptoms in chronic pain patients. *Pain Med.* **2018**, *19*, 2515–2527. [CrossRef] [PubMed]
52. DeWall, C.N.; Giancola, P.R.; Bushman, B.J. Too insensitive to care: Alcohol increases human aggression by increasing pain threshold. *J. Stud. Alcohol. Drugs.* **2024**, *86*, 755–760. [CrossRef]
53. Henschke, N.; Maher, C.G.; Refshauge, K.M.; Herbert, R.D.; Cumming, R.G.; Bleasel, J.; York, J.; Das, A.; McAuley, J.H. Prognosis in patients with recent onset low back pain in Australian primary care: Inception cohort study. *BMJ* **2008**, *337*, a171. [CrossRef]
54. Hüllemann, P.; Keller, T.; Kabelitz, M.; Gierthmühlen, J.; Freynhagen, R.; Tölle, T.; Forstenpointner, J.; Baron, R. Clinical manifestation of acute, subacute, and chronic low back pain in different age groups: Low back pain in 35,446 patients. *Pain Pract.* **2018**, *18*, 1011–1023. [CrossRef]
55. GBD 2021 Low Back Pain Collaborators. Global, regional, and national burden of low back pain, 1990–2020, its attributable risk factors, and projections to 2050: A systematic analysis of the Global Burden of Disease Study 2021. *Lancet Rheumatol.* **2023**, *22*, 316–329.
56. Jacob, L.; Rathmann, W.; Koyanagi, A.; Haro, J.M.; Kostev, K. Association between type 2 diabetes and chronic low back pain in general practices in Germany. *BMJ Open Diabetes Res. Care* **2021**, *9*, e002426. [CrossRef]
57. Zhou, W.B.S.; Meng, J.; Zhang, J. Does Low Grade Systemic Inflammation Have a Role in Chronic Pain? *Front. Mol. Neurosci.* **2021**, *14*, 785214. [CrossRef]
58. Wang, R.; Peng, M.S.; Wang, Y.Z.; Chen, P.J.; Wang, X.Q. Influence of Depression on Pain and Disability in Patients with Chronic Low Back Pain after Physical Therapy: A Secondary Analysis of a Randomized Controlled Trial. *Depress. Anxiety* **2024**, *2024*, 9065325. [CrossRef]
59. Millan, M.J. Descending control of pain. *Prog. Neurobiol.* **2002**, *66*, 355–474. [CrossRef]
60. Szpalski, M.; Hayez, J.P. How many days of bed rest for acute low back pain? Objective assessment of trunk function. *Eur. Spine J.* **1992**, *1*, 29–31. [CrossRef]

Journal of
Clinical Medicine

MDPI

Article

Wrist Joint Restriction: Impact on Foot Pressure, Center of Gravity, and the Role of the Dominant Hand

Leire Cruz Gambero [1], Gabriel A. Gijón-Noguerón [2,*], Salvador Díaz Miguel [2], Javier Barón-López [3] and Cantero-Téllez Raquel [1]

1 Physiotherapy Department, Faculty of Health Sciences, University of Malaga, IBIMA Plataforma BIONAND Hand Research Group FE-17, C/Arquitecto Francisco Peñalosa (Ampliación Campus Teatinos), 29010 Malaga, Spain; leiregam@uma.es (L.C.G.); cantero@uma.es (C.-T.R.)
2 Department of Nursing and Podiatry, Faculty of Health Science, University of Malaga, C/Arquitecto Francisco Peñalosa (Ampliación Campus Teatinos), 29010 Malaga, Spain; salvadordiazm@uma.es
3 Department of Public Health and Psiquiatry, Faculty of Medicine, University of Malaga, Blvr Louis Pasteur, 32 (Campus Teatinos), 29010 Malaga, Spain; baron@uma.es
* Correspondence: gagijon@uma.es

Abstract: Background: Wrist immobilization is a common clinical intervention for wrist injuries; however, its repercussions on gait parameters and plantar support have not been extensively investigated. **Objectives**: The purpose of the study was to determine whether wrist immobilization causes alterations in foot pressure and center of gravity, considering hand dominance and visual conditions (eyes open or closed). **Methods**: The research experiment was conducted using the PodoPrint S4 platform. Basic descriptive statistics were calculated to summarize the variables. Additionally, in the mixed linear model (t-tests use Satterthwaite's method) an analysis of variance for repeated measures (ANOVA-RM) was conducted for the determination of the objectives of the study. **Results**: This study included a total of 44 participants (29 females and 15 males), with an average age of 36.5 years (SD = 17.5). Immobilization, independent of eye condition, resulted in significant alterations in antero-posterior oscillation and in a larger plantar support area. In addition, the results suggest that the eye state significantly influences plantar support, independent of limb immobilization or dominance. **Conclusions**: Our findings reveal significant alterations in antero-posterior oscillation and plantar support due to immobilization, suggesting a dynamic interplay between wrist function and lower limb biomechanics.

Keywords: wrist immobilization; foot pressure; gravity; foot support

1. Introduction

Wrist injuries, encompassing distal radius fracture (DRF), triangular fibrocartilage complex injury, instability, scaphoid fracture, and various orthopedic conditions, are commonplace in clinical practice [1,2]. Joint restriction constrains the ability to flexibly coordinate the joints and might lead to reduced balance stability when people perform different tasks or activities [3]. To promote wrist stability and facilitate the healing process, healthcare providers often employ wrist immobilization devices, such as casts or splints [4–6]. The potential secondary effects of this intervention on other aspects of an individual's biomechanics and functional mobility have received limited attention in the scientific literature.

One of the most immediate reactions to upper limb immobilization is an altered gait pattern [7] to compensate for the loss of upper limb function and maintain equilibrium [8]. When the wrist is immobilized, there is a shift in the body's center of mass. To counteract this shift and prevent falls, individuals may adjust their body posture and engage their core and lower limbs more actively. This adaptive response helps in stabilizing the body's center of mass during walking [9].

Ford MP et al. [10] confirmed that constraining one arm resulted in an adaptation in trunk and inter-limb coordination when walking at higher velocities in healthy adults, but no specific upper limb extremity movement disorders participants have been included, and studies did not evaluate possible changes in plantar pressure distribution when there is immobilization and consequently no use of the upper limb. This potential alteration in statics could cause postural changes during daily activities that do not involve walking or any form of displacement. Arm swing is a natural component of walking that aids in balance and stability [11]. When upper limb function is compromised due to immobilization, there may be a compensatory reduction or modification in arm swing. Steven H. Collins et al. [11] conducted a series of simulations and human subject experiments with the goal of elucidating the role of arm swinging and its underlying mechanisms in human gait.

Other investigations [11–14] have concluded that normal arm swing indeed leads to a reduced vertical angular momentum when compared to walking without arm swing. These studies emphasized the imperative to identify alterations in plantar support following wrist or hand immobilization and how these changes may impact not only the movement of the upper limbs but also plantar support. This, in turn, can affect gait cadence and balance, potentially causing challenges or modifications in movement patterns during everyday activities.

Despite the presence of various factors that may affect plantar support following wrist or hand injuries requiring immobilization, such as fear of movement, pain, or catastrophizing, the specific influence of immobilization itself on plantar support remains inconclusive, leaving the potential impact on overall functional recovery uncertain.

The first aim of the present study was to analyze the intra-subject variability in antero-posterior oscillation (APO) and plantar pressure parameters in healthy subjects during the bipedal standing test under wrist–hand dominant and non-dominant immobilization, with both open-eye (OE) and closed-eye (CE) conditions. Based on this aim, we hypothesize that (1) wrist immobilization, regardless of hand dominance, will cause significant alterations in antero-posterior oscillation and plantar pressure distribution when compared to the non-immobilized condition, (2) the effects of wrist immobilization on these parameters will vary depending on hand dominance, and (3) visual conditions (eyes open vs. closed) will significantly influence plantar pressure parameters and postural stability, regardless of wrist immobilization or hand dominance.

2. Materials and Methods

2.1. Study Design and Participants

The study was performed in the Faculty of Health Science of the University of Málaga. The study was approved by the local ethics committee with the number CEUMA: 97-2022-H and was carried out according to the Helsinki Declaration on ethical principles for research involving human subjects [15]. A convenience sample of 44 participants was selected during November 2022 and December 2023. Informed consent was obtained from all participants before their inclusion in the study.

The inclusion criteria were age $\geq$ 18 years. The exclusion criteria included cognitive or neurological impairments that could interfere with the instructions, any previously diagnosed musculoskeletal disorders, recent acute injuries (<1 year) in any limb, immobilization within the previous 6 months, and balance problems.

2.2. Procedure

Participants were recruited through an open call via social media posts to ensure a diverse and representative sample within the study's eligibility criteria. Volunteers who expressed interest were invited to participate, provided they met the predefined inclusion criteria outlined in the study protocol. Additionally, all participants received detailed information about the study's objectives and procedures before providing their informed consent.

Firstly, a questionnaire (designed by the authors) was provided to the participants to obtain the demographic variables, such as age, sex, occupation, physical activity, and hand dominance. The platform pressure data were collected by a researcher who was familiar with the instrument and software, and all measurements were taken by the same evaluator to avoid discrepancies.

The baropodometric measurements were carried out using a baropodometric platform called PodoPrint® S4, a reliable tool for evaluating the distribution of plantar pressures in the dynamic study of the barefoot gait of healthy individuals. The ICCs showed moderate to good repeatability (greater than 0.81 and less than 0.93) [16]. The dimensions of this platform are 57 cm × 57 cm × 9 mm, and it has 1600 sensors. The data were sent digitally to a computer and then processed using software that shows the parameters of plantar pressure, center of pressure, and postural sway. All measurements were taken twice to make data more precise and eliminate possible bias. Assessment was performed in a soundproof room with absolute silence and with no visual distractions. Each participant had to take off any ornaments on their wrists or objects that they had in their pockets, and they had to be barefoot (with no socks). A foot positioning template was used to position the feet at an angle of 30°, with a separation of 2 cm between heels. For every measurement, the participant had to be standing, with resting arms along the body and looking straight ahead at a color signal that was previously placed on the wall. In this position, the following data were obtained for each subject: total foot support surface, measured in cm^2; average foot pressure in static support, measured in gr/cm^2; body sway length and body sway area, both in static support; and center of pressures on the X-axis (COP X) and Y-axis (COP Y), which represent the position of the center of foot pressure compared to the theoretical one.

At first, a quiet stance test was performed for each subject with open eyes (OEs), followed by a second measurement with the same procedure but with closed eyes (CEs). Secondly, a posture–stabilometric test was also performed with OEs and CEs. This procedure was repeated in the same order, immobilizing the wrist of the dominant arm and then immobilizing the other wrist. Dominance was determined by asking the patient which hand they use for writing. We immobilized the wrist with a thermoplastic splint that put the wrist in a neutral position [17,18]. Also, the splint did not cover any fingers or elbow. If the participant coughed, sneezed, turned his/her head, talked, or performed a sudden movement, the measurements were repeated to avoid possible bias.

2.3. Data Analysis

The data were processed with R version 4.3.2 for statistical study [19]. The validity conditions (sphericity and normality) were checked. Mauchly tests for sphericity and Greenhouse–Geisser and Huynh–Feldt corrections for departure from sphericity. The Shapiro–Wilk test for normality was used. A mixed linear model (t-tests use Satterthwaite's method) and an analysis of variance for repeated measures (ANOVA-RM) were conducted for the determination of the objectives of the study. Post hoc comparisons with Holm methods were used. For all statistical analyses, the significance level was set at 5%.

3. Results

This study included a total of 44 participants, composed of 29 females and 15 males, with an average age of 36.5 years (SD = 17.5). An initial exploration of the data revealed that the antero-posterior oscillation (APO) varies significantly with the state of the eyes (open vs. closed), as illustrated in Figure 1.

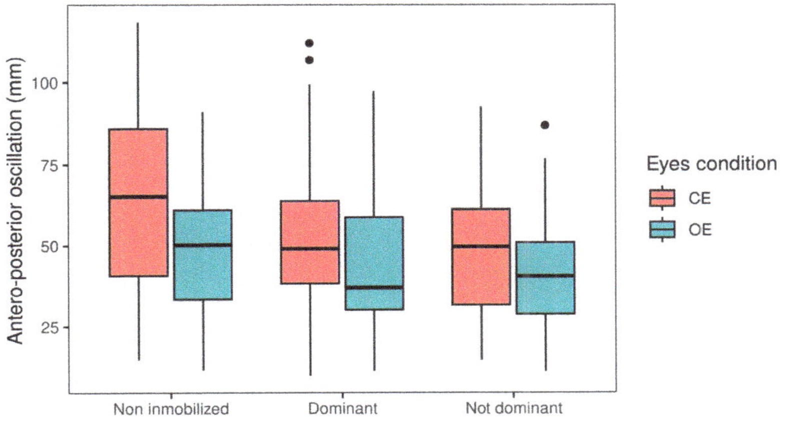

Figure 1. Antero-posterior oscillation associated with state of eyes (open vs. closed).

Notably, immobilization alone, independent of eye condition, resulted in significant alterations in APO ($p < 0.001$), as detailed in Table 1.

Table 1. Summary of the statistical significance of APO alterations due to immobilization alone.

		Value	
Predictors	Estimates	CI	p
(Intercept)	61.39	55.11–67.68	<0.001
Eyes [OE]	−9.51	−12.42–−6.60	<0.001
Dominant	−8.48	−12.05–−4.92	<0.001
Not dominant	−11.17	−14.74–−7.61	<0.001
Random effects			
σ^2	134.31		
$\tau_{00\ DNI}$	327.79		
ICC	0.71		
N_{DNI}	41		
Observations	246		
Marginal R^2/Conditional R^2	0.090/0.735		

Further analysis using an interaction model to assess the effects of eye condition (open vs. closed) separately revealed that immobilization impacts APO irrespective of eye condition ($p < 0.001$), without significant differences between immobilization of the dominant or non-dominant limb (Figure 2a).

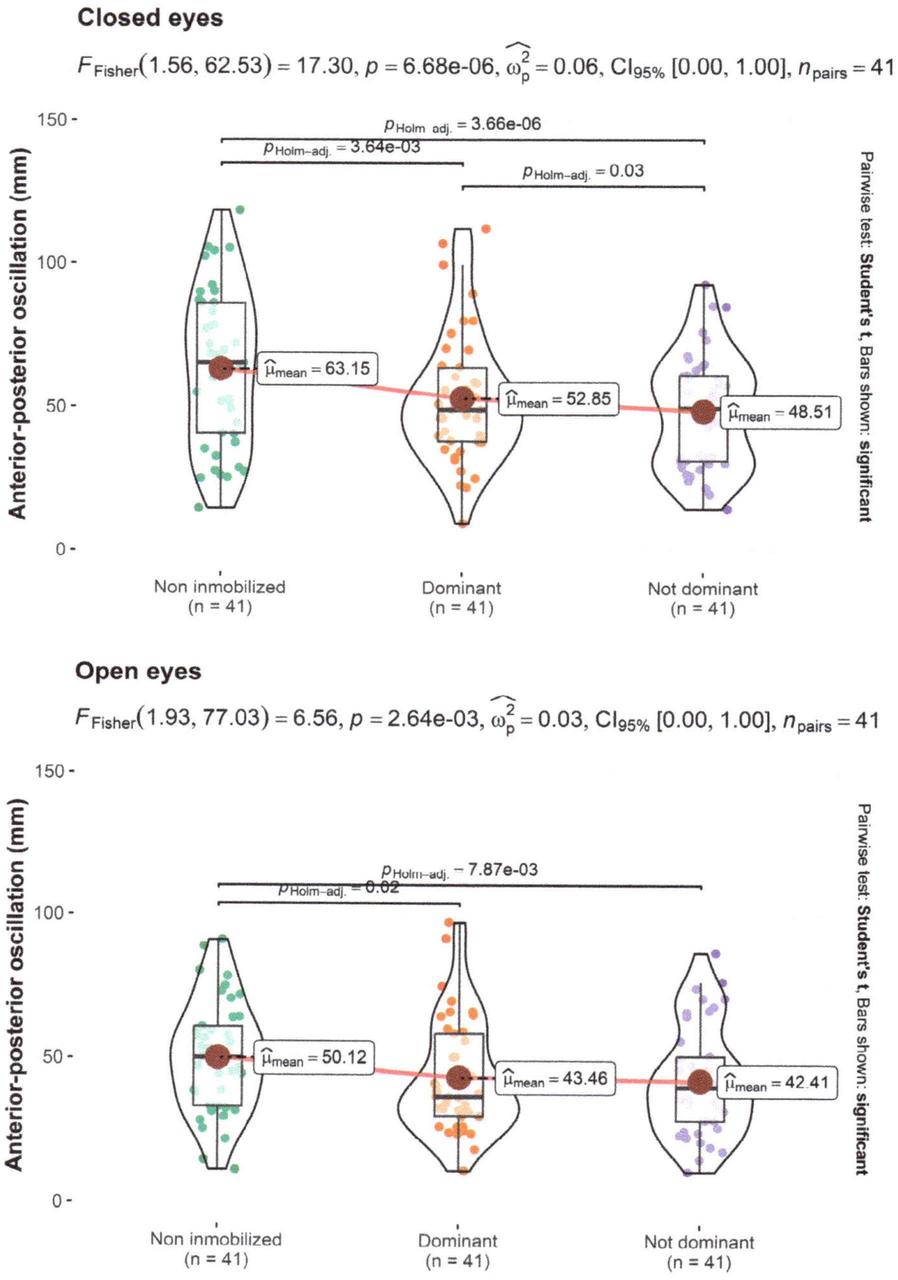

(a)

Figure 2. *Cont.*

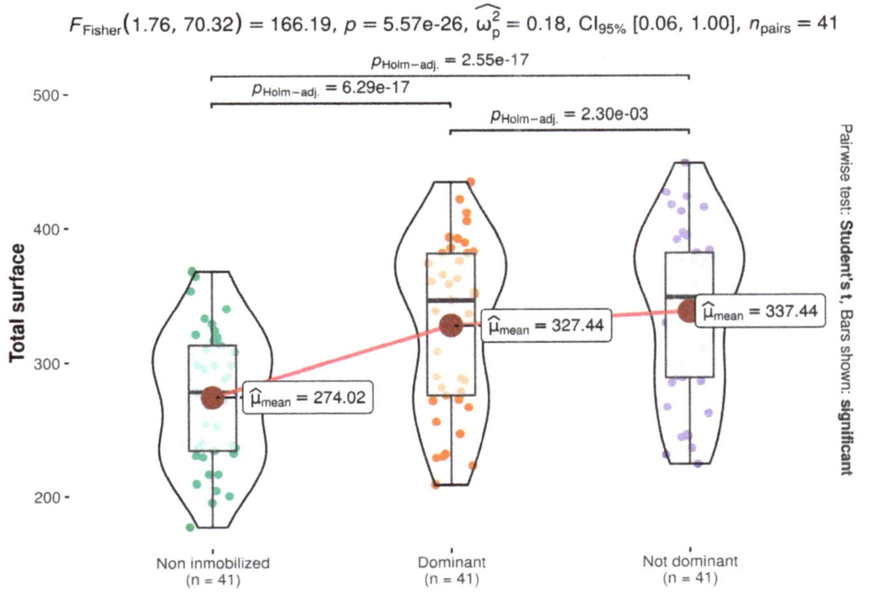

(**b**)

Figure 2. (**a**) Immobilization impacts APO irrespective of eye condition. (**b**). Differences between dominant and non-dominant sides.

Table 2 presents the effects of wrist and hand immobilization on the total plantar support area. The findings indicate a larger plantar support area during immobilization compared to non-immobilization, regardless of the dominance of the immobilized limb ($p < 0.001$), with discernible differences between the dominant and non-dominant sides (Figure 2b).

Table 2. Data on the impact of wrist and hand immobilization on total plantar support area.

	Value		
Predictors	Estimates	CI	p
(Intercept)	63.15	56.55–69.76	<0.001
Eyes [OE]	−13.03	−18.05–−8.01	<0.001
Dominant	−10.30	−15.32–−5.28	<0.001
Not dominant	−14.64	−19.66–−9.62	<0.001
Eyes [OE] x Dominant	3.64	−3.46–10.74	0.314
Eyes [OE] x Not dominant	6.93	−0.17–14.03	0.056
Random effects			
σ^2	133.19		
$\tau_{00\ DNI}$	327.97		
ICC	0.71		
N_{DNI}	41		
Observations	246		
Marginal R^2/Conditional R^2	0.093/0.738		

Additionally, when disregarding immobilization and limb dominance, the impact of eye state (open vs. closed) on plantar support was evaluated. The results suggest that the eye state significantly influences plantar support, independent of limb immobilization or dominance (Table 3).

Table 3. Exploring the effect of eye state on plantar support, disregarding immobilization and limb.

	Value		
Predictors	Estimates	CI	*p*
(Intercept)	27.60	20.37–34.82	<0.001
Eyes [OE]	−4.56	−8.88–−0.23	0.039
Dominant	−1.66	−6.95–3.63	0.537
Not dominant	−4.45	−9.74–0.84	0.099
Random effects			
σ^2	296.04		
$\tau_{00\ DNI}$	354.05		
ICC	0.54		
N_{DNI}	41		
Observations	246		
Marginal R^2/Conditional R^2	0.013/0.551		

4. Discussion

Despite the importance of proprioception in long-term functional outcomes after wrist–hand immobilization [20], no previous studies have examined the effect that wrist or hand immobilization may have on plantar support and, consequently, on the disruptions in the development of daily activities. Our study aimed to investigate the impact of wrist immobilization on postural control, specifically examining antero-posterior oscillation and plantar pressure distribution, while also considering the roles of hand dominance and visual conditions. In line with our hypotheses, the results revealed that wrist immobilization, regardless of hand dominance, led to significant changes in both postural sway and plantar pressure parameters when compared to the non-immobilized condition. These findings suggest that even distal upper limb constraints can influence body balance.

There are several plantar pressure measurement systems, such as Footscan® [21], TekScan® [22], Emed® [23], Pedar® [24], WalkinSense® [25], and Medicapteurs S-Plate® [26], among others. There have been some foot-related research studies that have used the PodoPrint® platform [27,28]. Reliability and repeatability of the PodoPrint® system have been demonstrated, and normal values of plantar foot pressure have also been identified in a healthy population [16].

We already knew that the immobilization of the wrist or hand had consequences on the shoulder [29], and increased time of immobilization of the wrist was associated with an increase in shoulder pain in patients after wrist fracture. However, we were unaware of the potential effects that immobilizing the wrist or hand could have on plantar support, gait development, balance, and consequently, on the sensation of movement and agility during locomotion. The results of this study could have clinical implications in patients with conditions involving wrist immobilization, highlighting the importance of a global rehabilitation approach. Specifically, the findings elucidated on the relationship between wrist immobilization and various postural parameters revealed not only the dynamic interplay between upper limb function and lower limb biomechanics but also the influence of wrist–hand immobilization on these parameters [30]. Our results indicate that wrist immobilization alone induces changes in antero-posterior oscillation (APO), regardless of whether the immobilized hand is dominant or non-dominant and independent of visual conditions (eyes open or closed). However, when the eyes are closed, the length of APO increases, likely due to the involvement of the vestibular system [31].

Previous studies concluded that plantar pressure parameters can be modulated in response to different visual inputs [31,32]. Effects of visual stimuli on plantar pressure parameters were also reported in open-eye (OE) condition by Fullin et al. [33]. Similarly, P. De Blasiis et al. [34] investigated the impact of visual stimuli on postural stability and plantar pressure parameters in a healthy population, analyzing changes under both OE and closed-eye (CE) conditions. Their results confirm that the coefficient of variation was lower than 20% in CEs and OEs across all parameters, except for the right arch index, which suggests a greater dynamic role of the dominant foot with respect to the postural adaptations occurring with closed eyes. Also, Hébert-Losier, K et al. [33,35] concluded that plantar pressure parameters do not seem to be affected by the different visual conditions. These studies partially differ from our results, as we observed differences in participants depending on whether their eyes were open or closed. This discrepancy may be attributed to wrist immobilization, a variable not considered in previous studies. Our findings suggest that eye condition (open vs. closed) significantly impacts the distribution of plantar load, regardless of limb immobilization or dominance. Nevertheless, it is important to emphasize that irrespective of the eye condition or dominance, it is the immobilization itself that induces effects on both antero-posterior oscillation and the area of plantar support.

Upper extremity limitations impact gait, balance, and overall functionality [36,37]. This redistribution of plantar pressure may be indicative of an attempt to redistribute body weight in response to compromised upper limb function. Our study also revealed significant changes in plantar pressure distribution in individuals due to wrist immobilization. It is conceivable that individuals with wrist immobilization, either consciously or subconsciously, engage their lower limbs to a greater extent to compensate for reduced upper limb functionality during walking, as interlimb neural coupling influences muscle recruitment [7]. It is not the first time that some investigators reported the correlation between the hand and the foot; for example, Slobounov, S et al. reported referred differences between the parameters of hand strength and plantar pressure distribution [38,39]. Other studies that have focused on postural control have shown the right hemisphere's pivotal role on balance control and body posture in healthy subjects [40,41]. In the same line, Rosario Emanuele Bonaventura et al. [42] investigated the effect of prismatic adaptation (PA) on handgrip strength and plantar pressure. They concluded that the PA effects on body posture are probably related to modulation of body representation.

Focus on body representation, and in concordance with our results, there are many results that converge on the conclusion that maintaining an upright posture requires the nervous system to integrate information from the somatosensory, visual, and vestibular systems. Therefore, any external factor that may influence this perception (such as wrist immobilization in our study) could impact the motor and sensory systems, leading to a series of mechanical and proprioceptive adjustments that are crucial for effective rehabilitation. These objective findings, which highlight the correlation between wrist immobilization and plantar support, could be the way for new research focused on clinical applications for upper limb injury rehabilitation.

However, our results are based on a healthy population; consequently, the impact of factors, such as kinesiophobia or post-injury wrist pain, on plantar support remains unknown. Moreover, a potential limitation of this study is the possibility of evaluator bias, as the evaluator was aware of the conditions being tested. Although efforts were made to ensure objective assessments, the lack of blinding may have introduced an unintended source of bias. Future research should address this limitation by implementing a double-blind design to enhance the reliability of the findings. Future research should integrate clinical assessments to strengthen the interpretation and clinical relevance of our findings. Additionally, further studies should explore the impact of various factors influencing plantar support following wrist immobilization, identifying both predictive and confounding variables, as well as potential changes occurring throughout the progression of the pathology.

5. Conclusions

Wrist–hand immobilization alone, independent of eye status (open or closed), resulted in significant alterations in antero-posterior oscillation and plantar pressure, with discernible differences between the dominant and non-dominant sides. The eye state significantly influenced plantar support, independent of limb immobilization or dominance.

Author Contributions: L.C.G.: conceptualization, methodology, investigation, and writing—original draft; G.A.G.-N.: validation, formal analysis, and writing—review and editing; S.D.M.: methodology, investigation, and resources; J.B.-L.: formal analysis; C.-T.R.: conceptualization, methodology, formal analysis, writing—review and editing, visualization, and supervision. All authors have read and agreed to the published version of the manuscript.

Funding: This research received no external funding.

Institutional Review Board Statement: The study was conducted in accordance with the Declaration of Helsinki and approved by the Ethics Committee of the University of Málaga with CEUMA: 97-2022-H.

Informed Consent Statement: Informed consent was obtained from all subjects involved in the study.

Data Availability Statement: The original contributions presented in this study are included in the article. Further inquiries can be directed to the corresponding author.

Acknowledgments: The University of Malaga.

Conflicts of Interest: The authors declare no conflicts of interest.

References

1. Kim, B.S.; Cho, C.H.; Lee, K.J.; Lee, S.W.; Byun, S.H. Pathomechanism of Triangular Fibrocartilage Complex Injuries in Patients with Distal-Radius Fractures: A Magnetic-Resonance Imaging Study. *J. Clin. Med.* **2022**, *11*, 6168. [CrossRef] [PubMed]
2. Rundgren, J.; Bojan, A.; Mellstrand Navarro, C.; Enocson, A. Epidemiology, Classification, Treatment and Mortality of Distal Radius Fractures in Adults: An Observational Study of 23,394 Fractures from the National Swedish Fracture Register. *BMC Musculoskelet. Disord.* **2020**, *21*, 88. [CrossRef]
3. Hsu, W.L. Adaptive Postural Control for Joint Immobilization during Multitask Performance. *PLoS ONE* **2014**, *9*, 108667. [CrossRef]
4. Rios-Russo, J.L.; Lozada-Bado, L.S.; De Mel, S.; Frontera, W.; Micheo, W. Ulnar-Sided Wrist Pain in the Athlete: Sport-Specific Demands, Clinical Presentation, and Management Options. *Curr. Sports Med. Rep.* **2021**, *20*, 312–318. [CrossRef]
5. Sprouse, R.A.; McLaughlin, A.M.; Harris, G.D. Braces and Splints for Common Musculoskeletal Conditions. *Am. Fam. Physician* **2018**, *98*, 570–576.
6. Howell, D.M.; Bechmann, S.; Underwood, P.J. Wrist Splint. In *Interventions, Controls, and Applications in Occupational Ergonomics*; CRC Press: Boca Raton, FL, USA, 2023. [CrossRef]
7. Hong, S.H.; Jung, S.Y.; Oh, H.K.; Lee, S.H.; Woo, Y.K. Effects of the Immobilization of the Upper Extremities on Spatiotemporal Gait Parameters during Walking in Stroke Patients: A Preliminary Study. *Biomed. Res. Int.* **2020**, *2020*, 6157231. [CrossRef]
8. Cooper, J.E.; Shwedyk, E.; Quanbury, A.O.; Miller, J.; Hildebrand, D. Elbow Joint Restriction: Effect on Functional Upper Limb Motion during Performance of Three Feeding Activities. *Arch. Phys. Med. Rehabil.* **1993**, *74*, 805–809. [CrossRef] [PubMed]
9. Boström, K.J.; Dirksen, T.; Zentgraf, K.; Wagner, H. The Contribution of Upper Body Movements to Dynamic Balance Regulation during Challenged Locomotion. *Front. Hum. Neurosci.* **2018**, *12*, 8. [CrossRef]
10. Ford, M.P.; Wagenaar, R.C.; Newell, K.M. Arm Constraint and Walking in Healthy Adults. *Gait Posture* **2007**, *26*, 135–141. [CrossRef]
11. Collins, S.H.; Adamczyk, P.G.; Kuo, A.D. Dynamic Arm Swinging in Human Walking. *Proc. Biol. Sci.* **2009**, *276*, 3679–3688. [CrossRef]

12. Umberger, B.R. Effects of Suppressing Arm Swing on Kinematics, Kinetics, and Energetics of Human Walking. *J. Biomech.* **2008**, *41*, 2575–2580. [CrossRef]
13. Ortega, J.D.; Fehlman, L.A.; Farley, C.T. Effects of Aging and Arm Swing on the Metabolic Cost of Stability in Human Walking. *J. Biomech.* **2008**, *41*, 3303–3308. [CrossRef] [PubMed]
14. De Graaf, M.L.; Hubert, J.; Houdijk, H.; Bruijn, S.M. Influence of Arm Swing on Cost of Transport during Walking. *Biol. Open* **2019**, *8*, bio039263. [CrossRef]
15. Manzini, J.L. DECLARACIÓN DE HELSINKI: PRINCIPIOS ÉTICOS PARA LA INVESTIGACIÓN MÉDICA SOBRE SUJETOS HUMANOS. *Acta Bioethica* **2000**, *6*, 321–334. [CrossRef]
16. Cobos-Moreno, P.; Astasio-Picado, Á.; Martínez- Nova, A.; Sánchez- Rodríguez, R.; Escamilla-Martínez, E.; Gómez-Martín, B. The Podoprint® Plantar Pressure Platform: Evaluation of Reliability and Repeatability, and Determination of the Normality Parameters. *J. Tissue Viability* **2022**, *31*, 619–624. [CrossRef] [PubMed]
17. Sayudo, I.F.; Sudarman, J.P.; Fernandes, A.; Park, J.Y.; Leibovitch, L.; Machinski, E.; Mahmoud, M.O. Short Versus Regular Periods of Cast Immobilization for Distal Radial Fractures: A Systematic Review and Meta-Analysis. *Cureus* **2024**, *16*, e54704. [CrossRef] [PubMed]
18. de Bruijn, M.A.N.; van Ginkel, L.A.; Boersma, E.Z.; van Silfhout, L.; Tromp, T.N.; van de Krol, E.; Edwards, M.J.R.; Stirler, V.M.A.; Hermans, E. Cast Immobilization Duration for Distal Radius Fractures, a Systematic Review. *Eur. J. Trauma. Emerg. Surg.* **2024**, *50*, 1621–1636. [CrossRef]
19. Patil, I. Visualizations with Statistical Details: The "ggstatsplot" Approach. *J. Open Source Softw.* **2021**, *6*, 3167. [CrossRef]
20. Cantero-Téllez, R. A Global Proprioception Concept after Hand Injury-Patient Report. *J. Hand Ther.* **2024**, *37*, 293–295. [CrossRef]
21. Xu, C.; Wen, X.X.; Huang, L.Y.; Shang, L.; Cheng, X.X.; Yan, Y.B.; Lei, W. Normal Foot Loading Parameters and Repeatability of the Footscan® Platform System. *J. Foot Ankle Res.* **2017**, *10*, 30. [CrossRef]
22. Zammit, G.V.; Menz, H.B.; Munteanu, S.E. Reliability of the TekScan MatScan® System for the Measurement of Plantar Forces and Pressures during Barefoot Level Walking in Healthy Adults. *J. Foot Ankle Res.* **2010**, *3*, 11. [CrossRef] [PubMed]
23. Maetzler, M.; Bochdansky, T.; Abboud, R.J. Normal Pressure Values and Repeatability of the Emed® ST2 System. *Gait Posture* **2010**, *32*, 391–394. [CrossRef] [PubMed]
24. Ramanathan, A.K.; Kiran, P.; Arnold, G.P.; Wang, W.; Abboud, R.J. Repeatability of the Pedar-X® in-Shoe Pressure Measuring System. *Foot Ankle Surg.* **2010**, *16*, 70–73. [CrossRef]
25. Castro, M.P.D.; Meucci, M.; Soares, D.P.; Fonseca, P.; Borgonovo-Santos, M.; Sousa, F.; Machado, L.; Vilas-Boas, J.P. Accuracy and Repeatability of the Gait Analysis by the WalkinSense System. *Biomed. Res. Int.* **2014**, *2014*, 348659. [CrossRef]
26. Izquierdo-Renau, M.; Pérez-Soriano, P.; Ribas-García, V.; Queralt, A. Intra and Intersession Repeatability and Reliability of the S-Plate® Pressure Platform. *Gait Posture* **2017**, *52*, 224–226. [CrossRef]
27. Sánchez-Sáez, J.M.; Palomo-López, P.; Becerro-De-bengoa-vallejo, R.; Calvo-Lobo, C.; Losa-Iglesias, M.E.; López-Del-amo-lorente, A.; López-López, D. Stability of Three Different Sanitary Shoes on Healthcare Workers: A Cross-Sectional Study. *Int. J. Environ. Res. Public Health* **2019**, *16*, 2126. [CrossRef]
28. Pereiro-Buceta, H.; Calvo-Lobo, C.; Becerro-De-bengoa-vallejo, R.; Losa-Iglesias, M.E.; Romero-Morales, C.; López-López, D.; Martínez-Jiménez, E.M. Intra and Intersession Repeatability and Reliability of Dynamic Parameters in Pressure Platform Assessments on Subjects with Simulated Leg Length Discrepancy. A Cross-Sectional Research. *Sao Paulo Med. J.* **2021**, *139*, 424–434. [CrossRef] [PubMed]
29. Shepherd, R.B.; Gentile, A.M. Sit-to-Stand: Functional Relationship between Upper Body and Lower Limb Segments. *Hum. Mov. Sci.* **1994**, *13*, 817–840. [CrossRef]
30. Cantero-Téllez, R.; Orza, S.G.; Bishop, M.D.; Berjano, P.; Villafañe, J.H. Duration of Wrist Immobilization Is Associated with Shoulder Pain in Patients with after Wrist Immobilization: An Observational Study. *J. Exerc. Rehabil.* **2018**, *14*, 694–698. [CrossRef]
31. Nishiike, S.; Okazaki, S.; Watanabe, H.; Akizuki, H.; Imai, T.; Uno, A.; Kitahara, T.; Horii, A.; Takeda, N.; Inohara, H. The Effect of Visual-Vestibulosomatosensory Conflict Induced by Virtual Reality on Postural Stability in Humans. *J. Med. Investig.* **2013**, *60*, 236–239. [CrossRef]
32. Stoffregen, T.A.; Pagulayan, R.J.; Bardy, B.G.; Hettinger, L.J. Modulating Postural Control to Facilitate Visual Performance. *Hum. Mov. Sci.* **2000**, *19*, 203–220. [CrossRef]
33. Fullin, A.; Caravaggi, P.; Picerno, P.; Mosca, M.; Caravelli, S.; De Luca, A.; Lucariello, A.; De Blasiis, P. Variability of Postural Stability and Plantar Pressure Parameters in Healthy Subjects Evaluated by a Novel Pressure Plate. *Int. J. Environ. Res. Public Health* **2022**, *19*, 2913. [CrossRef]
34. De Blasiis, P.; Caravaggi, P.; Fullin, A.; Leardini, A.; Lucariello, A.; Perna, A.; Guerra, G.; De Luca, A. Postural Stability and Plantar Pressure Parameters in Healthy Subjects: Variability, Correlation Analysis and Differences under Open and Closed Eye Conditions. *Front. Bioeng. Biotechnol.* **2023**, *11*, 1198120. [CrossRef]
35. Hébert-Losier, K.; Murray, L. Reliability of Centre of Pressure, Plantar Pressure, and Plantar-Flexion Isometric Strength Measures: A Systematic Review. *Gait Posture* **2020**, *75*, 46–62. [CrossRef]

36. Trehan, S.K.; Wolff, A.L.; Gibbons, M.; Hillstrom, H.J.; Daluiski, A. The Effect of Simulated Elbow Contracture on Temporal and Distance Gait Parameters. *Gait Posture* **2015**, *41*, 791–794. [CrossRef]
37. Leblebici, G.; Tarakcı, E.; Kısa, E.P.; Akalan, E.; Kasapçopur, Ö. The Effects of Improvement in Upper Extremity Function on Gait and Balance in Children with Upper Extremity Affected. *Gait Posture* **2024**, *110*, 41–47. [CrossRef] [PubMed]
38. Slobounov, S.; Hallett, M.; Stanhope, S.; Shibasaki, H. Role of Cerebral Cortex in Human Postural Control: An EEG Study. *Clin. Neurophysiol.* **2005**, *116*, 315–323. [CrossRef] [PubMed]
39. Siemionow, V.; Yue, G.H.; Ranganathan, V.K.; Liu, J.Z.; Sahgal, V. Relationship between Motor Activity-Related Cortical Potential and Voluntary Muscle Activation. *Exp. Brain Res.* **2000**, *133*, 303–311. [CrossRef]
40. Cioncoloni, D.; Rosignoli, D.; Feurra, M.; Rossi, S.; Bonifazi, M.; Rossi, A.; Mazzocchio, R. Role of Brain Hemispheric Dominance in Anticipatory Postural Control Strategies. *Exp. Brain Res.* **2016**, *234*, 1997–2005. [CrossRef]
41. Zhavoronkova, L.A.; Zharikova, A.V.; Kushnir, E.M.; Mikhalkova, A.A. EEG Markers of Upright Posture in Healthy Individuals. *Hum. Physiol.* **2012**, *38*, 604–612. [CrossRef]
42. Bonaventura, R.E.; Giustino, V.; Chiaramonte, G.; Giustiniani, A.; Smirni, D.; Battaglia, G.; Messina, G.; Oliveri, M. Investigating Prismatic Adaptation Effects in Handgrip Strength and in Plantar Pressure in Healthy Subjects. *Gait Posture* **2020**, *76*, 264–269. [CrossRef] [PubMed]

Journal of
Clinical Medicine

MDPI

Article

Cervical Spine Screening Based on Movement Strategies Improves Shoulder Physical Variables in Neck-Related Shoulder Pain Patients: A Secondary Analysis from an Observational Study

Alberto Roldán-Ruiz [1,2,*], Javier Bailón-Cerezo [3,4], Deborah Falla [5] and María Torres-Lacomba [2,4,6]

1 Departamento de Fisioterapia, Facultad de Ciencias de la Salud, Universidad Francisco de Vitoria, Ctra. Pozuelo-Majadahonda Km 1800, Pozuelo de Alarcón, 28223 Madrid, Spain
2 Physiotherapy and Nursing Department, Faculty of Medicine and Health Sciences, University of Alcalá, Alcalá de Henares, 28805 Madrid, Spain; maria.torres@uah.es
3 Departamento de Fisioterapia, Centro Superior de Estudios Universitarios La Salle, Universidad Autónoma de Madrid, 28023 Madrid, Spain; javier.bailon@lasallecampus.es
4 Physiotherapy in Women's Health Research Group-FPSM, Physiotherapy Unit, University of Alcalá, Alcalá de Henares, 28805 Madrid, Spain
5 Centre of Precision Rehabilitation for Spinal Pain (CPR Spine), School of Sport, Exercise and Rehabilitation Sciences, College of Life and Environmental Sciences, University of Birmingham, Birmingham B15 2TT, UK; d.falla@bham.ac.uk
6 Ramón y Cajal Institute of Health Research-IRYCIS, University Hospital of Ramón y Cajal, 28034 Madrid, Spain
* Correspondence: alberto.roldan@ufv.es; Tel.: +34-65-760-8266

Abstract: Background: It is important to consider the cervical spine as a potential contributor to shoulder pain, indicating the paramount importance of screening the cervical spine in patients with shoulder pain. **Objectives:** To study the immediate effects of cervical spine screening (CSS) on the shoulder active range of motion, isometric strength and self-reported function in patients with neck-related shoulder pain. **Methods**: A secondary analysis was conducted on data from a previous study. A cervical contribution was considered if a ≥30% shoulder symptom modification of pain intensity (Numeric Pain Rating Scales) was recorded during the most painful shoulder movement after CSS. Pre–post measurements of the shoulder active range of motion (inclinometer) and shoulder isometric strength (dynamometer) were recorded in a single session. Self-reported shoulder function (Shoulder Pain and Disability Index) was assessed at a 1-week follow-up. **Results:** Among 60 participants, statistically significant changes were found for those with a cervical contribution (n = 30) for shoulder flexion and the abduction range of motion ($p < 0.001$), with a medium size effect (r = 0.55), and in internal rotation ($p = 0.02$) and external rotation at 0° abduction ($p = 0.008$), with a small size effect (r = 0.3 and 0.34, respectively). The self-reported shoulder function in those without a cervical contribution significantly declined from the pre to post measurements ($p = 0.002$), with a small size effect (r = 0.4). No statistically significant changes were found for the isometric strength in either group. **Conclusions**: In patients with shoulder pain classified as having a cervical contribution, CSS produces intrasession improvements in the active shoulder range of motion but not in the shoulder isometric strength or self-reported shoulder function.

Keywords: shoulder pain; cervical spine; neck; range of motion; strength; function

1. Introduction

Shoulder pain constitutes the third most prevalent musculoskeletal pain condition [1] and is the leading cause of atraumatic upper limb complaints [2]. The shoulder pain incidence has been reported to be 14.7–29.3 in every 1000 patients in primary care [3,4]. The prevalence ranged from 41.2 to 48.4 in every 1000 people between the years 1998 and 2007, being higher in women than in men [4]. Up to 66.7% of people may develop shoulder pain at least once in their lifetime [5] and the symptoms often persist even beyond 18 months in 50% of those affected [6].

Although still scarce, the scientific research considering a cervical contribution in shoulder pain presentations is experiencing growing momentum [7–10]. Regional interdependence may explain the cervical contribution, as impairments in a body region distinct from the painful one may be related with a patient's chief complaint [11,12]. Regarding the interaction between the neck and shoulder region, referred shoulder pain patterns have been observed from the cervical zygapophyseal joints [13–16], cervical intervertebral discs [17] and neck muscles [18].

Being guided by the anatomical region presenting with symptoms may therefore be misleading, as conditions of both the neck and shoulder region may overlap [19–22]. Moreover, shoulder orthopedic test results may turn into false positives in the presence of undiagnosed spinal disorders [23]. If pain of spinal origin is incorrectly interpreted, poor decision-making and inadequate patient management can result [24]. Similarly, directing treatment only over the shoulder in a patient with a cervical contribution might compromise the treatment effectiveness [8].

In that manner, from a clinical reasoning perspective, certain clinical findings may prompt a cervical spine evaluation to assess its potential contribution to shoulder pain. These include the presence of cervical pain prior the onset of shoulder symptoms [7], the coexistence of shoulder pain and cervical pain [16], a restricted cervical range of motion [25,26], symptom modification with cervical movements [25], the diagnosis of rotator-cuff-related shoulder pain [27], minimal or no reduction in shoulder range of motion [25,28], and a history of prior cervical surgery [29,30].

The effects of cervical treatment on shoulder symptoms have been examined, with the results showing that joint mobilization strategies such as postero-anterior or antero-posterior mobilizations, lateral glides and manipulations may enhance shoulder pain and disability [31–37], with different forms of manual therapy showing comparable effects [31]. Similarly, other cervical approaches, such as repeated movements [9,24,38,39] and spinal mobilization with arm movement [40], seem to be effective in managing shoulder symptoms. Despite the growing recognition of the potential role of the cervical spine in shoulder pain, and a recent Delphi study attempting to establish a consensus on spine screening in patients with shoulder pain—incorporating strategies such as assessing the changes in shoulder symptoms with neck movements or active cervical movements—[41], there is currently no standardized examination procedure to identify this clinical pattern [8].

The application of symptom modification strategies as both a diagnostic and a treatment-guiding approach has the potential to enhance clinical practice. By identifying specific structures or areas where treatment leads to symptom improvement, physical interventions can be more effectively directed [10]. Thus, the aim of this study was to investigate the immediate effects of cervical spine screening (CSS) based on movement strategies on the active shoulder range of motion, isometric shoulder strength, and self-reported shoulder function in patients with shoulder pain.

2. Methods

2.1. Study Design

This study constitutes a secondary analysis of a previous prospective observational study [7] approved by the Research Ethics Committee of Hospital Universitario Príncipe de Asturias, Spain (OE 25/2019) on 4 December 2019, conducted in compliance with the Declaration of Helsinki. The reporting adheres to the STROBE guidelines. Participants provided informed written consent prior to data collection.

2.2. Participants

Participants were recruited from two separate hospitals in Madrid and were consecutive eligible individuals seeking orthopedic/traumatology consultation for their shoulder pain. A total of 6 participants were recruited from Hospital Universitario Príncipe de Asturias and 54 from Clínica Cemtro, Madrid, Spain. From February 2020 to June 2022, participants were assessed by the same physiotherapist, who had six years of expertise in the assessment and conservative treatment of patients with shoulder pain.

Participants were required to be over 18 years old, suffering from shoulder pain during movement and scoring ≥3/10 on the Numeric Pain Rating Scale (NPRS) for their shoulder pain intensity.

They were excluded if they:

- had prior shoulder surgery, pain at rest that improved with movement, history of trauma, shoulder fractures, systemic diseases, radiculopathy, peripheral neuropathy, or radicular pain (including a score of >11 on the S-LANSS scale);
- had received local analgesic or anti-inflammatory injections in the previous six months or taken those medications on the examination day.

2.3. Variables

Baseline demographic and descriptive information was recorded, including age, sex, and the Spanish version of the Central Sensitization Inventory (CSI) [42], along with clinical characteristics such as prior and concomitant neck pain, symptoms extending to the upper limb, duration of symptoms, and whether their pain was unilateral or bilateral. The physical therapist also recorded several dependent variables during the clinical examination of the participants, as detailed below. The primary outcomes were the pain intensity, active shoulder range of motion and isometric shoulder strength. Self-reported shoulder function was considered a secondary outcome.

The shoulder pain intensity was assessed during the most painful shoulder movement, which was rated using a Numeric Pain Rating Scale (NPRS), an 11-point numerical scale with scores from 0 (no pain) to 10 (worst imaginable pain). The NPRS has adequate test–retest reliability (ICC = 0.63–0.92) and internal consistency (alpha coefficient = 0.84–0.98) [43,44]. A diagnosis of cervical contribution was considered if a ≥30% modification of the shoulder pain intensity was recorded after CSS; as in previous studies, a ≥30% threshold was employed to determine a significant change in shoulder symptoms [45,46].

The shoulder active range of motion was assessed during the most painful shoulder movement using a smartphone inclinometer (www.plaincode.com, Plaincode Software Solutions, Gunzenhausen, Germany), where the use in shoulder flexion and abduction in a sitting position, external rotation at 0° abduction, external rotation at 90° abduction and internal rotation at 90° abduction in a supine position (Figure 1) has been validated, with results showing excellent inter-examiner reliability in symptomatic subjects (ICC > 0.80) [47].

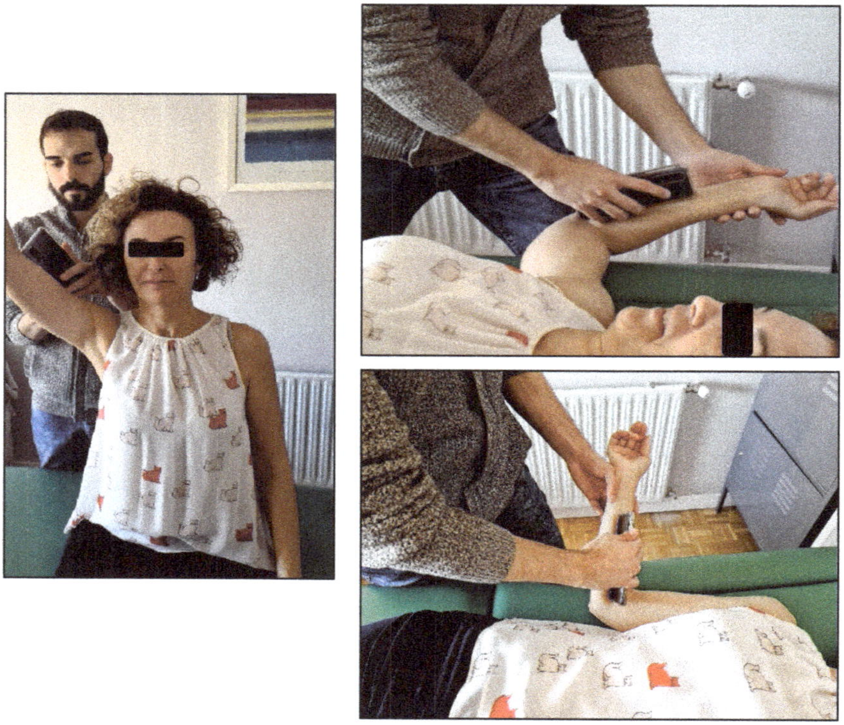

Figure 1. Shoulder external rotation in 90° abduction, external rotation in 0° abduction, and abduction measured with a smartphone inclinometer.

The isometric shoulder strength (Figure 2) was assessed using a hand-held dynamometer (MicroFET 2 MT Digital Handheld Dynamometer; Hoggan Health Industries, West Draper, UT, USA), which has been shown to have good to excellent intra-rater reliability for all shoulder strength tests (ICC = 0.87–0.99) [48,49]. As described by Roy et al., 2009 [50], the dynamometer was held over the anterior aspect of the humerus on the medial side for flexion and abduction, with the arm held at 90° and the participant in a seated position. For extension, the shoulder was at 0° of flexion–extension, and the dynamometer was placed over the posterior aspect of the humerus over the medial side. For external rotation, the dynamometer was held over the dorsal aspect of the forehand (or palmar aspect for internal rotation), close to the ulnar styloid process. Participants were asked to gradually increase their isometric force for 3 s, maintaining the contraction for a further 3 s and then relaxing. Two consecutive measurements with a 30 s rest period were carried out, with the mean force determined for each direction.

The self-reported shoulder function was assessed using the Shoulder Pain and Disability Index (SPADI), which is a questionnaire originally developed to measure shoulder pain and disability via 13 items [51]. It has been described as a questionnaire capable of adequately discriminating between patients with improving or worsening conditions [52]. The questionnaire was sent to the participants by email in Google Forms format prior to the CSS and after 1 week. A short-term follow-up was conducted for the self-reported shoulder function, given that substantial intrasession changes in this measure were not expected.

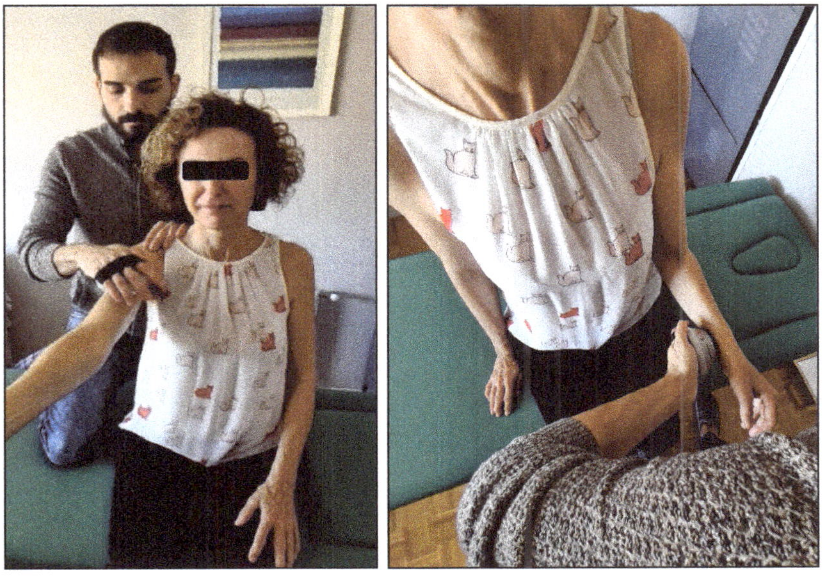

Figure 2. Shoulder flexion and internal rotation isometric strength measured with a dynamometer.

2.4. Procedure

The CCS consisted of different shoulder symptom modification strategies that were used with an evaluation approach to observe potential intrasession changes. After each intervention, the participant was asked to repeat the most painful movement and to report the pain intensity using the NPRS [43]. Immediately after completion of the CSS, the shoulder active range of motion and isometric strength were reassessed. The CSS was used to determine the presence of a cervical contribution, which was considered if a ≥30% modification of the shoulder pain intensity was recorded during the painful movement after the CSS. Based on this assessment, the included participants were then divided into the cervical contribution versus non-cervical contribution groups.

The CSS included the techniques presented in Table 1 (further detail is provided in Appendix A). All the strategies were applied to all the participants in the proposed order. If any strategy resulted in 100% symptom modification, the CSS was discontinued at that point.

Table 1. Proposed cervical spine screening.

Intervention	Included Variants
Postural change while performing painful movement	-
Repeated end-range movements	Cervical retraction, retraction plus extension and flexion
Spinal accessory mobilization with painful shoulder movement	Cervical global traction and lateral glide of C4 spinous process
Passive accessory mobilization	Posterior–anterior and anterior–posterior mobilizations and lateral glides
Neck flexor and extensor muscle activation	-

2.5. Data Analysis

Statistical analyses were performed using SPSS version 27.0 (IBM Corp, Armonk, NY, USA). Continuous variables were presented as the mean ± standard deviation or the median with interquartile range, depending on their distribution, which was evaluated using the Kolmogorov–Smirnov (K-S) test. Categorical variables were summarized as the absolute and relative frequencies. Inferential analyses were conducted with a 95% confidence interval, considering a p-value < 0.05 as the threshold for statistical significance. The association between the pre- and post-screening values was analyzed using the Wilcoxon test for paired samples, due to the non-parametric distribution of these variables. The effect size was measured with the correlation coefficient r, calculated as $r = Z/\sqrt{n}$. According to Cohen, 1988 [53], an r value of 0.1 to 0.3 indicates a small effect size, 0.3 to 0.5 indicates a moderate effect size, and ≥0.5 indicates a large effect size.

As this was an exploratory secondary analysis, the sample size was not established a priori and the power estimations were limited by the non-parametric nature of the data.

3. Results

A total of 60 participants were assessed from 2020 to 2022 (mean age: 40.78 ± 13.45 years), 26 women and 34 men. The baseline clinical characteristics of the sample are shown in Table 2.

Table 2. Baseline sample clinical characteristics. Absolute frequency—*n* (%).

Variables	Descriptive Data
Clinical characteristics. Absolute frequency—*n* (%)	
Painful shoulder (left)	28 (46.7)
Upper limb referred pain	27 (45)
Unilateral pain	49 (81.7)
Previous neck pain	22 (36.7)
Concomitant neck pain	23 (38.3)
Symptoms duration	
<3 months	16 (26.7)
3–6 months	9 (15)
>6 months	35 (58.3)
Clinimetrics	
Central sensitization (CSI), >40 points	12 (20)
Shoulder function (SPADI)—median [IQR]	38.57 [28]
Pain intensity (NPRS)—median [IQR]	6 [2]

Abbreviatures: SD—standard deviation, IQR—interquartile range, CSI—Central Sensitization Inventory, SPADI—Shoulder Pain and Disability Index, NPRS—Numeric Pain Rating Scale.

After the CSS, 30 out of the 60 participants experienced a ≥30% shoulder pain intensity modification, thus classifying 50% of the sample as having a cervical contribution.

3.1. Shoulder Range of Motion

When considering the whole sample and just those with a confirmed cervical contribution, the results revealed statistically significant changes after the CSS for all the shoulder range of motion variables except external rotation at 90° abduction (Table 3). The effect sizes were larger for those with a cervical contribution, especially for flexion and abduction ($p < 0.001$; r = 0.55).

Table 3. Pre–post changes in the shoulder active range of motion in the whole sample, those with a cervical contribution and those without a cervical contribution.

		V0 Median (IQR)	V1 Median (IQR)	*p*	Effect Size (r) *
Flexion	Whole sample (n = 60)	150.5 (37.25)	156.5 (34.25)	<0.001	0.46
	Cervical contribution (n = 30)	153.50 (30.50)	165 (27.75)	<0.001	0.55
	Non-cervical contribution (n = 30)	150 (42.75)	151 (46.25)	0.007	0.35
Abduction	Whole sample (n = 60)	155 (30)	160 (40.75)	<0.001	0.37
	Cervical contribution (n = 30)	155 (35.25)	170 (36.25)	<0.001	0.55
	Non-cervical contribution (n = 30)	155 (35)	155 (39.25)	0.833	0.03
External rotation at 0° abduction	Whole sample (n = 60)	62.43 (21.95) M (SD)	65.48 (20.29) M (SD)	0.010	0.23
	Cervical contribution (n = 30)	63.90 (18.76) M (SD)	69.43 (15.15) M (SD)	0.008	0.34
	Non-cervical contribution (n = 30)	61.06 (24.98) M (SD)	61.53 (23.99) M (SD)	0.461	0.10
External rotation at 90° abduction	Whole sample (n = 60)	84 (24.25)	85 (20.75)	0.363	0.08
	Cervical contribution (n = 30)	83 (24.25)	86 (19.25)	0.201	0.17
	Non-cervical contribution (n = 30)	84.5 (27.75)	83 (27.25)	0.843	0.03
Internal rotation at 90°	Whole sample (n = 60)	63.9 (18.73) M (SD)	66.95 (16.23) M (SD)	0.014	0.22
	Cervical contribution (n = 30)	64.97 (17.86) M (SD)	70.47 (13.63) M (SD)	0.020	0.30
	Non-cervical contribution (n = 30)	62.83 (19.81) M (SD)	63.43 (18.01) M (SD)	0.529	0.08

IQR—interquartile range; M—median; SD—standard deviation; V0—baseline mean values; V1—post-screening mean values; * r correlation coefficient [53].

Those without a cervical contribution did not show an improvement in the shoulder range of motion except for flexion, which was statistically significant ($p = 0.007$, r = 0.35). The effect sizes were small, except for flexion, which was moderate.

3.2. Shoulder Isometric Strength

The inferential analysis showed no statistically significant changes in the shoulder isometric strength immediately after the CSS in the whole sample or when people with or without a cervical contribution were considered separately. The effect sizes were small (Table 4).

Table 4. Pre–post changes in the shoulder isometric strength during the most painful movement in the whole sample, those with a cervical contribution and those without a cervical contribution.

	V0 Median (IQR)	V1 Median (IQR)	*p*	Effect Size (r) *
Whole sample (n = 60)	90 (77.87)	89 (61.75)	0.40	0.08
Cervical contribution (n = 30)	78.20 (44.93)	80.25 (46.25)	0.094	0.22
Non-cervical contribution (n = 30)	112 (67.75)	105 (66)	0.51	0.08

IQR—interquartile range; V0—baseline mean values; V1—post-screening mean values; * r correlation coefficient [53].

3.3. Shoulder Function (SPADI)

The self-reported shoulder function showed no statistically significant improvement when considering the whole sample or those with or without a cervical contribution. However, those without a cervical contribution did show a statistically significant worsening of the SPADI score after 1 week (Table 5).

Table 5. Pre–post changes in the self-reported shoulder function in the whole sample, those with a cervical contribution and those without a cervical contribution.

	V0 Median (IQR)	V1 Median (IQR)	p	Effect Size (r) *
Whole sample (n = 60)	38.57 (27.95)	39 (33.77)	0.868	0.02
Cervical contribution (n = 30)	37.7 (29.97)	29.63 (33.01)	0.088	0.22
Non-cervical contribution (n = 30)	39.35 (31.21)	43.5 (33.57)	0.002	0.40

IQR—interquartile range; SPADI—shoulder pain and disability index; V0—baseline mean values; V1—post-screening mean values; * r correlation coefficient [53].

4. Discussion

To the best of our knowledge, this research is the first study analyzing the intrasession effects of CSS on shoulder physical variables in patients classified as having a cervical contribution to their shoulder pain. The results show how CSS based on movement strategies may enhance shoulder mobility but not shoulder strength or short-term self-reported shoulder function. This could be analyzed in relation to the results of the study by Cook et al., 2014 [54], the only study that, to the best knowledge of the authors' knowledge, has shown the lack of value of cervical treatment in shoulder pathology, but without distinguishing between those with or without a cervical contribution to their shoulder pain condition.

4.1. Shoulder Range of Motion

Regarding the results of the active shoulder range of motion, it was observed that flexion, abduction, internal rotation, and external rotation at 0° of abduction obtained statistically significant changes when studying the whole sample and those with a confirmed cervical contribution. None of the similar studies analyzing cervical involvement in shoulder pain [9,10,24,38,39] have assessed the changes in the shoulder range of motion. Only Pheasant, 2016 [39], measured the baseline shoulder mobility in their case reports, but this was performed with a visual estimation and the post-intervention changes were not specifically described. However, improvements have been reported in the ROM, external rotation strength and abduction painful arc after cervical lateral glides [34,35], with this being a technique included in the current CSS.

It has been described that sustained or repeated cervical movements may modify shoulder symptoms, and if this is found to be a significant finding in the examination, cervical involvement can be considered a valid diagnosis [24,55]. In fact, given the difficulty of establishing a diagnosis based on the source or nociceptive structure responsible of the symptoms, this approach should be reserved for academic discussion, while in clinical practice, principles of reasoning based on the symptomatic response to mechanical stimuli during evaluation and treatment should be applied [55]. Nonetheless, the few studies considering the potential cervical spine involvement in shoulder pain have been based on examination and treatment under the premise of the McKenzie Mechanical Diagnosis and Therapy system [9,24,28,38,39], thus including only one part (repeated movements) of the CSS procedure that has been utilized in the current study.

4.2. Shoulder Isometric Strength

The shoulder isometric strength did not change following the CSS. There have been some reports of improvement in the shoulder strength and muscle activation after the implementation of treatment of the cervical spine, specifically with C5–C6 passive mobilization and C5–C6–C7 manipulation [32,33]. However, understandably, improvements in strength usually require a period of active exercise in order to induce neuromuscular adaptations to training, resulting in improved motor output. To assess the immediate changes, it may have been more relevant to assess the motor control, which is more likely to change immediately with an intervention [56].

The lack of change in the shoulder strength may be due to the assessment method. As manual therapy likely affects the pain-limited strength rather than the maximum contraction force, evaluating the pain-free contraction force, defined as the force generated up to the onset of pain, might have revealed different results.

4.3. Shoulder Function

The score on the SPADI questionnaire showed a statistically significant change for those without a cervical contribution to their shoulder pain, but the change [medians pre–post: 39.35 (31.21)–43.5 (33.57)] was below the minimal clinically important difference of this index, which is eight points [57]. In addition, the direction of change implied a worsening of the scores on the SPADI. However, measuring self-reported shoulder function within a single session may have limited value.

The absence of significant changes in the isometric strength or self-reported function raises questions about the clinical impact of CSS beyond mobility improvements. In this manner, the primary benefit of CSS may be restricted to an enhanced range of motion rather than broader functional improvements. Further research is needed to determine whether the intrasession changes derived from cervical screening may last in the long term. Similarly, longer-term interventions, rather than evaluations, might reveal additional benefits of addressing the cervical spine in shoulder physical variables in neck-related shoulder pain patients.

4.4. Strengths, Limitations and Future Research

This research used comprehensive CSS to classify whether or not people presenting with shoulder pain have a cervical contribution to their pain; previous studies have generally utilized repeated movements as the sole assessment strategy [9,24,38,39]. Considering the possibility of a cervical contribution in the symptomatic presentation of nontraumatic shoulder pain patients could enhance the overall management of this condition, since an approach based on the pathoanatomical model appears to be limited [56,58–62].

This is the first study to report the intrasession changes associated with a screening approach, rather than implementing treatment. However, the observed modifications in the physical variables could be influenced by unmeasured patient-specific factors, such as expectations, or placebo effects derived from the applied intervention. Future research should evaluate the role of these variables to determine whether the improvements reflect true physiological responses or expectancy-driven effects. Despite these limitations, the use of symptom modification strategies as a diagnostic, treatment, and reassessment method might be an option that aligns with clinical practice to guide treatment toward areas or structures that produce improvements [10]. Indeed, it has been reported that the intrasession changes in the pain intensity and range of motion may predict the future intersession changes in patients with neck disorders, and the same could happen with centralization phenomenon, i.e., distal symptoms diminish their expansion or disappear [63]. Likewise, it has been shown that intrasession changes higher than 36% are strongly associated with >50% changes in the Neck Disability Index after 96 h in patients with mechanical neck pain [64].

Nonetheless, this study has several noteworthy limitations. One significant concern is the representativeness of the sample, which may not adequately capture the diversity of a larger population as there was no sample size calculation. Additionally, the initial observational study that provided the dataset was not specifically designed to address the objectives of this research, leading to some inherent constraints in the data collection process. The reliance on secondary data also introduces challenges, such as the limited control over key variables and the possibility of missing or outdated information, so as not being able to control for confounding factors. These elements may impact the validity of the study's conclusions, necessitating a cautious interpretation of the results. On the other hand, the short-term follow-up prevents us from drawing clear conclusions about whether the effects of cervical spine screening persist in the long term. Finally, it is necessary to mention that an unblinded assessor was not possible, as well as the assessor and treating therapist being the same person, which could lead to observer bias. To overcome these limitations, future research should focus on developing more robust and targeted study designs that address these challenges and enhance the reliability of the findings.

Future research observing the shoulder symptom changes when directing specific treatment to patients responding positively to CSS is needed. Similarly, studies with larger sample sizes with prospective designs and longer-term follow-ups are needed.

5. Conclusions

In people with shoulder pain with a cervical contribution, CSS produces intrasession improvements in the active shoulder range of motion but not in the shoulder isometric strength nor self-reported shoulder function. Future research with larger samples and longer follow-ups is required.

Author Contributions: Conceptualization, A.R.-R. and J.B.-C.; writing—original draft preparation, A.R.-R.; writing—review and editing, J.B.-C., D.F. and M.T.-L.; supervision, D.F. and M.T.-L. All authors have read and agreed to the published version of the manuscript.

Funding: This research received no external funding.

Institutional Review Board Statement: Research Ethics Committee of the Hospital Universitario Príncipe de Asturias, Spain (OE 25/2019), on 4 December 2019.

Informed Consent Statement: Informed consent was obtained from all the subjects involved in this study.

Data Availability Statement: The raw data supporting the conclusions of this article will be made available by the authors on request.

Conflicts of Interest: The authors declare no conflicts of interest.

Abbreviation

The following abbreviation is used in this manuscript:

CSS   Cervical spine screening

Appendix A

Appendix A.1. Cervical Spine Screening

After each strategy, patients were asked to repeat their most painful movement to reassess the pain intensity. After the completion of the whole CSS, the remaining dependent variables were also reevaluated.

1. Postural adjustment during painful movement: forward head posture and thoracic/lumbar slump were corrected. By maintaining this neutral cervical spine position, the participant performed the painful or restricted movement.
2. Repeated end-range movements: cervical retraction, retraction plus extension and flexion were performed 10 times, followed by reassessment of the painful or restricted movement. If the participant was unable to reach the end range, passive overpressure

was applied by the examiner. Repeated end-range movements were conducted in all directions in the specified sequence unless a technique resulted in complete symptom resolution.

3. Spinal mobilization with shoulder movement:
    a. Cervical global traction: with the participant seated, the examiner positioned behind them applied gentle upward traction at the occiput using a bimanual grip. The participant then performed the painful or restricted movement while maintaining this mobilization.
    b. C4 lateral glide: with the participant seated, the examiner applied lateral pressure to the C4 spinous process in the direction opposite to the painful shoulder. This mobilization was maintained while the participant performed the painful or restricted movement.
4. Passive accessory mobilizations: techniques included posterior–anterior, anteroposterior, and lateral glides. The cervical segment selected for mobilization was the one that elicited symptom reproduction after three posterior–anterior mobilizations. If no symptoms were provoked, the segment associated with the greatest local discomfort was chosen [54]. Each mobilization was performed for 1 min.
5. Neck flexor (a) and extensor muscle (b) exercises while performing sets of contractions.
    a. Double chin movement (cranio-cervical flexion) was taught to the participant in a supine position. After this, he/she was placed standing with his/her back and head against a wall. A tennis ball was put between his/her head and the wall as feedback to better understand the exercise, and the subject was asked to perform the double chin movement while avoiding the ball falling. This was repeated 10 times.
    b. In a seated position, the subject was asked to place a band in his/her occiput and holding it forwards with his hands. Then, he/she was asked to perform a cervical retraction against the resistance of the band. This was repeated 10 times.
    c. As the CSS was an accumulation of strategies that could improve or worsen the subject's baseline status, the possibility of stopping the CSS if the subject experienced an increase of $\geq$2 points in the NPRS score was contemplated.

References

1. Urwin, M.; Symmons, D.; Allison, T.; Brammah, T.; Busby, H.; Roxby, M.; Simmons, A.; Williams, G. Estimating the burden of musculoskeletal disorders in the community: The comparative prevalence of symptoms at different anatomical sites, and the relation to social deprivation. *Ann. Rheum. Dis.* **1998**, *57*, 649–655. [CrossRef] [PubMed]
2. Tejera-Falcón, E.; Toledo-Martel, N.d.C.; Sosa-Medina, F.M.; Santana-González, F.; Quintana-de la Fe, M.d.P.; Gallego-Izquierdo, T.; Pecos-Martín, D. Dry needling in a manual physiotherapy and therapeutic exercise protocol for patients with chronic mechanical shoulder pain of unspecific origin: A protocol for a randomized control trial. *BMC Musculoskelet. Disord.* **2017**, *18*, 400.
3. van der Windt, D.A.; Koes, B.W.; de Jong, B.A.; Bouter, L.M. Shoulder disorders in general practice: Incidence, patient characteristics, and management. *Ann. Rheum. Dis.* **1995**, *54*, 959–964. [CrossRef] [PubMed]
4. Greving, K.; Dorrestijn, O.; Winters, J.; Groenhof, F.; van der Meer, K.; Stevens, M.; Diercks, R.L. Incidence, prevalence, and consultation rates of shoulder complaints in general practice. *Scand. J. Rheumatol.* **2012**, *41*, 150–155.
5. Luime, J.J.; Koes, B.W.; Hendriksen, I.J.M.; Burdorf, A.; Verhagen, A.P.; Miedema, H.S.; Verhaar, J.A.N. Prevalence and incidence of shoulder pain in the general population; a systematic review. *Scand. J. Rheumatol.* **2004**, *33*, 73–81. [CrossRef]
6. Croft, P.; Pope, D.; Silman, A. The clinical course of shoulder pain: Prospective cohort study in primary care. *Prim. Care Rheumatol. Soc. Shoulder Study Group BMJ* **1996**, *313*, 601–602.
7. Roldán-Ruiz, A.; Bailón-Cerezo, J.; Falla, D.; Torres-Lacomba, M. The prevalence of cervical contribution in patients reporting shoulder pain. An observational study. *Musculoskelet. Sci. Pract.* **2024**, *73*, 103158.
8. Walker, T.; Salt, E.; Lynch, G.; Littlewood, C. Screening of the cervical spine in subacromial shoulder pain: A systematic review. *Shoulder Elb.* **2018**, *11*, 305–315.

9. Heider Abady, A.; Rosedale, R.; Chesworth, B.M.; Rotondi, M.A.; Overend, T.J. Application of the McKenzie system of Mechanical Diagnosis and Therapy (MDT) in patients with shoulder pain; a prospective longitudinal study. *J. Man. Manip. Ther.* **2017**, *9817*, 1–9.
10. Karel, Y.H.J.M.; Scholten-Peeters, G.G.M.; Thoomes-de Graaf, M.; Duijn, E.; van Broekhoven, J.B.; Koes, B.W.; Verhagen, A.P. Physiotherapy for patients with shoulder pain in primary care: A descriptive study of diagnostic- and therapeutic management. *Physiotherapy* **2017**, *103*, 369–378.
11. Sueki, D.G.; Cleland, J.A.; Wainner, R.S. A regional interdependence model of musculoskeletal dysfunction: Research, mechanisms, and clinical implications. *J. Man. Manip. Ther.* **2013**, *21*, 90–102. [CrossRef] [PubMed]
12. Wainner, R.S.; Whitman, J.M.; Cleland, J.A.; Flynn, T.W. Regional Interdependence: A Musculoskeletal Examination Model Whose Time Has Come. *J. Orthop. Sports Phys. Ther.* **2007**, *37*, 658–660. [CrossRef] [PubMed]
13. Dwyer, A.; Aprill, C.; Bogduk, N. Cervical zygapophyseal joint pain patterns. I: A study in normal volunteers. *Spine* **1990**, *15*, 453–457.
14. Aprill, C.; Dwyer, A.; Bogduk, N. Cervical zygapophyseal joint pain patterns. II: A clinical evaluation. *Spine* **1990**, *15*, 458–461. [CrossRef]
15. Fukui, S.; Ohseto, K.; Shiotani, M.; Ohno, K.; Karasawa, H.; Naganuma, Y.; Yuda, Y. Referred pain distribution of the cervical zygapophyseal joints and cervical dorsal rami. *Pain* **1996**, *68*, 79–83. [CrossRef]
16. Cooper, G.; Bailey, B.; Bogduk, N. Cervical zygapophysial joint pain maps. *Pain Med.* **2007**, *8*, 344–353. [CrossRef]
17. Friedenberg, Z.B.; Miller, W.T. Degenerative Disc Disease of the Cervical Spine. *J. Bone Jt. Surg. Am.* **1963**, *45*, 1171–1178. [CrossRef]
18. Bogduk, N.; Simons, D.G. Neck pain: Joint pain or trigger points. In *Progress in Fibromyalgia and Myofascial Pain*; Vaeroy, H., Merskey, H., Eds.; Elsevier: Amsterdam, The Netherlands, 1993; pp. 267–273.
19. Katsuura, Y.; Bruce, J.; Taylor, S.; Gullota, L.; Kim, H.J. Overlapping, Masquerading, and Causative Cervical Spine and Shoulder Pathology: A Systematic Review. *Glob. Spine J.* **2020**, *10*, 195–208. [CrossRef]
20. Boksman, S.L.; DePasse, J.M.; Eltorai, A.E.M.; Paxton, E.S.; Green, A.; Daniels, A.H. An Evidence-Based Approach to Differentiating the Cause of Shoulder and Cervical Spine Pain. *Am. J. Med.* **2016**, *129*, 913–918. [CrossRef]
21. Holmes, R.E.; Barfield, W.R.; Woolf, S.K. Clinical evaluation of nonarthritic shoulder pain: Diagnosis and treatment. *Phys. Sportsmed.* **2015**, *43*, 262–268. [CrossRef]
22. Throckmorton, T.Q.; Kraemer, P.; Kuhn, J.E.; Sasso, R.C. Differentiating cervical spine and shoulder pathology: Common disorders and key points of evaluation and treatment. *Instr. Course Lect.* **2014**, *63*, 401–408. [PubMed]
23. Heidar Abady, A.; Rosedale, R.; Chesworth, B.M.; Rotondi, M.A.; Overend, T.J. Consistency of commonly used orthopedic special tests of the shoulder when used with the McKenzie system of mechanical diagnosis and therapy. *Musculoskelet. Sci. Pract.* **2018**, *33*, 11–17. [PubMed]
24. Rosedale, R.; Rastogi, R.; Kidd, J.; Lynch, G.; Supp, G.; Robbins, S.M. A study exploring the prevalence of Extremity Pain of Spinal Source (EXPOSS). *J. Man. Manip. Ther.* **2020**, *28*, 222–230.
25. Rastogi, R.; Rosedale, R.; Kidd, J.; Lynch, G.; Supp, G.; Robbins, S.M. Exploring indicators of extremity pain of spinal source as identified by Mechanical Diagnosis and Therapy (MDT): A secondary analysis of a prospective cohort study. *J. Man. Manip. Ther.* **2022**, *30*, 172–179.
26. Norlander, S.; Aste-Norlander, U.; Nordgren, B.; Sahlstedt, B. Mobility in the cervico-thoracic motion segment: An indicative factor of musculo-skeletal neck-shoulder pain. *Scand. J. Rehabil. Med.* **1996**, *28*, 183–192.
27. Roldán-Ruiz, A.; Bailón-Cerezo, J.; Torres-Lacomba, M. The prevalence of subclassification-based diagnoses when considering cervical contribution in shoulder pain patients: A secondary analysis from a previous research. *J. Man. Manip. Ther.* **2024**, 1–9. [CrossRef]
28. Maccio, J.R.; Carlton, L.; Levesque, K.; Maccio, J.G.; Egan, L. Directional preference of the extremity: A preliminary investigation. *J. Man. Manip. Ther.* **2018**, *26*, 272–280.
29. Khan, S.; Hameed, N.; Mazar, S.; Hashmi, I.A.; Rafi, M.S.; Shah, M.I.; Baloch, N.A.; Shah, M. Persistent Shoulder Pain After Anterior Cervical Discectomy and Fusion (ACDF): Another Dual Pathology. *Cureus* **2021**, *13*, e13709.
30. Khoinne, E.; Kwak, J.; Sun, Y.; Lee, H.; Koh, K.H.; Jeon, I. Risk Factors for Persistent Shoulder Pain After Cervical Spine Surgery. *Orthop. Surg.* **2019**, *11*, 845–849.
31. Hauswirth, J.; Ernst, M.J.; Preusser, M.L.; Meichtry, A.; Kool, J.; Crawford, R.J. Immediate effects of cervical unilateral anterior-posterior mobilisation on shoulder pain and impairment in post-operative arthroscopy patients. *J. Back Musculoskelet. Rehabil.* **2017**, *30*, 615–623.
32. Wang, S.S.; Meadows, J. Immediate and Carryover Changes of C5-6 Joint Mobilization on Shoulder External Rotator Muscle Strength. *J. Manip. Physiol. Ther.* **2010**, *33*, 102–108.
33. Suter, E.; McMorland, G. Decrease in elbow flexor inhibition after cervical spine manipulation in patients with chronic neck pain. *Clin. Biomech.* **2002**, *17*, 541–544.

34. Mintken, P. Shoulder Pain and Regional Interdependence: Contributions of the Cervicothoracic Spine. *J. Yoga Phys. Ther.* **2014**, *05*, 1–2.
35. McClatchie, L.; Laprade, J.; Martin, S.; Jaglal, S.B.; Richardson, D.; Agur, A. Mobilizations of the asymptomatic cervical spine can reduce signs of shoulder dysfunction in adults. *Man. Ther.* **2009**, *14*, 369–374.
36. Bergman, G.J.D.; Winters, J.C.; Groenier, H.; Pool, J.J.M.; Meyboom-de Jong, B. Article Manipulative Therapy in Addition to Usual Medical Care for Patients with Shoulder Dysfunction and Pain. *Am. Coll. Physicians* **2004**, *21*, 432–440.
37. Schneider, G. Restricted Shoulder Movement: Capsular Contracture or Cervical Referral—A Clinical Study. *Aust. J. Physiother.* **1989**, *35*, 97–100.
38. Hathcock, J.A.; Boyer, C.W.; Morris, J.B. Shoulder Pain of Spinal Source in the Military: A Case Series. *Mil. Med.* **2022**, *187*, e1240–e1246.
39. Pheasant, S. Cervical Contribution to Functional Shoulder Impingement: Two Case Reports. *Int. J. Sports Phys. Ther.* **2016**, *11*, 980–991.
40. Seo, Y.; Lee, J.; Han, D. The effects of spinal mobilization with arm movements on shoulder muscle strengthening. *J. Phys. Ther. Sci.* **2015**, *27*, 11–13.
41. Requejo-Salinas, N.; Fernández-Matías, R.; Cadogan, A.; Chester, R.; Roy, J.-S.; Struyf, F.; Bateman, M.; Balster, S.; Haik, M.N.; Seitz, A.L.; et al. Neck or Shoulder? Establishing Consensus for Spine Screening in Patients with Shoulder Pain: An International Modified Delphi Study. *Phys. Ther.* **2024**, *105*, pzae133.
42. Cuesta-Vargas, A.I.; Roldan-Jimenez, C.; Neblett, R.; Gatchel, R.J. Cross-cultural adaptation and validity of the Spanish central sensitization inventory. *Springerplus* **2016**, *5*, 1837. [CrossRef] [PubMed]
43. Jensen, M.P.; McFarland, C.A. Increasing the reliability and validity of pain intensity measurement in chronic pain patients. *Pain* **1993**, *55*, 195–203. [CrossRef] [PubMed]
44. Jensen, M.P.; Karoly, P.; Braver, S. The measurement of clinical pain intensity: A comparison of six methods. *Pain* **1986**, *27*, 117–126. [CrossRef]
45. Bahat, H.S.; Kerner, O. The Shoulder Symptom Modification Procedure (SSMP): A Reliability Study. *J. Nov. Physiother.* **2016**, *S3*, 1–6. [CrossRef]
46. Lewis, J.S. Rotator cuff tendinopathy/subacromial impingement syndrome: Is it time for a new method of assessment? *Br. J. Sports Med.* **2009**, *43*, 259–264. [CrossRef]
47. Werner, B.C.; Holzgrefe, R.E.; Griffin, J.W.; Lyons, M.L.; Cosgrove, C.T.; Hart, J.M.; Brockmeier, S.F. Validation of an innovative method of shoulder range-of-motion measurement using a smartphone clinometer application. *J. Shoulder Elb. Surg.* **2014**, *23*, e275–e282. [CrossRef]
48. McLaine, S.J.; Ginn, K.A.; Kitic, C.M.; Fell, J.W.; Bird, M.-L. The Reliability of Strength Tests Performed in Elevated Shoulder Positions Using a Handheld Dynamometer. *J. Sport Rehabil.* **2016**, *25*, jsr.2015-0034. [CrossRef]
49. Holt, K.L.; Raper, D.P.; Boettcher, C.E.; Waddington, G.S.; Drew, M.K. Hand-held dynamometry strength measures for internal and external rotation demonstrate superior reliability, lower minimal detectable change and higher correlation to isokinetic dynamometry than externally-fixed dynamometry of the shoulder. *Phys. Ther. Sport.* **2016**, *21*, 75–81. [CrossRef]
50. Roy, J.S.; MacDermid, J.C.; Orton, B.; Tran, T.; Faber, K.J.; Drosdowech, D.; Athwal, G.S. The Concurrent Validity of a Hand-held versus a Stationary Dynamometer in Testing Isometric Shoulder Strength. *J Hand Ther.* **2009**, *22*, 320–327. [CrossRef]
51. Breckenridge, J.D.; McAuley, J.H. Shoulder Pain and Disability Index (SPADI). *J. Physiother.* **2011**, *57*, 197. [CrossRef]
52. Beaton, D.E.; Richards, R.R. Measuring function of the shoulder. A cross-sectional comparison of five questionnaires. *J. Bone Jt. Surg. Am.* **1996**, *78*, 882–890. [CrossRef] [PubMed]
53. Cohen, J. *Statistical Power Analysis for the Behavioral Sciences (2. Auflage)*; Erlbaum: Hillsdale, NJ, USA, 1988.
54. Cook, C.; Learman, K.; Houghton, S.; Showalter, C.; O'Halloran, B. The addition of cervical unilateral posterior-anterior mobilisation in the treatment of patients with shoulder impingement syndrome: A randomised clinical trial. *Man. Ther.* **2014**, *19*, 18–24. [PubMed]
55. Menon, A.; May, S. Shoulder pain: Differential diagnosis with mechanical diagnosis and therapy extremity assessment—A case report. *Man. Ther.* **2013**, *18*, 354–357. [CrossRef] [PubMed]
56. Shelke, A.; Kumaran, S.D. Immediate effect of craniocervical flexion exercise and Mulligan mobilisation in patients with mechanical neck pain—A randomised clinical trial. *Hong Kong Physiother. J.* **2023**, *43*, 137–147.
57. Paul, A.; Lewis, M.; Shadforth, M.F.; Croft, P.R.; Van Der Windt, D.A.W.M.; Hay, E.M. A comparison of four shoulder-specific questionnaires in primary care. *Ann. Rheum. Dis.* **2004**, *63*, 1293–1299. [CrossRef]
58. Schibany, N.; Zehetgruber, H.; Kainberger, F.; Wurnig, C.; Ba-Ssalamah, A.; Herneth, A.M.; Lang, T.; Gruber, D.; Breitenseher, M.J. Rotator cuff tears in asymptomatic individuals: A clinical and ultrasonographic screening study. *Eur. J. Radiol.* **2004**, *51*, 263–268. [CrossRef]
59. Somerville, K.; Walston, Z.; Marr, T.; Yake, D. Treatment of shoulder pathologies based on irritability: A case series. *Physiother. Theory Pract.* **2020**, *36*, 1266–1274.

60. Beaudreuil, J.; Nizard, R.; Thomas, T.; Peyre, M.; Liotard, J.P.; Boileau, P.; Marc, T.; Dromard, C.; Steyer, E.; Bardin, T.; et al. Contribution of clinical tests to the diagnosis of rotator cuff disease: A systematic literature review. *Jt. Bone Spine* **2009**, *76*, 15–19. [CrossRef]
61. Walton, D.M.; Sadi, J. Identifying SLAP lesions: A meta-analysis of clinical tests and exercise in clinical reasoning. *Phys. Ther. Sport* **2008**, *9*, 167–176.
62. Cadogan, A.; Laslett, M.; Hing, W.; McNair, P.; Williams, M. Interexaminer reliability of orthopaedic special tests used in the assessment of shoulder pain. *Man. Ther.* **2011**, *16*, 131–135. [CrossRef]
63. Tuttle, N. Do changes within a manual therapy treatment session predict between-session changes for patients with cervical spine pain? *Aust. J. Physiother.* **2005**, *51*, 43–48.
64. Cook, C.; Lawrence, J.; Michalak, K.; Dhiraprasiddhi, S.; Donaldson, M.; Petersen, S.; Learman, K. Is there preliminary value to a within- and/or between-session change for determining short-term outcomes of manual therapy on mechanical neck pain? *J. Man. Manip. Ther.* **2014**, *22*, 173–180.

Journal of
Clinical Medicine

MDPI

Article

Impact of Sarcopenia and Functional Relationships Between Balance and Gait After Total Hip Arthroplasty

So-Yeong Kim [1,2], Woon-Su Cho [3], Chi-Bok Park [3] and Byeong-Geun Kim [3,*]

1 Department of Physical Therapy, Graduate School, Nambu University, Gwangju 62271, Republic of Korea
2 Rehabilitation Center, Gwangju 365 Rehabilitation Hospital, Gwangju 62232, Republic of Korea
3 Department of Physical Therapy, Nambu University, Gwangju 62271, Republic of Korea
* Correspondence: qudrms_92@naver.com

Abstract: Background/Objectives: Total hip arthroplasty (THA) is an effective surgical intervention for restoring hip function and alleviating pain caused by osteoarthritis, femoral head avascular necrosis, or fractures. Despite its benefits, postoperative recovery is influenced by various factors, among which sarcopenia plays a critical role. This study aimed to analyze the characteristics of sarcopenia in THA patients admitted to a convalescent rehabilitation hospital and examine its relationship with functional variables such as balance and gait independence. **Methods**: This cross-sectional study included 84 THA patients, categorized into sarcopenia and non-sarcopenia groups using the Asian Working Group for Sarcopenia 2019 criteria. Data were collected on demographic characteristics (e.g., age, gender, height, weight, range of motion (ROM), manual muscle test (MMT)) and functional variables, including balance (Berg Balance Scale, BBS) and gait independence (Functional Ambulation Category, FAC). **Results**: The prevalence of sarcopenia among THA patients was 44.05%. Significant differences were observed between the sarcopenia and non-sarcopenia groups in sex, age, height, weight, ROM, MMT, BBS, and FAC ($p < 0.05$). Logistic regression analysis showed that advanced age increased the likelihood of sarcopenia (OR: 1.072, $p < 0.05$), whereas higher body weight reduced it (OR: 0.784, $p < 0.05$). However, sarcopenia was not significantly associated with balance (BBS: $p = 0.710$) or gait independence (FAC: $p = 0.990$). Instead, a significant positive correlation was found between FAC and BBS (OR: 0.413, $p < 0.001$), as well as BBS and FAC (OR: 0.467, $p < 0.001$), indicating that better balance was associated with greater gait independence and vice versa. Additionally, patients who underwent THA due to fractures had a lower FAC compared to those with osteoarthritis (OR: −0.276, $p = 0.018$). **Conclusions**: Sarcopenia is prevalent among THA patients, and functional variables such as balance and gait independence are closely associated. Additionally, age and body weight were identified as key factors related to sarcopenia. These findings emphasize the importance of early detection and management of sarcopenia in rehabilitation hospital settings and highlight the significance of functional variables in recovery.

Keywords: total hip arthroplasty; sarcopenia; balance; gait

1. Introduction

Total hip arthroplasty (THA) is an effective surgical procedure performed to restore hip function and alleviate pain. It serves as a treatment method for replacing damaged hip joints caused by various conditions, such as osteoarthritis, avascular necrosis of the femoral head, and fractures [1,2]. This procedure significantly improves patients' physical function and quality of life, and its prevalence is expected to continue increasing in the future [3].

However, successful postoperative recovery and long-term functional maintenance depend on multiple factors, among which sarcopenia has been identified as a major limiting factor.

Sarcopenia is characterized by a decline in muscle mass, muscle strength, and physical performance and is commonly observed in older adults and various patient populations [4–7]. Among the key factors of sarcopenia, muscle mass plays a crucial role. In older adults, reduced muscle mass is closely associated with decreased muscle strength, which in turn contributes to impaired balance and slower gait speed [8–10]. This condition can lead to multiple complications, including reduced physical function, an increased risk of falls, and a decline in the ability to perform independent daily activities, all of which may also affect patients undergoing THA [11–13]. Recent studies have reported that sarcopenia negatively impacts functional recovery and prognosis across various patient groups, underscoring the importance of strategies to prevent and manage this condition [14–16]. Therefore, exercise and nutritional interventions should be considered as key strategies for mitigating the effects of sarcopenia and promoting recovery [17].

The prevalence of sarcopenia in THA patients varies depending on diagnostic criteria and surgical indications, with some studies reporting rates ranging from 23.2% to 37.6% [18,19]. In patients undergoing THA, sarcopenia is closely linked not only to reductions in muscle mass and strength but also to key functional variables, such as balance and gait [20,21]. These functional variables are critical indicators for determining a patient's ability to maintain independent living and achieve successful rehabilitation. Identifying sarcopenia and its associated characteristics in patients admitted to a convalescent rehabilitation hospital can provide valuable insights for optimizing recovery strategies. Therefore, this study aimed to analyze the characteristics of sarcopenia in THA patients admitted to a convalescent rehabilitation hospital and examine its relationship with functional variables, specifically balance and gait independence. By identifying key factors associated with sarcopenia, this study seeks to emphasize the importance of early detection and management to improve rehabilitation outcomes.

2. Materials and Methods

2.1. Study Design

This study was a cross-sectional analysis of the relationship between sarcopenia status and functional parameters in patients who had undergone THA. The study was conducted on patients hospitalized in a rehabilitation facility, and prior to its commencement, approval was obtained from the Institutional Review Board (IRB) of Nambu University (IRB: 1041478-2023-HR-033). Data collection was conducted from February 2024 to November 2024. The participants were patients who had undergone THA at other hospitals and were subsequently transferred to the research institution for post-acute rehabilitation. Assessments were conducted after obtaining informed consent from the participants upon hospital admission. All collected data were anonymized, and participant confidentiality was strictly maintained in accordance with ethical guidelines.

2.2. Study Participants

Participants were selected based on predefined inclusion and exclusion criteria. The inclusion criteria were as follows: patients who had undergone THA, were receiving rehabilitation treatment, and had provided informed consent to participate in the study. Patients were excluded if they had a neurological disorder, were in an acute inflammatory state that made functional assessment difficult or had cognitive impairments that prevented them from complying with the study procedures. Sarcopenia was diagnosed based on the 2019 criteria of the Asian Working Group for Sarcopenia (AWGS), and participants were categorized into either the sarcopenia or non-sarcopenia group accordingly. In this study, bioelectrical impedance analysis (BIA) was used to assess skeletal muscle mass, as recommended by the AWGS 2019 guidelines [4]. BIA was chosen over dual-energy X-ray absorptiometry due to its greater accessibility, lower cost, and ease of use in clinical settings, particularly in rehabilitation hospitals where routine body composition assessments are required.

2.3. Outcome Measures and Variables

In this study, the variables were categorized into general characteristics and functional parameters. General characteristics included age, sex, height, weight, reason for surgery (fracture, osteoarthritis, or avascular necrosis of the femoral head), surgical site (left, right, or bilateral), range of motion (ROM), and manual muscle test (MMT). These data were obtained from the electronic medical record, while the ROM and MMT were assessed using methods adapted for functional evaluation in convalescent rehabilitation patients in Korea.

The ROM was measured using a goniometer for both sides of the body, assessing the shoulder (flexion, extension, abduction, external rotation, and internal rotation), elbow (flexion and extension), wrist (flexion and extension), hip (flexion, extension, and abduction), knee (flexion and extension), and ankle (dorsiflexion and plantarflexion). Assessments were conducted with patients positioned for optimal safety and comfort. The upper extremity (shoulder, elbow, and wrist) and ankle ROM were measured in a sitting position. The hip ROM assessment varied depending on the surgical approach: patients who underwent anterior approach THA did not undergo hip extension assessment due to postoperative restrictions (recorded as 0 points), whereas those who underwent posterolateral approach THA were assessed for hip extension in a side lying position. Knee flexion was measured in a supine position instead of the standard prone position, as some post-surgical patients experienced discomfort and fear in the prone position. The scoring system assigned 2 points for normal motion and 1 point for restricted motion, with a total possible score of 64 points.

The MMT was evaluated for both sides of the body, assessing the shoulder (flexion and abduction), elbow (flexion and extension), wrist (flexion and extension), hip (flexion and extension), knee (flexion and extension), and ankle (dorsiflexion and plantarflexion). Assessments were conducted in the same positions as the ROM measurements to ensure consistency. The upper extremity and ankle MMT were evaluated in a sitting position, while the hip extension MMT was assessed in a side lying position for patients with a posterolateral surgical approach and not assessed for those with an anterior approach. The knee flexion MMT was performed in a supine position to accommodate post-surgical patient comfort. The grading system assigned 6 points for the "Normal" grade and 1 point for the "Zero" grade, with a total possible score of 144 points.

Sarcopenia was diagnosed when both the skeletal muscle mass index (SMI) and grip strength were below the established criteria. The SMI was measured using a BIA device (BWA 2.0, InBody, Seoul, Korea), with a threshold of <7.0 kg/m^2 for men and <5.7 kg/m^2 for women, according to the 2019 criteria of the AWGS. The grip strength was assessed using a handgrip dynamometer, recording the maximum grip strength of each hand, with a cut-off value of <28 kg for men and <18 kg for women.

Functional parameters were evaluated based on the balance ability and gait independence. The balance ability was assessed using the Berg Balance Scale (BBS), a widely used tool for assessing balance performance in clinical and rehabilitation settings. The BBS consists of 14 items, each scored from 0 (unable to perform the task) to 4 (able to perform the task independently) [22]. The total possible score was 56, with higher scores indicating better balance ability. The BBS was selected for this study due to its ability to evaluate functional balance tasks relevant to daily activities, making it particularly suitable for assessing THA patients recovering in rehabilitation hospitals. Gait independence was assessed using the Functional Ambulation Category (FAC), a validated tool for classifying gait independence based on the level of assistance required during ambulation [23]. The FAC classifies gait independence into six levels, ranging from 0 to 5, with higher scores indicating greater independence in ambulation. The FAC was chosen because it allows for a simple yet effective classification of ambulation ability, making it an appropriate measure for evaluating gait recovery in THA patients.

2.4. Statistical Analysis

The collected data were analyzed using Statistical Package for Social Sciences (SPSS) for Windows (Version 23.0, IBM Corp., Armonk, NY, USA) statistical software. Differences between groups were examined using independent sample t-tests and chi-square tests. Multiple regression analysis was performed to assess the impact on functional parameters, while logistic regression analysis was conducted to identify factors influencing the likelihood of sarcopenia. The level of statistical significance was set at $p < 0.05$.

3. Results

A total of 84 patients who underwent THA participated in this study, among whom 37 were diagnosed with sarcopenia, resulting in a sarcopenia prevalence rate of 44.05%. Comparisons between the sarcopenia and non-sarcopenia groups revealed significant differences in the sex, reason for surgery, age, height, weight, ROM, MMT, BBS, and FAC ($p < 0.05$) (Table 1). The analysis of the effects of the general and functional characteristics on sarcopenia in THA patients indicated that each additional year of age increased the likelihood of belonging to the sarcopenia group by 1.072 times ($p < 0.05$) (Table 2). In contrast, each 1 Kg increase in body weight reduced the likelihood of being classified in the sarcopenia group by 0.784 times ($p < 0.05$) (Table 2).

Table 1. Comparison of characteristics between the sarcopenia and non-sarcopenia groups.

Variables	Total	Sarcopenia Group	Non-Sarcopenia Group	p
Sex (male/female)	21/63	5/32	16/31	0.031 *
Surgery side (left/right/both)	44/34/6	23/13/1	21/21/5	0.174
Reason for surgery (AVN/FX/OA)	7/47/30	2/30/5	5/17/25	<0.001 *
Age (year)	68.38 ± 14.49	75.30 ± 12.63	62.94 ± 13.61	<0.001 *
Height (cm)	158.46 ± 8.84	155.22 ± 7.68	161.02 ± 8.92	0.002 *
Weight (kg)	57.10 ± 10.75	49.98 ± 7.59	62.71 ± 9.53	<0.001 *
ROM (score)	58.67 ± 4.28	57.46 ± 4.99	59.62 ± 3.40	0.021 *
MMT (score)	129.64 ± 13.92	124.57 ± 18.22	133.64 ± 7.25	0.006 *
BBS (score)	24.11 ± 12.88	18.24 ± 12.38	28.72 ± 11.40	<0.001 *
FAC (score)	1.17 ± 0.67	0.95 ± 0.62	1.34 ± 0.67	0.007 *

*: $p < 0.05$, AVN: avascular necrosis; FX: fractures; OA: osteoarthritis; ROM: range of motion; MMT: manual muscle test; BBS: Berg balance scale; FAC: functional ambulation category.

Table 2. Analysis of the effects of THA patient characteristics on sarcopenia.

Variables	B	OR	95%CI	p
Male	1.733	5.657	0.374~85.546	0.211
Reason for surgery (AVN: OA)	2.422	11.265	0.779~162.953	0.076
Reason for surgery (FX: OA)	1.490	4.439	0.840~23.467	0.079
Age	0.069	1.072	1.012~1.135	0.017 *
Height	0.018	1.018	0.890~1.165	0.792
Weight	−0.243	0.784	0.679~0.905	0.001 *
ROM	−0.047	0.954	0.753~1.208	0.695
MMT	−0.045	0.956	0.882~1.036	0.273

Table 2. *Cont.*

Variables	B	OR	95%CI	p
BBS	−0.013	0.987	0.920~1.059	0.710
FAC	0.010	1.010	0.227~4.496	0.990

*: $p < 0.05$, AVN: avascular necrosis; FX: fractures; OA: osteoarthritis; ROM: range of motion; MMT: manual muscle test; BBS: Berg balance scale; FAC: functional ambulation category.

The analysis of the impact of the general characteristics on the functional parameters (BBS and FAC) in THA patients showed that higher FAC scores were associated with higher BBS scores (OR: 0.413, $p < 0.05$). Similarly, higher BBS scores were associated with higher FAC scores (OR: 0.467, $p < 0.05$) (Table 3). Regarding the reason for surgery, patients who underwent THA due to fractures had lower FAC scores compared to those with osteoarthritis (OR: −0.276, $p < 0.05$) (Table 3).

Table 3. Analysis of the association between THA patient characteristics and functional variables.

Variables		B	OR	p
BBS	Sarcopenia	−1.186	−0.046	0.705
	Female	1.416	0.048	0.720
	Reason for surgery (AVN: OA)	3.689	0.080	0.402
	Reason for surgery (FX: OA)	1.712	0.066	0.553
	Age	−0.145	−0.163	0.131
	Height	0.010	0.007	0.965
	Weight	0.214	0.179	0.182
	ROM	0.527	0.175	0.058
	MMT	0.147	0.159	0.093
	FAC	7.892	0.413	<0.001 *
FAC	Sarcopenia	0.030	0.022	0.863
	Female	−0.409	−0.265	0.059
	Reason for surgery (AVN: OA)	−0.047	−0.019	0.849
	Reason for surgery (FX: OA)	−0.372	−0.276	0.018*
	Age	0.000	−0.008	0.942
	Height	−0.021	−0.280	0.077
	Weight	0.004	0.071	0.621
	ROM	−0.010	−0.063	0.527
	MMT	0.000	0.008	0.936
	BBS	0.024	0.467	<0.001 *

*: $p < 0.05$, AVN: avascular necrosis; FX: fractures; OA: osteoarthritis; ROM: range of motion; MMT: manual muscle test; BBS: Berg balance scale; FAC: functional ambulation category.

4. Discussion

The prevalence of sarcopenia in THA patients was 44.05%, which is similar to previous studies on total knee arthroplasty and THA [24–26]. This finding suggests that sarcopenia is a common condition in older adults undergoing joint replacement surgery. Given that THA is primarily performed in elderly populations, and sarcopenia is closely related to aging; the observed prevalence aligns with prior research findings [27,28]. Additionally, this study identified significant differences between sarcopenia and non-sarcopenia groups in terms of sex, age, weight, ROM, MMT, BBS, and FAC, indicating that sarcopenia may be associated with impaired functional outcomes in this population.

Given the high prevalence of sarcopenia in this population, it is important to understand its association with functional deficits. Comparisons between the sarcopenia and non-sarcopenia groups revealed significant differences in sex, age, height, weight, ROM, MMT, BBS, and FAC. Furthermore, differences in sex and body weight between the sarcopenia and non-sarcopenia groups are consistent with findings from previous studies. Sarcopenia is more prevalent in women, due to lower baseline muscle mass and hormonal changes associated with aging, which may contribute to greater muscle degradation compared to men [29,30]. Additionally, body weight has been identified as a protective factor against sarcopenia, as individuals with higher body weight generally have greater muscle mass [31]. However, excessive body weight may also contribute to obesity-related sarcopenia, necessitating careful evaluation of body composition rather than relying solely on weight as an indicator [32].

Previous studies have reported similar findings, indicating that sarcopenia is associated with poor functional outcomes in older adults undergoing orthopedic surgery. Sarcopenia can develop at any stage, either before or after surgery. Although this study did not specifically account for this aspect, previous research investigating the impact of sarcopenia on THA outcomes found that patients with sarcopenia exhibited significantly reduced gait ability at discharge and increased reliance on assistive devices [33]. These findings are consistent with the results observed in our study population. One possible explanation for these impairments is that sarcopenia leads to deficits in muscle strength, neuromuscular control, and proprioception, all of which are essential for balance and gait stability. Decreased lower limb strength reduces the ability to generate adequate push-off force during walking, leading to a slower gait speed and impaired dynamic stability [34]. Additionally, sarcopenia is associated with neuromuscular degradation, resulting in delayed motor responses and decreased coordination, which further contribute to balance deficits and a higher fall risk [35,36]. These mechanisms may explain why patients with sarcopenia in this study demonstrated significantly lower BBS and FAC scores compared to non-sarcopenic patients. These results suggest that sarcopenia contributes to impaired post-surgical recovery, further emphasizing the importance of early identification and management.

Logistic regression analysis identified sarcopenia risk factors. Age and body weight were significant predictors of sarcopenia occurrence. The positive association between older age and sarcopenia risk is consistent with the natural aging process, which involves a progressive decline in muscle mass [37]. Meanwhile, the negative association between body weight and sarcopenia risk aligns with previous studies suggesting that increased body weight may be linked to greater muscle mass [31]. However, higher body weight does not necessarily indicate healthy muscle mass gain, as obesity-related sarcopenia, where sarcopenia and obesity coexist, must also be considered, particularly in obese individuals [38]. Therefore, a more comprehensive evaluation is necessary.

Multiple regression analysis demonstrated a significant positive association between balance ability and gait independence in THA patients. This suggests that enhancing balance may contribute to improved gait independence [39]. Consequently, rehabilitation programs should incorporate both gait and balance training rather than focusing solely on ambulation. Additionally, patients who underwent surgery due to fractures had lower FAC scores compared to those with osteoarthritis, indicating that fractures may have a more detrimental impact on postoperative recovery [40]. This may be explained by age-related musculoskeletal deterioration, including reduced bone and muscle integrity. The loss of osteocytes and decreased osteoprogenitor activity impair the bone's response to mechanical stimuli, while muscle aging is characterized by reduced fiber size, decreased protein synthesis, and increased fatty infiltration, all of which compromise contractile function and may hinder recovery following THA [41]. Previous studies have also reported that THA patients with fractures experience delayed functional recovery compared to those with osteoarthritis [42]. These findings align with our results, further supporting the notion that surgical indication influences postoperative functional outcomes in THA patients.

The findings of this study suggest that while sarcopenia may not have a direct impact on balance and gait independence, it is associated with other physical characteristics, such as age and muscle mass, that influence post-THA recovery. Given these associations, rehabilitation programs for THA patients should prioritize strength training, neuromuscular exercises, and proprioceptive training to enhance functional recovery. Additionally, nutritional interventions, including adequate protein intake and supplementation when necessary, may support muscle preservation and improve overall rehabilitation outcomes. A multidimensional approach incorporating strength training and tailored rehabilitation strategies may help optimize mobility and independence in THA patients, particularly those at risk of sarcopenia.

This study has several limitations. First, as a cross-sectional study conducted in a single medical institution, its ability to establish causal relationships is limited, and the generalizability of the findings may be restricted. To address this limitation, prospective studies that track the long-term interaction between sarcopenia and functional changes across multiple centers are needed. Second, the social, cultural, and healthcare characteristics of the participants may have influenced the results; therefore, multicenter studies including more diverse populations are necessary. Third, while this study focused on key functional indicators such as BBS and FAC, other important clinical variables such as fall risk, quality of life, and activities of daily living were not included. Future research should incorporate these variables to provide a more comprehensive assessment of the impact of sarcopenia on overall patient function and quality of life.

5. Conclusions

This study examined the prevalence of sarcopenia and its association with functional outcomes in THA patients. Sarcopenic patients exhibited poorer functional status, with age and body weight identified as key predictors. Additionally, fracture as a surgical indication was linked to lower gait independence, and balance ability was positively associated with gait function. These findings highlight the need for targeted rehabilitation strategies in THA patients with sarcopenia. Future prospective studies should explore the long-term impact of sarcopenia on recovery. Additionally, interventions such as resistance training and nutritional support may help mitigate sarcopenia-related functional decline and should be further investigated.

Author Contributions: Conceptualization, S.-Y.K. and B.-G.K.; methodology, S.-Y.K. and B.-G.K.; software, W.-S.C. and C.-B.P.; validation, W.-S.C. and C.-B.P.; formal analysis, W.-S.C. and C.-B.P.; investigation, S.-Y.K.; resources, W.-S.C. and C.-B.P.; data curation, W.-S.C. and C.-B.P.; writing—original draft preparation, S.-Y.K. and B.-G.K.; writing—review and editing, S.-Y.K. and B.-G.K.; visualization, W.-S.C. and C.-B.P.; supervision, B.-G.K.; project administration, B.-G.K. All authors have read and agreed to the published version of the manuscript.

Funding: This research received no external funding.

Institutional Review Board Statement: The study was conducted in accordance with the Declaration of Helsinki and approved by the Institutional Review Board of Nambu University (IRB: 1041478−2023-HR-033 and date of approval: 20 February 2024).

Informed Consent Statement: Informed consent was obtained from all subjects involved in the study.

Data Availability Statement: The data can be requested from the corresponding author and will be released on reasonable request.

Conflicts of Interest: The authors declare no conflicts of interest.

Abbreviations

The following abbreviations are used in this manuscript:

THA	Total hip arthroplasty
AVN	Avascular necrosis
FX	Fractures
OA	Osteoarthritis
AWGS	Asian working group for sarcopenia
BIA	Bioelectrical impedance analysis
SMI	Skeletal muscle mass index
ROM	Range of motion
MMT	Manual muscle test
BBS	Berg balance scale
FAC	Functional ambulation category

References

1. Coomber, R.; Porteous, M.; Hubble, M.J.W.; Parker, M.J. Total hip replacement for hip fracture: Surgical techniques and concepts. *Injury* **2016**, *47*, 2060–2064. [CrossRef] [PubMed]
2. Salman, L.A.; Hantouly, A.T.; Khatkar, H.; Al-Ani, A.; Abudalou, A.; Al-Juboori, M.; Ahmed, G. The outcomes of total hip replacement in osteonecrosis versus osteoarthritis: A systematic review and meta-analysis. *Int. Orthop.* **2023**, *47*, 3043–3052. [CrossRef] [PubMed]
3. Kurtz, S.; Ong, K.; Lau, E.; Mowat, F.; Halpern, M. Projections of primary and revision hip and knee arthroplasty in the United States from 2005 to 2030. *J. Bone Jt. Surg. Am.* **2007**, *89*, 780–785. [CrossRef]
4. Chen, L.K.; Woo, J.; Assantachai, P.; Auyeung, T.W.; Chou, M.Y.; Iijima, K.; Jang, H.C.; Kang, L.; Kim, M.; Kim, S.; et al. Asian Working Group for Sarcopenia: 2019 Consensus Update on Sarcopenia Diagnosis and Treatment. *J. Am. Med. Dir. Assoc.* **2020**, *21*, 300–307.e2. [CrossRef]
5. Park, H.S.; Yoon, J.H.; Oh, J.K. Impact of Resistance Exercise and Nitrate Supplementation on Muscle Function and Clinical Outcomes After Knee Osteoarthritis Surgery in Middle-Aged Women with Sarcopenia: A Randomized, Double-Blind, Placebo-Controlled Clinical Trial. *J. Clin. Med.* **2025**, *14*, 615. [CrossRef]
6. Tsai, C.C.; Wang, P.C.; Hsiung, T.; Fan, Y.H.; Wu, J.T.; Kan, W.C.; Shiao, C.C. Sarcopenia in Chronic Kidney Disease: A Narrative Review from Pathophysiology to Therapeutic Approaches. *Biomedicines* **2025**, *13*, 352. [CrossRef]
7. van Bakel, S.I.J.; Gosker, H.R.; Langen, R.C.; Schols, A.M.W.J. Towards Personalized Management of Sarcopenia in COPD. *Int. J. Chronic Obstr. Pulm. Dis.* **2021**, *7*, 25–40. [CrossRef]
8. Goodpaster, B.H.; Park, S.W.; Harris, T.B.; Kritchevsky, S.B.; Nevitt, M.; Schwartz, A.V.; Simonsick, E.M.; Tylavsky, F.A.; Visser, M.; Newman, A.B. The loss of skeletal muscle strength, mass, and quality in older adults: The health, aging and body composition study. *J. Gerontol. A Biol. Sci. Med. Sci.* **2006**, *61*, 1059–1064. [CrossRef]
9. Lanza, M.B.; Arbuco, B.; Ryan, A.S.; Shipper, A.G.; Gray, V.L.; Addison, O. Systematic Review of the Importance of Hip Muscle Strength, Activation, and Structure in Balance and Mobility Tasks. *Arch. Phys. Med. Rehabil.* **2022**, *103*, 1651–1662. [CrossRef]
10. Stotz, A.; Hamacher, D.; Zech, A. Relationship between Muscle Strength and Gait Parameters in Healthy Older Women and Men. *Int. J. Environ. Res. Public Health* **2023**, *20*, 5362. [CrossRef]
11. Lang, T.; Streeper, T.; Cawthon, P.; Baldwin, K.; Taaffe, D.R.; Harris, T.B. Sarcopenia: Etiology, clinical consequences, intervention, and assessment. *Osteoporos. Int.* **2010**, *21*, 543–559. [CrossRef]
12. Senior, H.E.; Henwood, T.R.; Beller, E.M.; Mitchell, G.K.; Keogh, J.W. Prevalence and risk factors of sarcopenia among adults living in nursing homes. *Maturitas* **2015**, *82*, 418–423. [CrossRef] [PubMed]
13. Sumbal, R.; Abbas, M.; Sheikh, S.M.; Sumbal, A. Prevalence and Clinical Impact of Sarcopenia in Patients Undergoing Total Joint Arthroplasty: A Systematic Review and a Meta-Analysis. *J. Arthroplast.* **2024**, *39*, 3128–3135.e3. [CrossRef]
14. Kim, S.Y.; Cho, W.S.; Park, C.B.; Kim, B.G. Effect of Sarcopenia on Functional Recovery in Acute Stroke Patients Admitted for Standard Rehabilitation Program. *Medicina* **2024**, *60*, 1716. [CrossRef]
15. Yoshimura, Y.; Wakabayashi, H.; Bise, T.; Nagano, F.; Shimazu, S.; Shiraishi, A.; Yamaga, M.; Koga, H. Sarcopenia is associated with worse recovery of physical function and dysphagia and a lower rate of home discharge in Japanese hospitalized adults undergoing convalescent rehabilitation. *Nutrition* **2019**, *61*, 111–118. [CrossRef] [PubMed]
16. Yamasaki, Y.; Honda, Y.; Inoue-Umezaki, M.; Makieda, R.; Endo, Y.; Hanayama, K.; Sakaue, H.; Teramoto, F. The association between sarcopenia and functional outcomes in patients undergoing convalescent rehabilitation. *J. Med. Investig.* **2023**, *70*, 457–463. [CrossRef]

17. Park, S.H.; Lee, H. Effectiveness of Combined Exercise and Nutrition Interventions in Preventing and Improving Sarcopenia in Frail or Healthy Older Adults: A Systematic Review. *Res. Gerontol. Nurs.* **2023**, *16*, 312–320. [CrossRef] [PubMed]
18. Tanaka, S.; Kayamoto, A.; Terai, C.; Nojiri, S.; Fugane, Y.; Mori, T.; Nagaya, M.; Kako, M.; Iida, H.; Osawa, Y.; et al. Preoperative Sarcopenia Severity and Clinical Outcomes after Total Hip Arthroplasty. *Nutrients* **2024**, *16*, 2085. [CrossRef]
19. Kim, H.S.; Jang, G.; Park, J.W.; Lee, Y.K.; Koo, K.H. Vitamin D Deficiency and Sarcopenia in Hip Fracture Patients. *J. Bone Metab.* **2021**, *28*, 79–83. [CrossRef]
20. Morita, D.; Iwase, T.; Funahashi, H. Total hip arthroplasty improves systemic muscle atrophy in patients with hip osteoarthritis. *J. Orthop. Sci.* **2024**, *29*, 596–601. [CrossRef]
21. Wareńczak, A.; Lisiński, P. Does total hip replacement impact on postural stability? *BMC Musculoskelet. Disord.* **2019**, *20*, 229. [CrossRef] [PubMed]
22. Berg, K.; Wood-Dauphine, S.; Williams, J.I.; Gayton, D. Measuring balance in the elderly: Preliminary development of an instrument. *Physiother. Can.* **1989**, *41*, 304–311. [CrossRef]
23. Magaziner, J.; Fredman, L.; Hawkes, W.; Hebel, J.R.; Zimmerman, S.; Orwig, D.L.; Wehren, L. Changes in functional status attributable to hip fracture: A comparison of hip fracture patients to community-dwelling aged. *Am. J. Epidemiol.* **2003**, *157*, 1023–1031. [CrossRef] [PubMed]
24. Park, D.; Park, C.J.; Jung, M.G.; Choi, Y.H.; Park, K.S.; Koh, H.S. High prevalence of sarcopenia in Asian female patients awaiting primary total knee arthroplasty: Application of updated diagnostic tools from the Asian working group for sarcopenia. *J. Orthop. Surg.* **2022**, *30*, 10225536221113034. [CrossRef]
25. Babu, J.M.; Kalagara, S.; Durand, W.; Antoci, V.; Deren, M.E.; Cohen, E. Sarcopenia as a Risk Factor for Prosthetic Infection After Total Hip or Knee Arthroplasty. *J. Arthroplast.* **2019**, *34*, 116–122. [CrossRef]
26. Ueoka, K.; Kabata, T.; Kajino, Y.; Inoue, D.; Ohmori, T.; Ueno, T.; Yoshitani, J.; Yamamuro, Y.; Taninaka, A.; Kato, S.; et al. The prevalence and impact of sarcopenia in females undergoing total hip arthroplasty: A prospective study. *Mod. Rheumatol.* **2022**, *32*, 193–198. [CrossRef]
27. Bayliss, L.E.; Culliford, D.; Monk, A.P.; Glyn-Jones, S.; Prieto-Alhambra, D.; Judge, A.; Cooper, C.; Carr, A.J.; Arden, N.K.; Beard, D.J.; et al. The effect of patient age at intervention on risk of implant revision after total replacement of the hip or knee: A population-based cohort study. *Lancet* **2017**, *389*, 1424–1430. [CrossRef] [PubMed]
28. Sayer, A.A.; Cruz-Jentoft, A. Sarcopenia definition, diagnosis and treatment: Consensus is growing. *Age Ageing* **2022**, *51*, afac220. [CrossRef]
29. Yang, Y.; Zhang, Q.; He, C.; Chen, J.; Deng, D.; Lu, W.; Wang, Y. Prevalence of sarcopenia was higher in women than in men: A cross-sectional study from a rural area in eastern China. *PeerJ* **2022**, *10*, e13678. [CrossRef]
30. Collins, B.C.; Laakkonen, E.K.; Lowe, D.A. Aging of the musculoskeletal system: How the loss of estrogen impacts muscle strength. *Bone* **2019**, *123*, 137–144. [CrossRef]
31. Park, C.; Kim, S.; Cho, W.; Kim, B. Characteristics and Predictors of Sarcopenia in Patients with Stroke: A Cross-Sectional Study. *J. Int. Acad. Phys. Ther. Res.* **2024**, *15*, 3205–3210. [CrossRef]
32. Zamboni, M.; Mazzali, G.; Fantin, F.; Rossi, A.; Di Francesco, V. Sarcopenic obesity: A new category of obesity in the elderly. *Nutr. Metab. Cardiovasc. Dis.* **2008**, *18*, 388–395. [CrossRef] [PubMed]
33. Su, Y.; Peng, L.; Dong, D.; Ma, Z.; Gu, X. Impact of sarcopenia in elderly patients undergoing elective total hip arthroplasty on postoperative outcomes: A propensity score-matched study. *BMC Anesthesiol.* **2024**, *24*, 158. [CrossRef]
34. Browne, M.G.; Franz, J.R. Does dynamic stability govern propulsive force generation in human walking? *R. Soc. Open Sci.* **2017**, *4*, 171673. [CrossRef]
35. Sorock, G.S.; Labiner, D.M. Peripheral neuromuscular dysfunction and falls in an elderly cohort. *Am. J. Epidemiol.* **1992**, *136*, 584–591. [CrossRef]
36. Lim, S.K.; Kong, S. Prevalence, physical characteristics, and fall risk in older adults with and without possible sarcopenia. *Aging Clin. Exp. Res.* **2022**, *34*, 1365–1371. [CrossRef]
37. Cruz-Jentoft, A.J.; Sayer, A.A. Sarcopenia. *Lancet* **2019**, *393*, 2636–2646. [CrossRef] [PubMed]
38. Diago-Galmés, A.; Guillamon-Escudero, C.; Tenías-Burillo, J.M.; Soriano, J.M.; Fernández-Garrido, J. Sarcopenic Obesity in Community-Dwelling Spanish Adults Older than 65 Years. *Nutrients* **2023**, *15*, 4932. [CrossRef]
39. Kubo, H.; Kanai, M.; Nozoe, M.; Inamoto, A.; Taguchi, A.; Mase, K.; Shimada, S. Different association between physical activity and physical function according to walking independence in hospital-based rehabilitation program patients with sub-acute stroke. *Clin. Neurol. Neurosurg.* **2022**, *215*, 107202. [CrossRef]
40. Charette, R.S.; Sloan, M.; Lee, G.C. Not all hip arthroplasties are created equal: Increased complications and re-admissions after total hip arthroplasty for femoral neck fractures compared with osteoarthritis. *Bone Jt. J.* **2019**, *101-B*, 84–90. [CrossRef]

41. Tarantino, U.; Baldi, J.; Scimeca, M.; Piccirilli, E.; Piccioli, A.; Bonanno, E.; Gasbarra, E. The role of sarcopenia with and without fracture. *Injury* **2016**, *47* (Suppl. S4), S3–S10. [CrossRef] [PubMed]
42. Obada, B.; Georgeanu, V.; Iliescu, M.; Popescu, A.; Petcu, L.; Costea, D.O. Clinical outcomes of total hip arthroplasty after femoral neck fractures vs. osteoarthritis at one year follow up-A comparative, retrospective study. *Int. Orthop.* **2024**, *48*, 2301–2310. [CrossRef] [PubMed]

Journal of Clinical Medicine

MDPI

Article

Rasch Measurement Model Supports the Unidimensionality and Internal Structure of the Arabic Oswestry Disability Index

Ali H. Alnahdi [1,2,*], Abdulrahman M. Alsubiheen [1] and Mishal M. Aldaihan [1,2]

[1] Department of Rehabilitation Sciences, College of Applied Medical Sciences, King Saud University, P.O. Box 10219, Riyadh 11433, Saudi Arabia; aalsubiheen@ksu.edu.sa (A.M.A.); mishaldaihan@ksu.edu.sa (M.M.A.)

[2] King Salman Center for Disability Research, Riyadh 11614, Saudi Arabia

* Correspondence: alialnahdi@ksu.edu.sa; Tel.: +966-14693595; Fax: +966-14693589

Abstract: Background/Objectives: The objective of this study was to assess the unidimensionality and internal structure of the Arabic version of the Oswestry Disability Index (ODI) in patients with lower back pain (LBP) using the Rasch measurement model. **Methods:** Patients with LBP (N = 113) completed the Arabic ODI during their first visit to physical therapy departments. The Arabic ODI was examined by assessing its fit to the requirements of the Rasch measurement model. Chi-square statistics for item–trait interaction alongside mean item and person fit residuals were used for overall model fit assessment. Additionally, the analysis included assessments for the fit of individual items, the sequence of thresholds, local dependency, unidimensionality using the *t*-test method, and differential item functioning (DIF) by sex, age, chronicity, and the presence of radiating pain. **Results:** The overall fit of the Arabic ODI to the Rasch measurement model was supported by non-significant Chi-square statistics ($\chi^2 = 25.32$, $p = 0.19$) and acceptable mean item and person fit residuals. All items showed acceptable fit (standardized fit residual -1.89 to 1.62) with no violation of local item independence. The t-test method supported the scale's unidimensionality. The ODI showed good internal consistency with a person separation index of 0.85, with good overall targeting of item thresholds to the participants' lower back function. Items 2, 7, and 10 showed disordered thresholds, and potential bias by sex was detected in item 9 (social life). **Conclusions:** The Arabic ODI is a unidimensional measure valid for assessing disability due to low back pain; however, indications of the inappropriate functioning of some response options along with potential bias by sex need to be revisited.

Keywords: psychometric; measurement property; structural validity; item response; patient-reported outcome measures

1. Introduction

Lower back pain (LBP) is a significant public health issue and a leading cause of disability worldwide, affecting approximately 8.2% of the global population [1,2]. As a result, various disability assessment tools have been developed, with the Oswestry Disability Index (ODI) being one of the most widely used instruments for measuring disability related to LBP [3–5]. The ODI assesses a patient's perceived limitations in daily activities, such as personal care, lifting, walking, and social life, and has been extensively validated across different languages and cultures [6–8].

The ODI's Arabic version has been introduced with evidence supporting its reliability and construct validity but with concerns regarding its unidimensionality [9,10]. A recently published study supported the unidimensionality of the Arabic ODI using confirmatory factor analysis [11]. However, the internal structure of the Arabic ODI has not yet been evaluated using more rigorous modern measurement models such as the Rash measurement model. The term internal structure is used to refer to aspects of internal characteristic of the scale items in terms of the fit of individual items to the expectation of the measurement model, the behavior and appropriateness of the items' response categories, local item independence, differential item functioning, and internal consistency. Additionally, no prior study has assessed the functioning of the scale response categories or the presence of item bias across important patient characteristics, nor delineated the hierarchy of item difficulty within the Arabic ODI and how Arabic-speaking patients with LBP perceive the difficulty of the different items.

Evaluating the internal structure of an assessment scale is crucial for ensuring its validity and fairness in measuring the intended construct. A well-defined internal structure guarantees that individual items align with the expectations of the measurement model, confirming that they collectively measure a single underlying trait rather than unrelated dimensions [12,13]. Proper response category functioning ensures that rating scales are interpreted consistently by respondents, minimizing ambiguity and enhancing measurement precision. Local item independence is vital, as dependencies between items can distort scores and lead to redundant information, compromising a scale's ability to provide distinct, meaningful results [14]. Additionally, assessing differential item functioning helps identify potential biases in how different subgroups (e.g., by sex, age) respond to items, ensuring the scale is equitable and applicable across diverse populations. Finally, adequate internal consistency indicates that all items contribute to a coherent and stable measurement of the construct, reinforcing the scale's reliability. Together, these elements of internal structure are essential for developing and validating a robust measurement tool that provides accurate, interpretable, and generalizable results across varied clinical and research settings [14,15].

The Rasch measurement model is a probabilistic measurement model that ensures that a scale measures a single underlying construct in a valid and reliable way [14,15]. It is based on the principle that an individual's response to an item is governed solely by the item's difficulty and the responder's ability, making it independent of sample characteristics. The Rasch measurement model is particularly suited for evaluating the structural validity of instruments like the ODI [16]. One of the model's key strengths is its ability to assess whether a scale's items fit a single underlying construct, thereby confirming unidimensionality. Additionally, the Rasch model evaluates the internal structure of the scale, including the scoring structure of individual items, ensuring that the response categories are properly ordered. It also assesses local item independence, meaning that the response to one item should not directly influence the response to another, a key assumption in many measurement theories [17,18]. Additionally, the Rasch measurement model is well suited to assess for any differential item function or item bias and allow for the transformation of ordinal scores into interval-level scores, providing a more precise and meaningful representation of the underlying construct [19,20].

Given the lack of examination of the Arabic ODI using rigorous modern measurement models, this study aimed to use the Rasch measurement model to assess the unidimensionality and internal structure of the Arabic ODI, including evaluations of unidimensionality, individual item fit, response category functioning, local item independence, and potential item bias. This study also aimed to determine item difficulty hierarchies and whether items' difficulty levels are well targeted to the disability level of patients with LBP.

2. Materials and Methods

2.1. Study Design

This cross-sectional study used the Rasch measurement model to evaluate the unidimensionality and internal structure of the Arabic version of the ODI. The study protocol was reviewed and approved by the institutional review boards at King Saud University (E-20-5529) and the Security Forces Hospital (22-601-37), and informed consent was obtained from all the participants.

2.2. Setting and Participants

This study was conducted across two physical therapy departments in the Security Forces Hospital and the Alrass General Hospital, which are located in the central region of Saudi Arabia, involving patients with LBP on their first clinic visit. Eligible participants were aged 18 years and older, had been referred to physical therapy for LBP, and were fluent in the Arabic language. Individuals were evaluated by specialist physicians in primary care, orthopedic, and spinal clinics and subsequently referred to physical therapy. Participants with systemic disease or neurological and cardiopulmonary disorders that were self-perceived to cause functional limitations were excluded from this study to exclude factors other than lower back pain causing functional limitation and disability. Participants who had previously undergone back surgery were also excluded from this study.

2.3. Procedure

Participants were asked to complete the Arabic ODI during their first physical therapy clinic visit. Relevant medical history, demographic data, including age and sex, chronicity of LBP (acute < 1 month; subacute 1–3 months; chronic > 3 months), and presence of radiating pain were also recorded at the same visit.

2.4. Outcome Measures

Oswestry Disability Index (ODI)

The Arabic version of the ODI was used as the primary outcome measure [9]. The ODI consists of 10 items, each scored on a 6-point Likert scale ranging from 0 to 5, where 0 represents no disability and 5 represents maximum disability. The recommended total scoring method for the ODI involves adding all items scores and then convert this sum into a percentage (0–100), with higher scores indicating greater disability [6,7]. Previous studies have examined the reliability and construct validity of the Arabic version of the ODI, supporting these measurement properties for the Arabic ODI [9,10].

2.5. Statistical Analysis

Rasch analysis in the current study was conducted using the partial credit model [21] and the specialized software RUMM2030 [22]. Rasch analysis addressed the objectives of this study by assessing the unidimensionality and internal structure (fit of individual items to the expectation of the measurement model, the appropriateness of items' response categories, local item independence, differential item functioning, and internal consistency) of the Arabic ODI. The details of how these aspects were assed are detailed below. The item–trait interaction was used to assess the overall fit of the observed data to the Rasch measurement model, with a non-significant Chi-square statistic ($p > 0.05$) was used to indicate good fit [16,22]. The overall fit was evaluated by examining the item and person fit residuals. Good overall fit to the Rasch measurement model was indicated when the mean item and person fit residuals were near zero, and the standard deviation was approximately one. Good overall fit of the Arabic ODI would support the notion that the Arabic ODI satisfies the requirement of the Rasch measurement model and that responses to the ODI items are governed solely by the item's difficulty and the responder's ability. In addition to the assessment of overall model fit, the fit of each item and person was evaluated by assessing the standardized fit residuals. Standardized fit residuals exceeding $\pm$ 2.5, along with significant Chi-square statistics (adjusted using Bonferroni correction), were considered indicators of poor fit of an individual item to the Rasch measurement model [16,22]. The scoring structure of Arabic ODI items was assessed to ensure that each response category functioned as intended. Threshold ordering was evaluated by assessing individual item category characteristic curves, with disordered thresholds indicating that participants could not distinguish between adjacent response categories [16,18,23]. To check for local item independence, the residual correlations between items were analyzed. Items with residual correlations exceeding 0.2 were flagged for potential local dependency [12,24]. To assess the unidimensionality of the Arabic ODI, the t-test method was applied [16,25,26]. The process began with a principal component analysis (PCA) of the residuals. The loadings of the first component were then used to classify the items into two groups: those with positive loadings and those with negative loadings. Using these groups, the participants' LBP-related disability was estimated twice, once for each set of items. The two estimates were then compared through a t-test. The Arabic ODI was deemed unidimensional if the proportion of significant differences between the estimates did not exceed 5% [16,25]. The performance of the Arabic ODI's items was analyzed to determine whether they functioned consistently across different patient subgroups [13,16]. Differential item functioning (DIF) was assessed based on sex (male vs. female), age (younger than 28 vs. 28 or older, based on the median), chronicity (acute and subacute vs. chronic), and the presence of radiating pain (yes vs. no). To identify both uniform and non-uniform DIF, residuals were analyzed using two-way ANOVAs, factoring in class intervals and subject characteristics. The person separation index was used to examine the internal consistency of the ODI. Targeting of the ODI items to the ability level of the participants was examined by assessing the person–item threshold plot where, in a well-targeted test, the range of item thresholds should overlap with the range of a person's abilities.

2.6. Sample Size Estimation

The necessary sample size was established in accordance with the COSMIN guidelines [27]. A cohort of 100 individuals was deemed sufficient by the COSMIN criteria for the assessment of structural validity (unidimensionality) utilizing Rasch analysis; therefore, a minimum sample size of 100 was employed in the present investigation.

3. Results

A total of 113 patients with LBP were recruited in the current study. The characteristics of the participants are summarized in Table 1. In the present investigation, the analysis was performed utilizing the partial credit model, as the likelihood ratio test [22] had yielded a significant result ($p < 0.001$), suggesting that the partial credit model [21] would be more suitable than the rating scale model [28].

The first two runs of the analysis identified misfitting individuals that were then removed from the analysis (Table 2). Assessments of the Arabic ODI's overall fit after the removal of misfitting individuals indicated good fit to the Rasch measurement model (Table 2). The Chi-square statistics for item–trait interactions was non-significant, indicating a good overall fit to the Rasch model. The mean item and person fit residuals were close to zero, with acceptable standard deviations near 1 supporting the overall fit the ODI to the Rasch model (Table 2).

Table 1. Characteristics of the participants (N = 113).

Variable	Mean ± SD or N (%)
Age (year)	30.45 ±12.07
Age group	
≤28 years	57 (50.44)
>28 years	56 (49.56)
Sex	
Male	54 (47.8)
Female	59 (52.2)
Height (m)	1.67 ± 0.10
Mass (Kg)	71.54 ±12.14
Body mass index (Kg/m^2)	25.96 ± 5.61
LBP duration	
Acute (<1 month)	17 (15.04)
Subacute (1–3 months)	19 (16.81)
Chronic (>3 months)	77 (68.14)
Radiating pain	
Yes	78 (69.03)
No	35 (30.97)
Oswestry Disability Index (0–100)	25.27 ± 15.38

LBP = Lower back pain.

Table 2. ODI Rasch analysis results at each run.

Run	Analysis	N	Item Fit Residual		Person Fit Residual		Item–Trait Interaction		PSI	Unidimensionality T-Tests	
			Mean	SD	Mean	SD	χ^2 (df)	p		% of Significant Tests	Lower Limit of 95% CI *
1	Initial analysis	113	0.249	1.329	−0.228	1.098	26.02 (20)	0.165	0.86	8.85%	4.80%
2	Delete 4 misfit persons	109	0.205	1.26	−0.193	0.973	25.94 (20)	0.168	0.85	7.34%	3.20%
3	Delete 1 misfit person	108	0.191	1.242	−0.187	0.945	25.32 (20)	0.189	0.85	6.48%	2.40%

ODI = Oswestry Disability Index; SD = standard deviation; χ^2 = Chi-square; df = degrees of freedom; and PSI = person separation index. * Represents the lower limit of the binomial 95% confidence interval for the percentage of significant *t*-tests.

The individual ODI items showed good fit to the requirements of the Rasch measurement model. This was supported by the acceptable individual item standardized fit residuals, ranging from −1.89 to 1.62, with non-significant Chi-square statistics (Table 3). The t-test methodology revealed that a relatively low proportion of the subjects exhibited a statistically significant distinction between the two estimates of the disability level (derived from the two test sets), thereby corroborating the unidimensional nature of the scale (Table 2). This conclusion was based on the lower limit of the binomial 95% confidence interval for the percentage of significant t-tests, which was less than 5%. (Table 2). The assessment of residual correlations between items revealed no two pairs with residual correlation above the pre-determined threshold (0.2), suggesting no breach of the local dependency between these items. The highest residual correlation was observed between item 4 (walking) and item 6 (standing) (r = 0.169).

Table 3. Items' hierarchy and calibration of the ODI after removing misfit individuals (items arranged from the most difficult to the easiest).

Item	Location	SE	Fit Residual	χ^2	p	Ordered Thresholds
1 (Pain intensity)	−1.15	0.10	1.46	3.01	0.22	✓
3 (Lifting)	−1.10	0.11	0.58	3.73	0.15	✓
6 (Standing)	−0.83	0.11	0.56	0.12	0.94	✓
10 (Traveling)	−0.53	0.12	0.35	2.49	0.29	×
5 (Sitting)	−0.17	0.12	1.62	1.41	0.49	✓
8 (Sex life)	0.12	0.12	−1.75	6.62	0.04	✓
9 (Social life)	0.16	0.12	−1.89	3.53	0.17	✓
7 (Sleeping)	0.57	0.13	1.41	1.96	0.37	×
2 (Personal care)	1.36	0.14	−0.37	2.08	0.35	×
4 (Walking)	1.58	0.12	−0.04	0.37	0.83	✓

ODI = Oswestry Disability Index; SE = standard error; and χ^2 = Chi-square. ✓ = indicate all thresholds were ordered; × = indicate the existence of disordered thresholds.

Despite the good fit of the Arabic ODI to the requirements of the Rasch measurement model, some deviations from the model were observed. Items 2 (personal care), 7 (lifting), and 10 (social life) exhibited some threshold disordering, suggesting the inappropriate use of the response categories for these items (Figure 1). A uniform DIF was detected for item 9 (social life) based on sex, with females perceiving greater difficulty in social life than males ($p < 0.001$) (Figure 2). The ODI showed good internal consistency with a person separation index of 0.85. The range of ODI item thresholds exhibited good spread and overlap with the range of person abilities, except in those with a very high level of function (lower than −5 logit), generally suggesting acceptable targeting to the intended population (Figure 3). ODI items' difficulty hierarchy is displayed in Table 3 with pain intensity and then lifting determined to be the most difficult items and walking, followed by personal care, being the easiest.

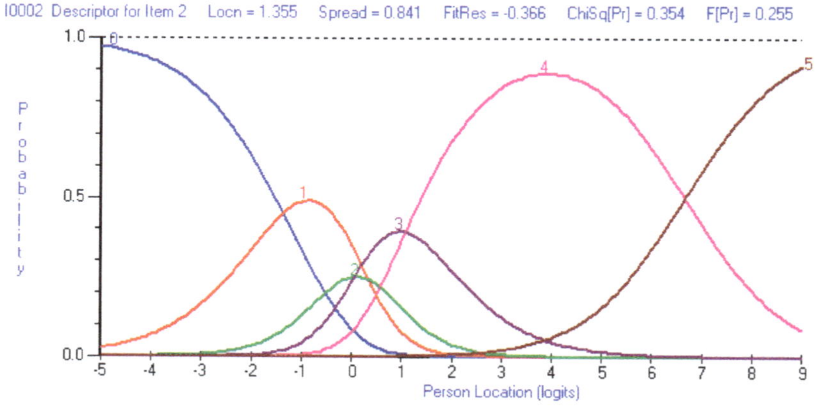

Figure 1. *Cont.*

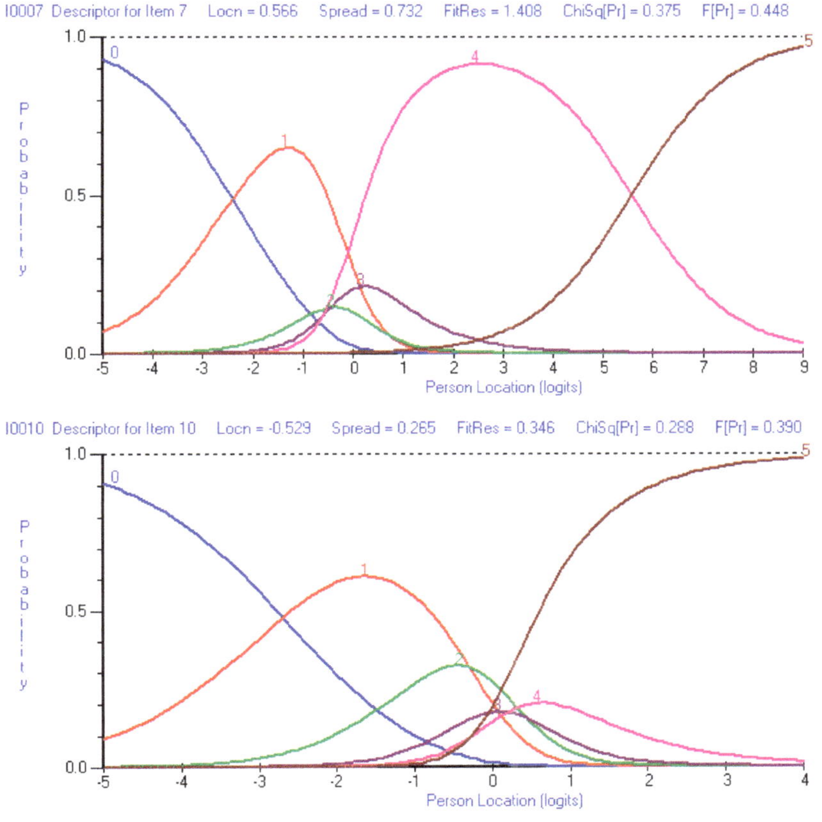

Figure 1. Category characteristic curves for the ODI items exhibiting disordered thresholds: item 2 (personal care, **top figure**); item 7 (sleeping, **middle figure**); and item 10 (traveling, **bottom figure**). Category characteristic curves were assessed for all items to examine whether the response categories displayed proper function and sequence. Lines 0 to 5 represents the six response categories for each ODI item with where 0 represents no disability and 5 represents maximum disability.

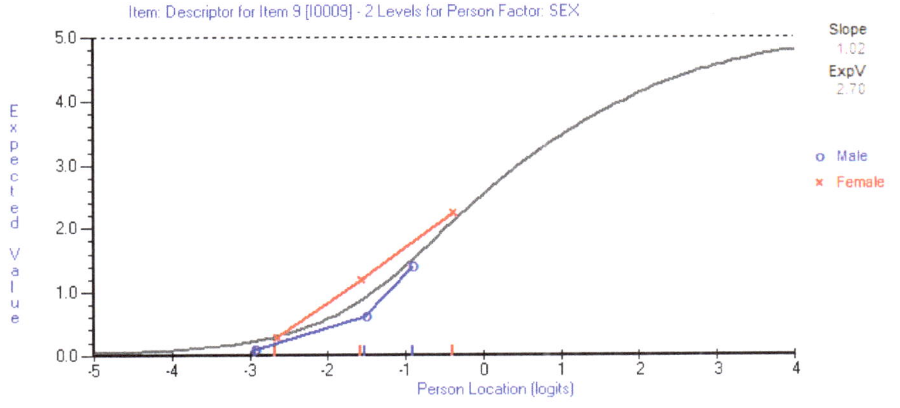

Figure 2. Item characteristic curves for item 9 (social life), showing the differential function of this item in male versus female respondents despite similar levels of lower back function.

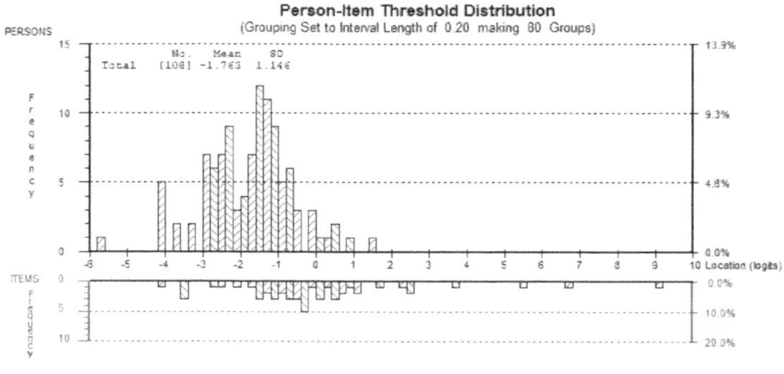

Figure 3. Person–item threshold plot showing the good spread of item thresholds and overlap with the range of person abilities, except in those with a very high level of lower back function (lower than −5 logit). This figure assessed the targeting of the ODI's items to the ability level of the participants.

4. Discussion

Using the Rasch measurement model, the current study confirmed the unidimensionality and appropriate internal structure of the Arabic ODI, indicating that it assesses a single underlying construct related to disability due to LBP. This finding suggested that Arabic ODI is a valid measure for assessing disability and functional limitations in Arabic-speaking patients with LBP, which aligns with the intended purpose of the instrument.

The Arabic ODI demonstrated an excellent overall fit with the Rasch measurement model. This fit suggests that the Arabic ODI could provide accurate interval-level measurement, allowing clinicians and researchers to capture lower back disability levels effectively across a spectrum of LBP severity. In Rasch models, item difficulties should ideally remain stable (invariant) across the entire range of person abilities, meaning that item performance should not vary for different ability groups [29]. The non-significant item–trait interaction reported in our study suggested that the Arabic ODI scale was functioning consistently across all levels of lower back function, with only a single underlying construct (lower back function) governing the functioning of all items [16]. A significant item–trait interaction, on the other hand, would have indicated potential misfit between the data and the Rasch model, suggesting that the given scale does not measure the construct consistently across different levels of disability [16]. This could result in measurement bias, where certain items function differently depending on the severity of the condition, ultimately affecting the reliability and validity of the instrument. The absence of such interaction in our findings reinforces the Arabic ODI's suitability for use in diverse clinical populations, ensuring that scores can be meaningfully compared across individuals with varying levels of lower back disability.

Individual items within the Arabic ODI exhibited acceptable standardized fit residuals suggesting that the functioning and scores of the ODI's individual items were only governed by one construct—lower back function—and that each item contributed effectively to assessing the overarching construct. The good fit exhibited by all the items within the Arabic ODI suggests that these item behaved in line with the expectation of the Rash measurement model, where the response to the item was governed by the individual's level of lower back function and the difficulty of the item, meaning that participants with lower back function higher than the difficulty of the item would end up reporting a higher probability of being able to perform the activity without difficulty. These findings are consistent with previous studies that explored the ODI's item-level fit and reported adequate fit to the Rasch measurement model [30–33]. Additional studies indicated that ODI items showed good fit to the Rasch model, except for the pain intensity item, which was determined to be misfitting [34,35]. The ODI's versions used in these studies contain a pain intensity item related to the use of painkillers and pain relief rather than pain intensity. This difference in item content suggests that variations in how pain is framed within the questionnaire may influence its measurement properties and overall model fit. Specifically, assessing pain intensity through medication use introduces additional factors, such as differences in prescription practices, medication accessibility, and individual responses to pain relief methods, which may not directly reflect the severity of the pain itself.

Threshold disordering in three items (items 2, 7, and 10) was observed in our study, suggesting potential issues with the response scale functioning for these items. Disordered thresholds often reflect difficulty in distinguishing between adjacent response categories, potentially compromising measurement precision for those items. This issue may arise if respondents struggle to differentiate between response options due to ambiguous wording, overlapping severity levels, or inconsistencies in how they interpret the scale. Disordered thresholds in ODI items have been reported in previous studies [30,32–35], but the number of items exhibiting disordered thresholds along with the specific dysfunctional response categories vary among these. To address the issue of disordered thresholds, a couple of previous studies recommended and implemented a general change to the ODI item-scoring scheme, from a six-point score to either a five-point score [32] or a four-point score [34,35]. A replication of the findings of the current study is needed to ensure consistency of the observed disordered thresholds before recommending and implementing changes to the scoring scheme of an established outcome measure such as the ODI. Ensuring that all items exhibit ordered thresholds will enhance the precision of the Arabic ODI, making it a more effective tool for assessing disability severity and tracking functional changes over time.

The current study detected DIF in item 9 (social life) based on sex, with female participants perceiving it as more challenging than their male counterparts at similar disability levels. This DIF could stem from cultural or societal factors influencing social engagement perceptions in Arabic-speaking populations, particularly among women. It should be made clear that the DIF analysis conducted in the current study should be considered a preliminary analysis with preliminary findings given that the number of participants within each subgroup was below the recommended sample size [27]. Thus, a larger sample is needed to draw a firmer conclusion regarding DIF in the Arabic ODI. Most previous studies did not examine for DIF in the ODI items by age, sex, or any other relevant patient characteristics [31,32,34,35]. Two previous studies reported no DIF by sex in the ODI items but reported uniform DIF by age in item 4 (walking) [33] and item 7 (sleeping) [30]. Based on these studies, it seems that there is no consistent DIF pattern among the published studies. Given these mixed findings, future research should prioritize more extensive DIF analyses with adequately powered samples to determine whether the DIF in item 9 is a stable characteristic of the Arabic ODI or a sample-specific occurrence. If confirmed, the presence of DIF in the social life item may indicate that modifications are necessary to enhance measurement fairness across sex groups, such as revising the item's wording or exploring alternative response formats. Additionally, DIF should be assessed across other demographic and clinical variables, such as age, education level, and pain duration, to ensure that the Arabic ODI functions equitably across diverse patient populations.

Pain intensity and lifting emerged as the most difficult items. Following these were items associated with prolonged standing and traveling, which were moderately difficult. Items related to sexual function, social life, and sleeping represented intermediate levels of difficulty. Meanwhile, items focused on personal care and walking were identified as the easiest in this hierarchy, suggesting that patients with LBP perceived these activities as more manageable. Similar to the current study, lifting was consistently reported in the literature to be among the most difficult items in the ODI and personal care was consistently reported to be among the easiest items [30,33–35]. Page et al. reported walking to be among the easiest items in the ODI, similarly to our finding [35]. We reported pain intensity to be the most difficult item, while two previous studies ranked pain intensity among the items with medium difficulty [30,33]. This indicates that the Arabic-speaking patients with LBP in our study perceived pain intensity to be a more difficult item in comparison to patients from different cultures. Further research is needed to explore whether these difficulty rankings remain consistent across different Arabic-speaking regions and whether factors such as the chronicity of LBP, occupational demands, and gender differences influence item difficulty perception. Understanding these variations can help refine the interpretation of ODI scores and improve the scale's applicability in diverse clinical settings. Additionally, examining how item difficulty rankings change over time with treatment interventions could provide valuable insights into the responsiveness of the Arabic ODI and its utility in tracking patient progress.

A major strength of this study was its rigorous Rasch analysis, which validated the Arabic ODI's structure and item fit. This validation supports clinical and research applications in Arabic-speaking populations with LBP, providing a valid tool for assessing disability. However, this study's limitations include its specific focus on patients within Saudi Arabia, which may limit generalizability to Arabic speakers from other regions. The findings of the DIF analysis in this study should be interpreted with caution giving that dividing the full sample into subgroups for DIF analysis (e.g., male and female) resulted in each subgroup having fewer participants than recommended for scale invariance assessment [27]. Furthermore, the disordered thresholds suggest potential response clarity issues, which could be addressed in future research. Recommendations for further studies include exploring refined response categories for items with disordered thresholds and evaluating the DIF findings to enhance the scale's universality and interpretative accuracy.

5. Conclusions

The Rasch measurement model confirmed the unidimensionality and appropriate internal structure of the Arabic ODI, indicating that it assesses a single underlying construct reflecting low back pain-related disability. However, the Arabic ODI demonstrated inappropriate functioning of response categories in three items and indication of bias by sex in one item.

Author Contributions: Conceptualization, A.H.A., A.M.A. and M.M.A.; methodology, A.H.A. and A.M.A.; validation, A.H.A. and M.M.A.; formal analysis, A.H.A. and M.M.A.; investigation, A.H.A. and A.M.A.; resources, A.H.A.; data curation, A.H.A., A.M.A. and M.M.A.; writing—original draft preparation, A.H.A., A.M.A. and M.M.A.; writing—review and editing, A.H.A., A.M.A. and M.M.A.; supervision, A.H.A.; project administration, A.H.A., A.M.A. and M.M.A.; and funding acquisition, A.H.A. All authors have read and agreed to the published version of the manuscript.

Funding: King Salman Center for Disability Research through Research Group no KSRG-2024-019.

Institutional Review Board Statement: This study was conducted according to the guidelines of the Declaration of Helsinki and approved by the institutional review boards of King Saud University (E-20-5529, date of approval: 22 December 2020) and the Security Forces Hospital (22-601-37, date of approval: 28 June 2022).

Informed Consent Statement: Informed consent was obtained from all the subjects involved in this study.

Data Availability Statement: The data presented in this study are available from the corresponding author upon reasonable request.

Acknowledgments: The authors extend their appreciation to the King Salman Center For Disability Research for funding this work through Research Group no KSRG-2024-019.

Conflicts of Interest: The authors declare no conflicts of interest.

References

1. GBD 2021 Low Back Pain Collaborators. Global, regional, and national burden of low back pain, 1990–2020, its attributable risk factors, and projections to 2050: A systematic analysis of the Global Burden of Disease Study 2021. *Lancet Rheumatol* **2023**, *5*, e316–e329. [CrossRef] [PubMed]
2. GBD 2021 Diseases and Injuries Collaborator. Global incidence, prevalence, years lived with disability (YLDs), disability-adjusted life-years (DALYs), and healthy life expectancy (HALE) for 371 diseases and injuries in 204 countries and territories and 811 subnational locations, 1990–2021: A systematic analysis for the Global Burden of Disease Study 2021. *Lancet* **2024**, *403*, 2133–2161.
3. Smeets, R.; Koke, A.; Lin, C.W.; Ferreira, M.; Demoulin, C. Measures of function in low back pain/disorders: Low Back Pain Rating Scale (LBPRS), Oswestry Disability Index (ODI), Progressive Isoinertial Lifting Evaluation (PILE), Quebec Back Pain Disability Scale (QBPDS), and Roland-Morris Disability Questionnaire (RDQ). *Arthritis Care Res.* **2011**, *63* (Suppl. 11), S158–S173.
4. Chapman, J.R.; Norvell, D.C.; Hermsmeyer, J.T.; Bransford, R.J.; DeVine, J.; McGirt, M.J.; Lee, M.J. Evaluating common outcomes for measuring treatment success for chronic low back pain. *Spine* **2011**, *36*, S54–S68. [CrossRef]
5. Clement, R.C.; Welander, A.; Stowell, C.; Cha, T.D.; Chen, J.L.; Davies, M.; Fairbank, J.C.; Foley, K.T.; Gehrchen, M.; Hagg, O.; et al. A proposed set of metrics for standardized outcome reporting in the management of low back pain. *Acta Orthop.* **2015**, *86*, 523–533. [CrossRef]
6. Roland, M.; Fairbank, J. The Roland-Morris Disability Questionnaire and the Oswestry Disability Questionnaire. *Spine* **2000**, *25*, 3115–3124. [CrossRef] [PubMed]
7. Fairbank, J.C.; Couper, J.; Davies, J.B.; O'Brien, J.P. The Oswestry low back pain disability questionnaire. *Physiotherapy* **1980**, *66*, 271–273.
8. Fairbank, J.C.; Pynsent, P.B. The Oswestry Disability Index. *Spine* **2000**, *25*, 2940–2952; discussion 2952. [CrossRef] [PubMed]
9. Algarni, A.S.; Ghorbel, S.; Jones, J.G.; Guermazi, M. Validation of an Arabic version of the Oswestry index in Saudi Arabia. *Ann. Phys. Rehabil. Med.* **2014**, *57*, 653–663. [CrossRef]
10. Guermazi, M.; Mezghani, M.; Ghroubi, S.; Elleuch, M.; Med, A.O.; Poiraudeau, S.; Mrabet, F.; Dammak, J.; Fermanian, J.; Baklouti, S.; et al. The Oswestry index for low back pain translated into Arabic and validated in a Arab population. *Ann. Readapt. Med. Phys.* **2005**, *48*, 1–10. [CrossRef]
11. Alnahdi, A.H. The Arabic Oswestry Disability Index is a Unidimensional Measure: Exploratory and Confirmatory Factor Analysis. *Spine* **2024**. [CrossRef] [PubMed]
12. Christensen, K.B.; Kreiner, S.; Mesbah, M. *Rasch Models in Health*; ISTE-Wiley: London, UK, 2013.
13. Hagquist, C.; Bruce, M.; Gustavsson, J.P. Using the Rasch model in nursing research: An introduction and illustrative example. *Int. J. Nurs. Stud.* **2009**, *46*, 380–393. [CrossRef]
14. Andrich, D.; Marais, I. *A Course in Rasch Measurement Theory: Measuring in the Educational, Social and Health Sciences*; Springer: Singapore, 2019.
15. Boone, W.J.; Staver, J.R.; Yale, M.S. *Rasch Analysis in the Human Sciences*; Springer: Dordrecht, The Netherlands, 2013.
16. Tennant, A.; Conaghan, P.G. The Rasch measurement model in rheumatology: What is it and why use it? When should it be applied, and what should one look for in a Rasch paper? *Arthritis Rheum.* **2007**, *57*, 1358–1362. [CrossRef]
17. Bond, T.G.; Fox, C.M. *Applying the Rasch Model: Fundamental Measurement in the Human Sciences*, 3rd ed.; Taylor & Francis: New York, NY, USA, 2015.
18. Pallant, J.F.; Tennant, A. An introduction to the Rasch measurement model: An example using the Hospital Anxiety and Depression Scale (HADS). *Br. J. Clin. Psychol.* **2007**, *46*, 1–18. [CrossRef] [PubMed]
19. Hobart, J.C.; Cano, S.J.; Zajicek, J.P.; Thompson, A.J. Rating scales as outcome measures for clinical trials in neurology: Problems, solutions, and recommendations. *Lancet Neurol.* **2007**, *6*, 1094–1105. [CrossRef] [PubMed]
20. Horton, M.; Tennant, A. Patient Reported Outcomes: Misinference from ordinal scales? *Trials* **2011**, *12*, A65. [CrossRef]
21. Masters, G.N. A Rasch Model for Partial Credit Scoring. *Psychometrika* **1982**, *47*, 149–174. [CrossRef]
22. Andrich, D.; Sheridan, B.E.; Luo, G. *RUMM2030-Professional Edition (Rasch Unidimensional Measurement Model, Version 5.4) [Computer Software]*; RUMM Laboratory: Perth, Australia, 2014.
23. Andrich, D.A. Category ordering and their utility. *Rasch Meas. Trans.* **1996**, *9*, 464.
24. Christensen, K.B.; Makransky, G.; Horton, M. Critical Values for Yen's Q(3): Identification of Local Dependence in the Rasch Model Using Residual Correlations. *Appl. Psychol. Meas.* **2017**, *41*, 178–194. [CrossRef] [PubMed]
25. Smith, E.V., Jr. Detecting and evaluating the impact of multidimensionality using item fit statistics and principal component analysis of residuals. *J. Appl. Meas.* **2002**, *3*, 205–231. [PubMed]

26. Prinsen, C.A.C.; Mokkink, L.B.; Bouter, L.M.; Alonso, J.; Patrick, D.L.; de Vet, H.C.W.; Terwee, C.B. COSMIN guideline for systematic reviews of patient-reported outcome measures. *Qual. Life Res.* **2018**, *27*, 1147–1157. [CrossRef] [PubMed]
27. Mokkink, L.B.; de Vet, H.C.W.; Prinsen, C.A.C.; Patrick, D.L.; Alonso, J.; Bouter, L.M.; Terwee, C.B. COSMIN Risk of Bias checklist for systematic reviews of Patient-Reported Outcome Measures. *Qual. Life Res.* **2018**, *27*, 1171–1179. [CrossRef]
28. Andrich, D. A rating formulation for ordered response categories. *Psychometrika* **1978**, *43*, 561. [CrossRef]
29. Engelhard, G. *Invariant Measurement: Using Rasch Models in the Social, Behavioral, and Health Sciences*; Routledge: New York, NY, USA, 2013.
30. Lu, Y.M.; Wu, Y.Y.; Hsieh, C.L.; Lin, C.L.; Hwang, S.L.; Cheng, K.I.; Lue, Y.J. Measurement precision of the disability for back pain scale-by applying Rasch analysis. *Health Qual. Life Outcomes* **2013**, *11*, 119. [CrossRef]
31. Brodke, D.S.; Goz, V.; Lawrence, B.D.; Spiker, W.R.; Neese, A.; Hung, M. Oswestry Disability Index: A psychometric analysis with 1610 patients. *Spine J.* **2017**, *17*, 321–327. [CrossRef] [PubMed]
32. Lochhead, L.E.; MacMillan, P.D. Psychometric properties of the Oswestry disability index: Rasch analysis of responses in a work-disabled population. *Work* **2013**, *46*, 67–76. [CrossRef]
33. Davidson, M. Rasch analysis of three versions of the Oswestry Disability Questionnaire. *Man. Ther.* **2008**, *13*, 222–231. [CrossRef]
34. White, L.J.; Velozo, C.A. The use of Rasch measurement to improve the Oswestry classification scheme. *Arch. Phys. Med. Rehabil.* **2002**, *83*, 822–831. [CrossRef]
35. Page, S.J.; Shawaryn, M.A.; Cernich, A.N.; Linacre, J.M. Scaling of the revised Oswestry low back pain questionnaire. *Arch. Phys. Med. Rehabil.* **2002**, *83*, 1579–1584. [CrossRef] [PubMed]

Journal of
Clinical Medicine

MDPI

Review

Frozen Shoulder as a Systemic Immunometabolic Disorder: The Roles of Estrogen, Thyroid Dysfunction, Endothelial Health, Lifestyle, and Clinical Implications

Santiago Navarro-Ledesma

Department of Physiotherapy, Faculty of Health Sciences, Campus of Melilla, University of Granada, Querol Street 5, 52004 Melilla, Spain; snl@ugr.es

Abstract: Frozen shoulder (FS), traditionally regarded as an idiopathic musculoskeletal disorder characterized by pain, stiffness, and capsular fibrosis, is increasingly recognized as the clinical manifestation of systemic endocrine, metabolic, vascular, and immunological dysfunctions. This narrative review reframes FS within a broader neuro–endocrine–immunometabolic model, emphasizing the central role of estrogen deficiency, resistance, and receptor-level disruption, together with their interactions with thyroid dysfunction, endothelial health, and lifestyle-related low-grade inflammation (LGI). Evidence from epidemiological, clinical, and mechanistic studies shows that estrogen signaling failure weakens anti-inflammatory, antifibrotic, and antioxidant defenses, predisposing peri- and postmenopausal women to more severe FS phenotypes. Thyroid dysfunction, particularly hypothyroidism, further contributes to fibrosis and pain sensitization. Endothelial dysfunction—driven by poor diet, advanced glycation end-products (AGEs), and oxidative stress—impairs vascular integrity and promotes local microvascular inflammation. In parallel, lifestyle factors such as sedentarism, circadian misalignment, psychosocial stress, and environmental exposures sustain systemic LGI and hormonal resistance. Together, these interconnected mechanisms suggest that FS is not merely a localized joint pathology but a systemic disorder requiring integrative clinical strategies that combine orthopedic management with endocrine evaluation, metabolic monitoring, dietary interventions, circadian health, and stress regulation. In addition, this review outlines specific clinical implications, highlighting how an integrative, personalized approach that targets hormonal, metabolic, vascular, and lifestyle dimensions may improve pain, function, and long-term prognosis in FS. This paradigm shift underscores the need for future research to focus on stratified patient profiling and interventional trials targeting hormonal, vascular, and lifestyle axes to improve outcomes, particularly in women who remain disproportionately affected by FS.

Keywords: frozen shoulder; lifestyle; inflammation; metabolic factors; pain; estrogen; thyroid; endothelial

1. Introduction

Frozen Shoulder (FS), also referred to as adhesive capsulitis, is a chronic and often debilitating musculoskeletal condition characterized by progressive pain, stiffness, and restricted range of motion in the glenohumeral joint [1,2]. It primarily affects the capsular structures of the shoulder, leading to capsular thickening, fibrosis, and chronic synovial inflammation [3,4]. Despite being a relatively common clinical entity, its etiopathogenesis remains poorly understood, and current treatment strategies are frequently limited to symptom management rather than targeting underlying mechanisms [4,5]. Epidemiological studies report a prevalence of 2–5% in the general population, which increases significantly in individuals with comorbidities such as diabetes mellitus, thyroid disorders, and autoimmune diseases [6–10]. Importantly, FS demonstrates a notable sex dimorphism, with a higher prevalence in women, particularly between the ages of 40 and 60, and a more prolonged and symptomatic course compared to men [11]. This sex-based disparity remains largely underexplored in clinical and mechanistic research [12,13].

Over time, FS has been referred to using various terms—adhesive capsulitis, primary idiopathic frozen shoulder, or simply FS—depending on the clinical context and presumed etiology [2]. While secondary FS may occur after trauma, surgery, or prolonged immobilization, primary FS appears spontaneously, often without a clear inciting factor, further complicating diagnosis and treatment planning [1,2]. Traditionally, FS has been considered a local mechanical and inflammatory disorder. However, emerging evidence supports a broader and more systemic conceptualization, implicating chronic low-grade inflammation (LGI), neuroimmune dysregulation, and metabolic dysfunction in its pathogenesis [5,8,14]. These perspectives open the door to integrative models that account for the influence of endocrine, nutritional, and psychosocial factors, particularly those related to female hormonal physiology.

Given the predominance of FS in women, especially around perimenopause and menopause—a period marked by a sharp decline in estrogen levels—the female sex hormonal axis emerges as a promising and under-investigated component in the etiological framework of FS [15]. Estrogens are known to exert anti-inflammatory, neuroprotective, and immunomodulatory effects, and their decline may create a systemic environment that favors fibrotic, inflammatory, and pain-sensitized states [16–18]. This hormonal transition may intersect with other metabolic and lifestyle factors (e.g., diet, stress, physical inactivity), contributing to the onset and progression of FS [14].

In this narrative review, our aim is to reframe FS as a systemic disorder rather than an isolated musculoskeletal condition. We explore the interconnected roles of the female sex hormonal axis—particularly estrogen deficiency, resistance, and receptor-level interference—alongside thyroid dysfunction, endothelial dysregulation, and lifestyle-driven low-grade inflammation. By integrating evidence from endocrinology, immunometabolism, vascular biology, and psychoneuroimmunology, we propose a comprehensive framework in which FS emerges as the clinical expression of hormonal, metabolic, and environmental imbalances. This perspective not only clarifies the marked female predominance and metabolic associations of FS but also highlights actionable targets for diagnosis, prognosis, and treatment. Ultimately, this review emphasizes the need for integrative and personalized strategies in physiotherapy and clinical care, bridging orthopedic, metabolic, and endocrine dimensions to improve outcomes in patients with FS.

2. Methods

This review was conducted as a narrative–scoping review aimed at synthesizing multidisciplinary evidence that reframes FS as a systemic, immuno-metabolic, endocrine-modulated disorder. The approach prioritized conceptual completeness and mechanistic triangulation across domains (endocrine, metabolic, vascular, neuroimmune, lifestyle) rather than exhaustive enumeration of all studies, consistent with scoping methodology, thus a PRISMA numerical flow diagram was not carried out. While not a systematic review, we prospectively defined the mechanistic domains, core questions, data sources, eligibility criteria, and an evidence-grading scheme to enhance transparency and reproducibility. Where applicable, reporting was informed by PRISMA-ScR guidance (without claiming full systematic compliance).

2.1. Sources and Time Frame

We searched the following databases: MEDLINE/PubMed, Embase, Scopus, Web of Science Core Collection, and the Cochrane Library. Searches covered January 2000 to May 2025, with English or Spanish language restrictions. Reference lists of key reviews and guidelines were back-snowballed to identify additional primary sources. Preprints were not included unless subsequently published in peer-reviewed journals. A full, domain-stratified search matrix (databases, exemplar queries, inclusions/exclusions) is provided in Supplementary Materials.

2.2. Eligibility Criteria

2.2.1. Inclusion

Clinical human studies (epidemiology, cross-sectional, cohort, case–control, RCTs) on FS and: sex hormones/estrogens, thyroid axis, metabolic biomarkers (HbA1c, lipids, AGEs), endothelial function/NO/ADMA, microbiome, sleep/circadian health, psychoneuroimmunology, lifestyle/exposome, and clinical interventions.

Mechanistic/experimental studies (in vitro, animal) when directly informative of pathways relevant to FS (e.g., estrogen receptor signaling, TGF-β/ECM remodeling, AGE-RAGE, endothelial biology), used to support biological plausibility.

High-quality reviews/consensus statements (narrative/systematic/metaanalysis) to contextualize domains and summarize clinical signals.

2.2.2. Exclusion

Non-FS shoulder conditions without explicit FS subgroup analysis; conference abstracts without full text; letters/editorials without primary data; non-English/Spanish full texts; preprints not peer-reviewed; duplicated cohorts; pediatric populations; pure surgical technique papers without pathophysiological content. Studies whose primary focus was unrelated to the predefined mechanistic domains were also excluded.

2.3. Study Selection and Data Handling

Given the single-author nature of this review, screening and selection were performed by the author using the pre-specified domains/criteria. To mitigate selection bias, the process followed a two-pass workflow: (1) title/abstract screen against domain questions; (2) full-text evaluation for eligibility and domain mapping. A screening log (retrieved, included, excluded with main reasons) was maintained. Data were extracted into structured evidence tables by domain (clinical vs. mechanistic signals) capturing design, population, exposure/biomarker, outcome, and level of evidence. Each record was explicitly tagged as Clinical (human), Translational (human tissue/biomarker), or Experimental (animal/in vitro). Clinical evidence was preferentially used for practice-oriented statements; experimental findings were used to explain mechanisms and are labeled to avoid over-extrapolation. Where evidence originated from animal/in vitro models, this is stated in text and in the tables.

2.4. Evidence Appraisal and Synthesis

We did not perform formal risk-of-bias scoring, consistent with scoping aims. Instead, we graded contributions as High (meta-analyses/RCTs or large human cohorts), Moderate (observational human studies or convergent multi-study signals), or Low (mechanistic/experimental or expert consensus). Narrative synthesis integrated human clinical signals with biological plausibility from experimental data, making explicit where inferences remain hypothesis-generating. Sections and summary tables clearly separate clinical versus experimental evidence lines. To strengthen interpretability, we distinguish throughout between established clinical associations, translational correlates, and emerging mechanistic hypotheses; recommendations tied primarily to mechanistic or consensus sources are identified as such. No ethics approval was required (secondary synthesis of published data); no protocol was registered given the narrative–scoping design.

3. Current Knowledge and Latest Hypotheses on Frozen Shoulder Pathophysiology

Traditionally, the pathophysiology of FS has been understood through the lens of localized inflammation, capsular fibrosis, and contracture of the glenohumeral joint, often associated with minor trauma, immobilization, or idiopathic onset [4,19]. Histologically, FS is characterized by chronic synovial inflammation, fibroblastic proliferation, and excessive collagen deposition, particularly in the rotator interval and coracohumeral ligament [20,21]. However, this conventional view has proven insufficient to explain several clinical observations—such as the prolonged and variable course, the incomplete recovery in many patients, and the clear female predominance, especially in peri- and postmenopausal women. Consequently, emerging evidence has led to a more integrative and systemic perspective on the etiology of FS [5,8,14].

Recent studies suggest that FS may be a manifestation of a broader systemic LGI and immunometabolic dysfunction, sharing mechanistic pathways with other fibrosing and pain-related disorders [14]. Elevated levels of pro-inflammatory cytokines such as IL-1β, TNF-α, and IL-6 have been observed in the synovial fluid and capsular tissue of FS patients, indicating an active immune-inflammatory component in the early and intermediate stages of the disease [22]. Additionally, FS has been strongly associated with systemic comorbidities including type 2 diabetes mellitus, dyslipidemia, thyroid dysfunction, and metabolic syndrome [9,23]. These conditions are known to promote oxidative stress, microvascular damage, and tissue fibrosis via AGEs, leptin resistance, and chronic activation of the HPA axis [5,24–28]. These systemic factors may interact with local joint environments, perpetuating inflammation and altering fibroblast behavior toward a profibrotic phenotype. Furthermore, chronic psychological stress, depression, and sleep disorders—conditions more prevalent in FS patients—have been implicated in the amplification of pain perception and central sensitization [3,29,30]. The chronic activation of stress-related neuroendocrine axes (particularly HPA and the autonomic nervous system) can exacerbate systemic inflammation and pain processing, linking FS to biopsychosocial models of chronic musculoskeletal conditions [5].

In this evolving framework, the female sex hormonal axis, particularly estrogen signaling, is gaining attention as a potentially crucial modulator of FS onset, severity, and prognosis [15]. The notably higher prevalence of FS in women, especially around menopause, has prompted hypotheses about the protective and regulatory roles of estrogens on joint inflammation, connective tissue integrity, and pain modulation [31]. These hormonal changes could act synergistically with metabolic and inflammatory imbalances, making postmenopausal women particularly vulnerable [15].

Therefore, the pathophysiology of FS may be better understood as a multifactorial condition, where hormonal, immunometabolic, psychosocial, and environmental factors converge to disrupt joint homeostasis, trigger chronic inflammation, and promote fibrotic remodeling. This integrative model paves the way for new therapeutic strategies that go beyond localized treatment and target systemic pathways involved in FS progression.

4. The Female Sex Hormonal Axis: Neuroendocrine, Immunologic, and Metabolic Dimensions

The female sex hormonal axis, primarily governed by estrogens, progesterone, and their regulatory interplay with the hypothalamic-pituitary-gonadal (HPG) axis, plays a critical role not only in reproductive physiology but also in systemic homeostasis—including immune function, pain perception, inflammatory control, and tissue remodeling [32,33]. In recent years, the understanding of this axis has expanded beyond its reproductive role, unveiling complex neuroendocrine and immunometabolic mechanisms that may be especially relevant in conditions such as FS [34,35].

4.1. Neuroendocrine Influence

Estrogens, particularly 17β-estradiol, exert significant effects on the central and peripheral nervous systems, modulating neurotransmitter release, neuronal plasticity, and pain signaling. Estrogen receptors (ERα and ERβ) are widely expressed in the brain, dorsal root ganglia, and spinal cord, where they regulate nociceptive pathways, stress responses, and mood [34,36]. Declining estrogen levels during menopause have been associated with increased central sensitization, decreased pain thresholds, and heightened responsiveness to inflammatory stimuli—factors that may exacerbate the chronic pain and stiffness observed in FS [37,38]. Moreover, estrogens interact with the HPA axis, modulating cortisol secretion and stress resilience [39,40]. In estrogen-deficient states, this axis may become dysregulated, contributing to pro-inflammatory neuroendocrine activity [41]. Chronic stress, in turn, can lower circulating estrogen levels, perpetuating a vicious cycle of neuroendocrine imbalance [40].

4.2. Immunologic Modulation

From an immunological perspective, estrogens possess biphasic effects: at low concentrations, they tend to promote pro-inflammatory activity, while at physiological or replacement levels, they often exert anti-inflammatory effects [42]. Estrogens enhance the function of regulatory T cells (Tregs), suppress pro-inflammatory macrophage phenotypes (M1), and reduce the expression of cytokines such as IL-1β, IL-6, and TNF-α—all of which are implicated in the pathogenesis of FS [43,44]. Additionally, estrogens stabilize mast cells and inhibit NF-κB signaling, a central inflammatory pathway activated by dietary and metabolic stressors [45]. This anti-inflammatory potential becomes particularly relevant in the context of low-grade systemic LGI, a common feature in FS patients with metabolic comorbidities [5]. Therefore, estrogen decline may shift the immune environment toward a pro-inflammatory and profibrotic state, favoring the activation of fibroblasts and excessive collagen production in the shoulder capsule [15,34].

4.3. Metabolic Regulation

Estrogens also play a crucial role in metabolic homeostasis, influencing lipid metabolism, glucose regulation, mitochondrial function, and oxidative stress resistance [46,47]. They promote insulin sensitivity, reduce visceral fat accumulation, and modulate adipokine release (e.g., leptin and adiponectin), all of which are known to impact systemic inflammation and joint health [48,49]. The decline in estrogen levels during menopause is associated with increased risk of metabolic syndrome, type 2 diabetes, and dyslipidemia, conditions highly prevalent in FS patients [7,9,19,50,51]. These metabolic alterations can create a systemic environment conducive to oxidative stress and vascular dysfunction, which in turn may impair tissue repair mechanisms and contribute to fibrosis [26,27,52].

One important connection lies in the role of cholesterol, both as a cardiovascular risk factor and a precursor to estrogen synthesis [53,54]. Cholesterol is converted into pregnenolone in mitochondria by the enzyme cytochrome P450scc (CYP11A1), a rate-limiting step in steroidogenesis, leading ultimately to the synthesis of estrogens [55,56]. Thus, adequate intracellular cholesterol availability is essential for maintaining estrogen levels, especially in postmenopausal women where adrenal and peripheral synthesis becomes more critical [55–57]. Importantly, recent evidence—including the latest meta-analysis on metabolic and inflammatory profiles in FS—has shown that elevated levels of HbA1c are a consistent feature in these patients, reflecting chronic hyperglycemia and poor glucose regulation [58]. Persistent high blood glucose can directly impair cholesterol transport mechanisms at the cellular level, particularly by glycation of apolipoproteins (e.g., ApoA1, ApoB100), dysfunction of LDL receptors, and increased oxidative modification of lipoproteins. These changes lead to decreased cholesterol uptake by cells, increased circulating LDL-C, and ultimately hypercholesterolemia [58–60].

This altered cholesterol metabolism not only reduces the substrate available for estrogen synthesis, potentially exacerbating hormonal imbalances, but also contributes to the formation of pro-inflammatory lipid species (e.g., oxidized LDL), which activate macrophages, endothelial cells, and fibroblasts via toll-like receptors and the NF-κB pathway [61,62]. The result is a sustained inflammatory response, fibrosis, and impaired tissue repair—a molecular landscape highly relevant to FS pathophysiology [63,64].

Furthermore, impaired glucose and cholesterol homeostasis can lead to mitochondrial dysfunction through increased production of reactive oxygen species (ROS), reduced ATP synthesis, and impaired cellular redox status [21,26,65,66]. In fibroblasts, these disruptions can activate fibrotic signaling cascades, including TGF-β1 and connective tissue growth factor (CTGF), promoting extracellular matrix (ECM) deposition and capsular thickening in the shoulder [64]. Therefore, the metabolic crosstalk between hyperglycemia, dyslipidemia, and hormonal decline may act synergistically to sustain the chronic inflammation, fibrosis, and pain characteristic of FS. Understanding and targeting this axis is crucial for developing future integrative interventions.

5. Estrogen Deficiency, Resistance, and Metabolic Disruption in FS

The biological relevance of estrogen in human physiology goes far beyond reproductive function [67,68]. As a pleiotropic hormone, estrogen exerts systemic effects on immune regulation, metabolism, tissue repair, vascular tone, and pain modulation [67,69,70]. These regulatory roles are especially relevant in conditions like FS, a disorder characterized by chronic capsular inflammation, fibrosis, and functional loss that disproportionately affects women, particularly during perimenopause and postmenopause (see Table 1) [5]. Despite this striking epidemiological pattern, the role of estrogen and the broader female hormonal axis has been largely overlooked in FS pathophysiology [5,15].

Emerging evidence suggests that the estrogen axis is not only vulnerable to deficiency states—as seen in menopause—but also to resistance mechanisms and metabolic interference that hinder receptor-level signaling [34,48,71]. In the context of FS, where metabolic disturbances such as chronic LGI, hyperglycemia, dyslipidemia, and adipose tissue dysfunction converge, estrogen signaling may be downregulated or altered in ways that exacerbate fibrosis, pain sensitization, and impaired tissue regeneration [21,22,24,28]. This section explores these complex interrelationships, aiming to reframe FS within a broader immunometabolic-endocrine model [14,72].

Table 1. Estrogen & Thyroid Axes in Frozen Shoulder.

Domain	Study Type	Core Finding	Implication for FS
Estrogen axis	Clinical (SR/MA, cohorts)	Higher prevalence and worse outcomes in peri/postmenopausal women; metabolic comorbidity associations; ER expression in glenohumeral capsule biopsies.	Estrogen deficiency/resistance may underlie inflammation, pain, and fibrosis.
Estrogen axis	Experimental (in vitro/animal)	E2 inhibits NF-κB, IL-1β, IL-6, TNF-α; modulates TGF-β1 and MMP/TIMP; antioxidant and antinociceptive effects.	Supports hypothesis of receptor-level resistance in FS.
Thyroid axis	Clinical (SR/MA, MR, cohorts)	Overt and subclinical hypothyroidism ↑ risk of FS; causal support from Mendelian randomization; weaker evidence for hyperthyroidism.	Thyroid dysfunction contributes to fibrosis and pain; screening recommended.
Thyroid axis	Experimental (animal/in vitro)	Low T3/T4 → ↓MMPs, ↑TGF-β, ECM accumulation, impaired collagen turnover.	Mechanistic link between hypothyroidism and capsular fibrosis.
Estrogen–Thyroid crosstalk	Translational	Hypothyroidism alters SHBG, insulin and leptin resistance → reduced estrogen bioavailability/action.	Functional estrogen resistance in thyroid dysfunction.

Note: FS = Frozen Shoulder; SR = Systematic Review; MA = Meta-analysis; MR = Mendelian Randomization; ER = Estrogen Receptor; E2 = 17β-estradiol; NF-κB = Nuclear Factor kappa-light-chain-enhancer of activated B cells; TGF-β = Transforming Growth Factor beta; MMP = Matrix Metalloproteinase; TIMP = Tissue Inhibitor of Metalloproteinases; ECM = Extracellular Matrix; SHBG = Sex Hormone–Binding Globulin.

5.1. Estrogen Resistance and Chronobiological Disruption

While hormonal deficiency—particularly the decline in estrogen during menopause—has been widely studied, less attention has been paid to the concept of hormonal resistance, including resistance to estrogen [73]. Hormonal resistance refers to a state in which circulating hormone levels may be adequate or only mildly reduced, yet tissue responsiveness is diminished due to defects at the receptor or post-receptor level [74,75]. In the case of estrogen, this can involve decreased receptor density, impaired receptor activation, altered cofactor binding, or interference by inflammatory or metabolic signals [34]. This phenomenon may be accentuated by chronobiological dysregulation. Estrogen follows a natural circadian and infradian rhythm, with cyclical acrophases and nadirs that coordinate immune and metabolic processes [76–78]. Disruption of this rhythm—through aging, stress, light pollution, or metabolic dysfunction—may desynchronize estrogen receptor activation and gene transcription [77–80]. In perimenopausal women, for instance, the amplitude of estrogen fluctuations increases while predictability declines, leading to episodic surges and troughs that confuse receptor signaling machinery [81]. In FS, such dysregulation may promote an inflammatory microenvironment where estrogen cannot exert its usual anti-inflammatory, anti-fibrotic, and analgesic effects. Receptor resistance or desensitization in synovial fibroblasts, immune cells, or endothelial tissue could thus contribute to unchecked fibrosis, nociceptive amplification, and impaired tissue remodeling.

5.2. Hyperglycemia and AGEs

Hyperglycemia represents a major source of metabolic stress and a key factor in estrogen signaling impairment [82,83]. Chronic elevations in blood glucose—commonly assessed via HbA1c—lead to the non-enzymatic glycation of proteins, forming advanced glycation end-products (AGEs) [82,83]. AGEs are known to accumulate in connective tissue, disrupt collagen homeostasis, and activate receptors such as RAGE (Receptor for Advanced Glycation End-products), which in turn stimulate the NF-κB pathway and the release of pro-inflammatory cytokines like IL-1β and TNF-α [45,84,85].

Importantly, AGEs also interfere with lipid transport and cholesterol homeostasis, impairing the availability of cholesterol as a precursor for steroidogenesis [86]. This is particularly relevant for estrogen synthesis, which relies on sufficient intracellular cholesterol [82,86]. The sustained presence of AGEs can also oxidize LDL particles, contributing to dyslipidemia and endothelial dysfunction, both of which have been associated with FS [87,88]. Moreover, hyperglycemia-induced oxidative stress downregulates estrogen receptor expression and functionality, leading to estrogen resistance at the cellular level, even in the presence of circulating hormone. In the context of FS, this may potentiate synovial fibroblast activation and perpetuate the fibrotic cascade [89,90].

5.3. Dyslipidemia and Cholesterol Overload

Cholesterol plays a central role in steroid hormone biosynthesis, acting as a precursor for estrogen and other sex steroids [91]. However, in metabolic disorders like insulin resistance and FS, this balance may be disrupted [29,58,92]. Hypercholesterolemia, particularly elevated LDL and total cholesterol, has been repeatedly observed in FS patients and may act as both a marker and contributor to disease pathogenesis [58].

Cholesterol overload in tissues can lead to membrane stiffness, impaired cellular signaling, and pro-inflammatory foam cell formation [91,93]. Excess cholesterol may inhibit estrogen biosynthesis by saturating feedback loops in steroidogenic tissues or by interfering with transport proteins and enzymes such as CYP19A1 (aromatase) [53]. This creates a vicious cycle where high cholesterol contributes to low estrogen bioavailability and signaling, exacerbating inflammation and fibrosis [94].

In FS, this dyslipidemic environment may further fuel capsular thickening, neoangiogenesis, and immune cell infiltration [8,58,59]. Furthermore, oxidized LDL can interact with estrogen receptors or compete for similar binding sites, contributing to receptor-level interference and functional resistance [95].

5.4. Adipose Tissue Dysfunction and Endocrine Crosstalk in FS

Adipose tissue, long considered a passive energy reservoir, is now recognized as a dynamic endocrine organ that exerts profound influences on inflammation, immunity, and hormonal signaling [96]. In FS, particularly among patients with central obesity or features of metabolic syndrome, adipose dysfunction may play a central role in modulating disease course [23,97].

Hypertrophic adipocytes secrete pro-inflammatory adipokines such as leptin, resistin, and visfatin, while reducing anti-inflammatory signals like adiponectin [98,99]. These changes foster systemic LGI, which in turn impairs estrogen receptor signaling by inducing serine phosphorylation, oxidative damage, or nuclear exclusion of receptor complexes [5,100,101]. Moreover, leptin resistance—frequently seen in insulin-resistant states—has been shown to downregulate estrogen receptor alpha (ERα) in various tissues [101].

This dysfunctional adipose secretome may also affect fibroblast activity, matrix remodeling, and synovial inflammation [96,102]. Visceral adiposity, in particular, has been associated with elevated TNF-α and IL-6 levels, key drivers of fibrosis in FS [22,58]. Simultaneously, reduced aromatase activity in dysfunctional adipose tissue may decrease peripheral estrogen synthesis, compounding the effects of systemic estrogen deficiency or resistance [103–105].

Additionally, adipose tissue expresses estrogen receptors, and their dysfunction contributes to a feedback loop of hormonal insensitivity, metabolic imbalance, and inflammatory activation [106,107]. This establishes a complex endocrine-immuno-metabolic network in FS, where estrogen resistance becomes both a cause and consequence of adipose dysfunction [108,109].

5.5. Clinical and Molecular Implications in FS

The cumulative effects of estrogen resistance, chronic inflammation, hyperglycemia, dyslipidemia, and adipose tissue dysfunction converge to create a pathological environment conducive to FS development and progression [8,58,59,92]. At the molecular level, impaired estrogen signaling reduces the transcription of anti-inflammatory cytokines (e.g., IL-10), increases M1 macrophage polarization, and enhances TGF-β-mediated fibroblast activation [110]. Estrogen receptor dysfunction in joint capsules may also impair angiogenesis, increase mast cell degranulation, and limit extracellular matrix turnover [15,73]. Clinically, this translates into a more severe and prolonged disease course, particularly in women undergoing perimenopausal transition or experiencing metabolic syndrome [46,81]. These patients often present with higher pain intensity, reduced mobility, and slower response to physical therapy [92]. Recognizing these molecular signatures could facilitate early identification of high-risk phenotypes and guide tailored interventions—for instance, combining hormonal modulation with anti-inflammatory diets, exercise, and insulin-sensitizing agents.

As the field progresses, integrating estrogen signaling pathways into FS management could offer a more comprehensive framework for understanding and treating this complex condition.

5.6. Estrogen Deficiency in Menopause: A Missing Link in FS

Estrogen deficiency has traditionally been considered one of the principal hormonal drivers behind the disproportionately high prevalence of FS in women, particularly during the perimenopausal and postmenopausal stages [46]. During this transitional period, ovarian estrogen production declines significantly, often to below 10% of premenopausal levels [15]. Far from being a solely reproductive hormone, estrogen plays a vital role in maintaining immune homeostasis, connective tissue remodeling, metabolic regulation, and nociceptive modulation [48,70,108]. Its absence introduces a cascade of dysregulated processes that can critically influence the onset and progression of FS [58].

At the molecular level, 17β-estradiol (E2), the most potent form of estrogen, performs several protective functions highly relevant to FS pathogenesis:

Anti-inflammatory effects: Estrogens inhibit key pro-inflammatory transcription factors, notably nuclear factor kappa B (NF-κB), thereby reducing the expression of cytokines such as IL-1β, IL-6, and TNF-α. These mediators are commonly elevated in synovial fluid and capsular biopsies from FS patients and are involved in promoting nociceptive sensitization and fibrotic responses [20,27,34,111].

Antifibrotic signaling: E2 modulates the transforming growth factor-beta (TGF-β1) pathway, a central orchestrator of fibrotic remodeling. In physiological conditions, estrogen limits fibroblast-to-myofibroblast transition and curbs collagen I/III synthesis. Its deficiency allows unopposed TGF-β1 activity, resulting in capsular thickening, contracture, and loss of joint range [31,48,49,69].

Antioxidant defense: Estrogen promotes the expression of antioxidant enzymes such as superoxide dismutase (SOD), catalase, and glutathione peroxidase, thereby reducing oxidative stress. The accumulation of reactive oxygen species (ROS) in low-estrogen environments exacerbates collagen cross-linking, impairs angiogenesis, and accelerates extracellular matrix stiffening [112].

Pain regulation: Estrogens modulate both central and peripheral pain pathways through their interaction with opioid receptors, TRPV1 channels, and NMDA receptors. Estrogen deficiency may lead to heightened pain sensitivity and decreased endogenous analgesia—hallmarks of FS symptomatology [41,113].

Histological studies have confirmed the presence of estrogen receptors (ERα and ERβ) in the glenohumeral joint capsule, particularly in fibroblasts, endothelial cells, and synovial lining. When estrogen is deficient, these receptors may remain unbound and inactive, disrupting normal gene transcription for anti-inflammatory and tissue-reparative processes [114].

The downstream consequences of this signaling void include: (i) Enhanced fibroblast proliferation and extracellular matrix deposition [31,115]; (ii) Sustained activation of pro-inflammatory M1 macrophages and reduced IL-10 production [116,117]; (iii) Altered expression of matrix metalloproteinases (MMPs) and their inhibitors (TIMPs), impairing collagen turnover [26,66]; (iv) Increased vascular permeability and neoangiogenesis, promoting synovial hyperplasia [118].

Clinically, estrogen deficiency is associated with greater FS severity in postmenopausal women, who often experience more intense pain, prolonged stiffness, and delayed response to rehabilitation. The correlation between low estrogen and other musculoskeletal disorders—such as osteoarthritis, tendinopathy, and sarcopenia—further reinforces its role as a central modulator of connective tissue health and repair [15]. Notably, estrogen deficiency seldom occurs in isolation. It often coexists with increased insulin resistance, visceral adiposity, and elevated LDL cholesterol, all of which converge to reinforce the fibrotic and inflammatory milieu [58]. Moreover, the decline in aromatase activity within dysfunctional adipose tissue reduces peripheral estrogen production, amplifying systemic deficiency [104]. However, it is also important to recognize that not all postmenopausal women develop FS, and cases in premenopausal women suggest that deficiency alone is insufficient to trigger the condition [15]. This observation has led to growing interest in the roles of estrogen resistance, receptor-level interference, and metabolic stress as complementary or alternative mechanisms—paving the way for more nuanced and integrative models of FS pathogenesis [5,8,58,59].

5.7. Receptor-Level Interference by Metabolic and Environmental Factors

In recent years, a growing body of evidence has emphasized that endocrine signaling—particularly estrogen signaling—can be profoundly disrupted not only by internal pathophysiological changes, but also by chronic exposure to environmental, dietary, and lifestyle factors [119,120]. This subclinical disruption can occur even in the presence of normal or mildly reduced estrogen levels, and is increasingly understood as a central mechanism in the pathogenesis of hormone-sensitive disorders such as FS [71,73].

5.7.1. Environmental Estrogen Disruptors and Receptor Occupancy

Modern industrial environments expose individuals to a wide range of endocrine-disrupting chemicals (EDCs) [121,122]. These include xenoestrogens, such as bisphenol A (BPA), phthalates, parabens, polychlorinated biphenyls (PCBs), and heavy metals (e.g., cadmium), which are ubiquitously found in plastics, food packaging, cosmetics, detergents, pesticides, and even indoor air [122]. These compounds mimic the structure of natural estrogens and bind to estrogen receptors (ERα and ERβ), acting as partial agonists or antagonists depending on the tissue [121]. Although some EDCs weakly activate estrogen receptors, their constant low-level presence leads to receptor desensitization, misactivation, or competitive inhibition, which interferes with the body's endogenous estrogen signaling [123]. In fibroblasts, immune cells, or endothelial cells within the glenohumeral capsule, this interference could blunt the normal anti-inflammatory and antifibrotic actions of estrogen, promoting unchecked cytokine release, immune cell recruitment, and matrix stiffening—hallmarks of FS pathology [124,125].

5.7.2. Chronic Low-Grade Inflammation (LGI) and Receptor Dysfunction

A pro-inflammatory lifestyle, characterized by poor diet, physical inactivity, chronic psychological stress, inadequate sleep, and environmental pollutant exposure, can induce a sustained state of LGI [126,127]. Unlike acute inflammation, LGI operates at subclinical levels, often undetected by routine diagnostics, but it exerts pervasive molecular effects [128]. LGI activates transcription factors such as NF-κB and AP-1, which not only promote cytokine and chemokine expression (e.g., IL-6, TNF-α, IL-1β), but also impair estrogen receptor signaling through multiple mechanisms [129]: (i) Serine phosphorylation of ERα, which reduces its transcriptional activity and may even convert it into a pro-inflammatory modulator; (ii) Nitrosative and oxidative stress, which modifies receptor structure, reducing ligand binding affinity and nuclear translocation; (iii) Downregulation of receptor expression, particularly in adipose, immune, and musculoskeletal tissues; (iv) This inflammatory-induced ER dysfunction renders peripheral tissues partially or fully resistant to estrogen, even in the presence of normal hormone concentrations. In FS, this would hinder estrogen's regulation of fibroblast activation, immune polarization, and vascular function, thereby fueling capsular fibrosis and pain sensitivity [72,125,126,130,131].

5.7.3. Metabolic Disruptors: Diet, Obesity, and Mitochondrial Stress

Modern dietary patterns—rich in ultra-processed foods, refined carbohydrates, trans fats, and artificial additives—are a major driver of metabolic dysregulation [132,133]. Diets with high glycemic load, poor fiber diversity, and excessive omega-6 to omega-3 ratios promote insulin resistance, adipose tissue dysfunction, and microbiota imbalances, all of which converge on inflammatory and endocrine axes [134–136]. These metabolic shifts result in: (i)Elevated leptin and decreased adiponectin, which impair ERα expression [137]; (ii) Mitochondrial dysfunction and ROS accumulation, damaging estrogen receptors and coactivators [138,139]; (iii) Reduced cholesterol bioavailability for steroidogenesis, particularly under conditions of dyslipidemia and AGE accumulation [51,140,141]. Moreover, high-fat, high-sugar diets exacerbate hepatic estrogen metabolism, leading to increased conjugation and excretion, thereby reducing systemic bioavailability of active estrogens [48,142,143]. The result is a state of functional estrogen deficiency, even without absolute hormonal decline [71].

5.7.4. Hormonal Crosstalk and Receptor Interference

Insulin, cortisol, leptin, and inflammatory cytokines all interact with estrogen signaling pathways, either by competing for shared coactivators (e.g., SRC-1, p300) or by modulating transcriptional responses at estrogen-responsive elements (EREs) [144]. Chronic insulin resistance and hypercortisolemia, common in FS patients with metabolic syndrome, may further inhibit estrogen action through: (i) Nuclear receptor crosstalk, where glucocorticoid receptor activation suppresses ER-mediated transcription [145]; (ii) Histone deacetylase activation, which closes chromatin at ER target sites [146]; (iii) Direct inhibition of aromatase, reducing local estrogen synthesis in tissues such as fat and muscle [147]. This complex hormonal crosstalk means that receptor functionality is not only a function of estrogen concentration, but also of the metabolic and inflammatory milieu, which can override or block hormonal effects [71].

6. A Paradigm Shift in FS Pathophysiology

The traditional understanding of FS has long centered on localized mechanical and inflammatory changes within the glenohumeral joint capsule—namely, synovitis, fibroblast proliferation, and collagen deposition [1,2,22]. While this model has clinical utility, it fails to account for the striking epidemiological, metabolic, and hormonal patterns increasingly observed in FS patients, particularly in women during the menopausal transition [46,58]. A growing body of evidence now calls for a paradigm shift: one that moves beyond joint-centric explanations and instead views FS as a systemic, immunoendocrine-metabolic disorder [5,8,14,25,50,58,124]. In this revised framework, the shoulder capsule becomes not the origin, but the target organ of upstream dysregulations involving sex hormones, chronic LGI, metabolic dysfunction, and environmental interference [5,8,14,25,50,58,124].

Estrogen, once considered solely a reproductive hormone, now emerges as a central regulatory signal for immune modulation, extracellular matrix remodeling, pain processing, and tissue repair [148,149]. Its deficiency, resistance, or receptor-level disruption—whether due to menopause, metabolic syndrome, or environmental exposures—sets the stage for a pathological cascade where tissue resilience is lost and [150,151] fibrosis prevails. At the same time, systemic factors such as hyperglycemia, dyslipidemia, mitochondrial stress, and adipokine imbalance exacerbate this hormonal vulnerability [152]. They promote fibro-inflammatory signaling through the activation of TGF-β, NF-κB, and pro-inflammatory macrophages, while simultaneously blunting protective pathways involving IL-10, antioxidant enzymes, and estrogen receptor signaling [153]. The result is a pro-fibrotic, pro-inflammatory phenotype, particularly evident in women with features of metabolic stress or hormonal transition [72,124]. Furthermore, the occupational burden of endocrine-disrupting chemicals (EDCs) and environmental stressors (e.g., sleep deprivation, circadian disruption, psychosocial stress) adds a previously overlooked dimension to FS pathogenesis [154,155]. These factors interfere with receptor binding, chronobiological hormone release, and intracellular signaling fidelity, making estrogen resistance a likely—and perhaps central—player in disease expression [121].

This integrative lens compels us to re-evaluate not only the causes of FS but also the way it is treated. If FS were, in part, a manifestation of disrupted estrogen signaling within a pro-inflammatory metabolic environment, then future therapeutic approaches must go beyond joint mobilization or corticosteroids. They should include: (i) Hormonal evaluation and, where appropriate, modulation (e.g., estrogen support, phytoestrogens); (ii) Anti-inflammatory nutritional interventions; (iii) Lifestyle optimization focused on circadian alignment, stress management, and physical activity; (iv) Environmental detoxification strategies to reduce EDC exposure; (v) Targeted metabolic interventions to restore insulin sensitivity, mitochondrial health, and lipid balance. Thus, the future of FS management lies not only in better understanding the joint capsule—but in restoring systemic balance at the intersection of hormones, metabolism, immunity, and environment. Such a paradigm shift holds promise for not only improved treatment outcomes but also for preventive strategies, particularly in high-risk female populations. To facilitate comprehension and provide a visual synthesis of the integrative model proposed, a summary figure (Figure 1) was developed. This schematic representation illustrates how lifestyle, endocrine, metabolic, vascular, and neuroimmune factors interact to create a systemic environment that culminates in capsular fibrosis, pain sensitization, and the clinical phenotype of frozen shoulder.

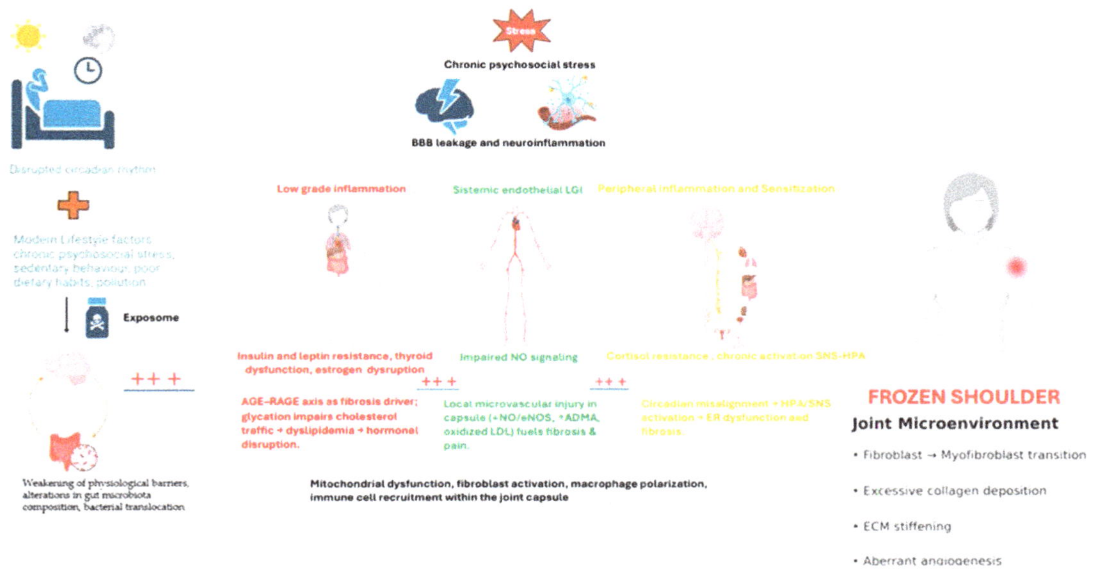

Figure 1. Integrative model of frozen shoulder pathophysiology. This figure illustrates the multifactorial cascade linking lifestyle, environmental, and systemic factors to the onset and persistence of FS. On the left, modern lifestyle influences—including circadian disruption, sedentarism, poor dietary habits, pollution, and broader exposome exposures—act as primary triggers of systemic dysregulation. These exposures weaken physiological barriers, alter gut microbiota composition, and promote bacterial translocation, thereby amplifying inflammatory signaling. In the central section, chronic psychosocial stress contributes to blood–brain barrier leakage and neuroinflammation, which interact with systemic pathways represented in three axes: (i) low-grade systemic inflammation (LGI), encompassing endocrine and metabolic alterations such as insulin and leptin resistance, thyroid dysfunction, and estrogen dysregulation (red text); (ii) systemic endothelial inflammation, marked by vascular injury, impaired nitric oxide (NO) signaling, and microvascular dysfunction (green text); and (iii) peripheral inflammation and sensitization, characterized by chronic activation of the sympathetic nervous system, hypothalamic–pituitary–adrenal axis, and cortisol resistance (yellow text). Collectively, these processes converge downstream to promote mitochondrial dysfunction, fibroblast activation, macrophage polarization, and immune cell recruitment within the joint capsule. The final right-hand representation highlights the clinical phenotype of FS, where fibroblast-to-myofibroblast transition, excessive collagen deposition, extracellular matrix stiffening, and aberrant angiogenesis result in capsular fibrosis, chronic pain, and restricted mobility.

6.1. Sleep, Circadian Rhythms, and Hormonal Crosstalk in FS

The endocrine system operates not in isolation but in harmony with the body's circadian architecture, governed by the suprachiasmatic nucleus (SCN) of the hypothalamus. This master clock orchestrates daily rhythms of hormonal release—including estrogen, melatonin, cortisol, thyroid hormones, and growth hormone (GH)—which in turn regulate immune tone, metabolic efficiency, tissue repair, and inflammatory resolution [156,157]. Disruption of these rhythms, particularly through poor sleep quality or altered light exposure, has profound implications for musculoskeletal health and may be a silent driver of FS pathogenesis [29,158].

Sleep is essential for hormonal synchronization, with specific peaks in anabolic and regulatory hormones occurring during nocturnal rest [159,160]. For instance: (i) Estrogen secretion, although modulated primarily by the ovarian axis, follows ultradian rhythms influenced by circadian cues. Fragmented or delayed sleep impairs estrogen receptor activation and downstream gene transcription [159]; (ii) Growth hormone, critical for collagen turnover and connective tissue repair, is secreted in pulses during slow-wave sleep. Poor sleep reduces GH amplitude, impairing tendon and capsular recovery [161]; (iii) Cortisol, with its diurnal peak in the early morning, may become chronically elevated with sleep disruption, contributing to insulin resistance, immunosuppression, and estrogen resistance [162,163]; (iv) Melatonin, the principal chronobiotic hormone, modulates estrogen receptor expression and has anti-fibrotic, antioxidant, and immune-regulating properties [164,165]. Light-at-night, especially from screens, suppresses melatonin production and indirectly derails hormonal coordination [166]; (v) Disrupted sleep architecture thus acts as a multisystemic stressor, capable of precipitating or worsening LGI, estrogen insensitivity, and metabolic imbalance—all of which converge in the FS phenotype [5,14,167].

6.2. *Thyroid Dysfunction in FS: A Key but Overlooked Axis*

Among the endocrine alterations associated with FS, thyroid dysfunction has received increasing attention [168]. Population-based and clinical studies have reported a higher prevalence of hypothyroidism in FS patients, with estimates ranging from 10% to 34% [168,169]. A recent systematic review and meta-analysis confirmed that both overt and subclinical hypothyroidism significantly increase the risk of FS, whereas the evidence for hyperthyroidism is less consistent [170]. Indeed, a Mendelian randomization study has provided causal support for the association between hypothyroidism and FS, suggesting a direct role of thyroid hormones in capsular pathophysiology [9].

Several mechanisms have been proposed. Hypothyroidism reduces basal metabolic rate and mitochondrial function, promotes the accumulation of glycosaminoglycans, and disrupts collagen turnover, thereby favoring capsular fibrosis [171]. In addition, reduced expression of matrix metalloproteinases (MMPs) and increased TGF-β have been reported, stimulating fibroblast-to-myofibroblast transition and extracellular matrix accumulation [171]. In parallel, thyroid hormone deficiency may induce insulin resistance and alterations in leptin and adiponectin, interfering with estrogen signaling and contributing to a systemic pro-inflammatory state. In patients with autoimmune thyroiditis (e.g., Hashimoto's disease), the presence of chronic inflammatory background may further amplify local fibrotic processes in the joint capsule [172,173]. Although hypothyroidism is the condition most frequently associated with FS, some recent studies suggest that a hypermetabolic state may also be implicated [8]. In this context, increased oxidative stress and metabolic demand could potentiate inflammatory responses and pain sensitization [8,59]. These findings indicate that both deficient and excessive thyroid hormone states may alter the capsular microenvironment, albeit through different mechanisms.

Clinically, the coexistence of FS and thyroid dysfunction is often associated with greater symptom severity and, in some cases, with poorer response to conventional treatment [58,170]. However, results remain inconsistent, and further studies are required to determine whether correcting thyroid dysfunction directly improves FS outcomes [168,170]. Importantly, both thyroid hormones (T3 and T4) and estrogens act in coordination to regulate metabolism, connective tissue remodeling, immune modulation, and pain perception [174,175]. When one of these axes is altered, the other is often secondarily affected, creating an environment favorable to chronic inflammation and fibrosis. In this context, the estrogen axis is deeply impacted [174,175]. Hypothyroidism alters the synthesis of sex hormone–binding globulin (SHBG), reducing estrogen bioavailability, while also inducing insulin and leptin resistance, which interfere with estrogen receptor signaling [174,176]. This combination can lead to functional estrogen resistance, even in the presence of relatively preserved serum estrogen levels [176]. Since estrogens exert anti-inflammatory, antioxidant, and antifibrotic properties—such as inhibiting NF-κB and negatively regulating TGF-β—their dysfunction leaves the joint microenvironment more vulnerable to damage [34,42,49,151,177].

The interaction between estrogen deficiency (due to menopause, resistance, or signaling alterations) and thyroid dysfunction creates a vicious cycle that exacerbates pain and fibrosis: (i) Hypothyroidism promotes fibrosis and pain sensitization through excessive TGF-β activity, impaired mitochondrial function, and systemic inflammation [178]; (ii) Estrogen deficiency or resistance prevents counteracting these mechanisms by limiting fibroblast regulation, reducing antioxidant activity (SOD, catalase, GPx), and diminishing central pain modulation [179]; (iii) Together, these dysfunctions converge into an inflammatory-fibrotic phenotype, characterized by M1 macrophage activation, excess ROS, and disrupted collagen metabolism [180,181].

Clinically, this scenario is particularly evident in peri- and postmenopausal women, where the prevalence of subclinical or overt hypothyroidism is higher and the decline in estrogen levels is more pronounced [9,15]. In this group, FS tends to present with more intense pain, greater capsular stiffness, and poorer response to conventional treatments [10,170]. Thus, the combined dysfunction of the thyroid and estrogen axes may constitute a central node in the pathogenesis of FS. Their disruption not only promotes the establishment of fibrosis and chronic pain, but also provides a plausible explanation for the strong female predominance of FS and its frequent association with metabolic comorbidities.

6.3. The Lifestyle Hypothesis: LGI as the Root Cause

An increasing body of evidence suggests that many endocrine and metabolic derangements in FS may originate from lifestyle-induced chronic LGI [127,132,182]. Modern behaviors—sedentarism, diets rich in ultra-processed foods and poor in micronutrients, excessive screen exposure and artificial light-at-night (ALAN), psychosocial stress, and sleep disruption—collectively impair circadian biology, induce persistent immune activation, and promote hormonal resistance across multiple axes [132].

LGI operates through sustained activation of stress axes (HPA, HPT, HPG) and inflammatory mediators [72,127]. This systemic inflammatory context leads to: (i) Insulin resistance, hyperglycemia, and AGEs, which desensitize estrogen receptors and enhance fibrotic signaling [48,183]; (ii) Leptin resistance, impairing hypothalamic–pituitary regulation and disrupting estrogen and GH rhythms [184,185]; (iii) Cortisol dysregulation, with chronic elevation suppressing melatonin and TSH, thereby compromising both thyroid and estrogen pathways [162,186,187]; (iv) Oxidative and nitrosative stress, driving receptor phosphorylation, conformational changes, and nuclear exclusion of estrogen–receptor complexes [188].

Psychoneuroimmunology research highlights how these contextual risk factors act as "lifestyle-associated molecular patterns" (LAMPs) that mimic pathogen or danger signals, thereby perpetuating immune activation even in the absence of acute threats [126]. This maladaptive response—robust in evolutionary terms but deleterious in modern environments—may explain why FS manifests as a systemic immunoendocrine disorder rather than a purely local musculoskeletal disease [5,8,14,58]. Thus, the FS phenotype could be reframed as the clinical expression of endocrine–metabolic disintegration rooted in lifestyle and environmental exposures. Recognizing this cascade underscores the urgency of adopting integrative interventions, such as sleep hygiene, stress resilience training, anti-inflammatory and phytonutrient-rich nutrition, regular physical activity, and targeted hormonal rebalancing. These strategies should not be considered ancillary, but rather core therapeutic pillars in the management and prevention of FS.

On the other hand, socio-emotional health and sustained psychosocial stress appear to play a significant role in both the onset and perpetuation of FS symptoms [8]. Recent systematic reviews have shown that pain-related fear and depression are prognostic for disability, function, and pain severity, while anxiety is consistently associated with worse self-reported pain and functional impairment [3]. In perioperative settings, prospective data indicate that preoperative anxiety increases the risk of developing FS after rotator cuff repair, underscoring the importance of psychological factors in secondary shoulder stiffness [30]. From a psychoneuroimmunological perspective, chronic stress sustains HPA axis activation and sympathetic nervous system drive, fostering neuroinflammation, LGI, and increased barrier permeability (e.g., intestinal), all of which amplify systemic immune activation [14]. In FS specifically, psychosocial stressors, circadian disruption, and lifestyle-related factors have been proposed as converging triggers of LGI, fibrotic signaling, and pain sensitization [5,8,14,25,58]. Practically, integrating psychological assessment and targeted interventions—addressing anxiety, depression, catastrophizing, and fear of movement—into rehabilitation may enhance treatment outcomes [3]. This is supported by evidence on the benefits of psychological strategies and pain neuroscience education in musculoskeletal pain and shoulder disorders [189–191].

The Lifestyle Hypothesis: Endothelial Health

Finally, another key pathway linking lifestyle factors to FS pathogenesis is endothelial inflammation and dysfunction [3,30,192,193]. Modern exposures such as poor nutrition, ultra-processed diets, sedentarism, chronic psychosocial stress, sleep disruption, and environmental pollutants elevate circulating inflammatory mediators, homocysteine, oxidized lipids, and particulate toxins [132,194,195]. These factors directly injure the vascular endothelium, leading to reduced nitric oxide (NO) bioavailability and impaired endothelial nitric oxide synthase (eNOS) activity [196,197]. The imbalance between vasodilatory and vasoconstrictive forces promotes oxidative and nitrosative stress, driving the generation of peroxynitrite and other reactive nitrogen species [198,199]. This state of endothelial dysfunction sustains systemic low-grade inflammation while simultaneously producing local microvascular alterations in the shoulder capsule, including impaired perfusion, increased vascular permeability, leukocyte recruitment, and aberrant angiogenesis [26,118]. These events create a permissive environment for fibroblast activation, excessive collagen deposition, and ultimately capsular fibrosis and persistent pain (see Table 2) [22,26].

Table 2. Vascular/Endothelial Dysfunction, NO/AGEs, and FS.

Domain	Study Type	Core Finding	Implication for FS
Endothelial dysfunction (ED)	Clinical (biomarkers/imaging)	ED associated with LGI, dyslipidemia, oxidative stress; impaired microvascular perfusion.	Local hypoperfusion and abnormal angiogenesis → fibrosis and pain.
Nitric oxide (NO) biology	Experimental/Translational	ADMA, homocysteine, ROS/RNS reduce eNOS activity; peroxynitrite ↑ tissue damage.	Impaired NO signaling favors pro-fibrotic environment.
AGEs–RAGE axis	Clinical (FS biopsies)	Elevated AGEs in FS capsules; RAGE/NF-κB activation confirmed.	AGEs act as active mediators of stiffness and fibrosis.
Lipids/inflamed lipoproteins	Clinical (SR/MA, cohorts)	↑ LDL and total cholesterol in FS; ICAM-1 upregulated in capsule.	Vascular inflammation and fibrosis link.

Note: FS = Frozen Shoulder; ED = Endothelial Dysfunction; LGI = Low-Grade Inflammation; ADMA = Asymmetric Dimethylarginine; ROS = Reactive Oxygen Species; RNS = Reactive Nitrogen Species; eNOS = Endothelial Nitric Oxide Synthase; AGEs = Advanced Glycation End-products; RAGE = Receptor for Advanced Glycation End-products; LDL = Low-Density Lipoprotein; ICAM-1 = Intercellular Adhesion Molecule 1.

In parallel, lifestyle-driven disturbances in the gut microbiota further amplify vascular and immune dysregulation [200–202]. Dysbiosis and increased intestinal permeability promote bacterial translocation and the systemic release of pro-inflammatory metabolites, such as lipopolysaccharides (LPS) and asymmetric dimethylarginine (ADMA), the latter being a potent endogenous inhibitor of eNOS [203,204]. Elevated ADMA levels have been strongly associated with impaired NO production, vascular inflammation, and collagen remodeling [204]. In FS, this may synergize with capsular hypoperfusion and aberrant angiogenesis, fostering extracellular matrix stiffening and reduced tissue resilience [118].

The role of AGEs adds another mechanistic layer to this process [82,83]. Chronic hyperglycemia and oxidative stress drive AGE accumulation in connective tissue, where they cross-link collagen fibers, reduce tissue elasticity, and impair remodeling [205]. AGEs also bind to their receptor (RAGE) on endothelial and immune cells, activating NF-κB signaling and perpetuating a cycle of cytokine release, vascular inflammation, and fibroblast proliferation [84,206]. Recent studies in idiopathic FS have confirmed elevated AGE deposition in the shoulder capsule, supporting their pathogenic contribution not only as markers of chronic metabolic imbalance but as active mediators of fibrosis [21,24].

Altogether, these interrelated mechanisms illustrate how lifestyle-related exposures converge at the vascular interface to initiate a primary inflammatory insult at the endothelium [199,207]. This "first hit" propagates into systemic LGI, disrupts hormonal and metabolic regulation, and establishes a molecular milieu favoring fibrosis, pain sensitization, and chronic joint dysfunction [72,127]. Within FS, the endothelial–immune axis therefore represents a critical but underrecognized bridge between lifestyle behaviors, metabolic stress, and the characteristic clinical phenotype of stiffness and pain (see Table 3) [14,58,83].

Table 3. Lifestyle, Psychoneuroimmunology, and Metabolic Drivers.

Domain	Study Type	Core Finding	Implication for FS
Diet & glycemic load	Clinical (SR/MA, cohorts)	HbA1c consistently elevated in FS; high-glycemic/ultra-processed diets → LGI, microbiota dysbiosis.	Diet as modifiable driver; supports anti-inflammatory strategies.
Physical inactivity & sleep	Clinical/Translational	Sedentarism and circadian disruption impair HPA, GH, pain modulation.	Exercise and sleep hygiene key for management.
Psychosocial stress	Clinical (cohorts, RCTs)	Anxiety/depression worsen FS prognosis; psychotherapies improve MSK outcomes.	Supports psychoneuroimmunology-based interventions.
Exposome/EDCs	Experimental/Human observational	BPA, phthalates, cadmium alter ER function and circadian release.	Exposome as overlooked contributor to FS pathogenesis.

Note: FS = Frozen Shoulder; LGI = Low-Grade Inflammation; HbA1c = Glycated Hemoglobin; HPA = Hypothalamic–Pituitary–Adrenal axis; GH = Growth Hormone; RCT = Randomized Controlled Trial; MSK = Musculoskeletal; EDCs = Endocrine-Disrupting Chemicals; BPA = Bisphenol A; ER = Estrogen Receptor.

7. Future Research Directions

The integration of hormonal, metabolic, vascular, and lifestyle factors into the pathophysiological framework of FS underscores the need for a paradigm shift in research. Historically, FS has been examined through orthopedic and localized inflammatory lenses; however, converging evidence supports FS as a systemic immuno–endocrine–metabolic condition—particularly in women—best studied with systems-biology approaches. To provide practical guidance to the field, we delineate short-term, feasible directions and long-term, exploratory programs.

7.1. Short-Term, Feasible Directions (12–24 Months)

(A) Longitudinal endocrine monitoring in routine care

Dynamic profiling of estradiol, progesterone, testosterone, cortisol, thyroid hormones (TSH, T3, T4), leptin, insulin, and melatonin across menopausal and metabolic states to reveal patterns that precede or accompany capsular fibrosis and pain chronification. Couple these measures to pain, function, ROM, and time-to-recovery to generate actionable phenotyping rules.

(B) Endothelial–vascular assessments in FS

Evaluate microvascular flow surrogates together with nitric-oxide metabolism (e.g., NO metabolites, asymmetric dimethylarginine [ADMA]) and endothelial inflammation (e.g., ICAM-1/VCAM-1). Clarify how lifestyle, dysbiosis, and metabolic stress converge on the endothelium to trigger capsular fibrosis.

(C) Sleep and circadian alignment pilots

Use actigraphy plus melatonin/cortisol rhythm analysis to quantify circadian misalignment and test pragmatic interventions (sleep hygiene, evening blue-light restriction, timed light therapy, melatonin where appropriate) on pain, function, and ROM.

(D) Diet-first pragmatic trials

Pilot integrative nutritional strategies—Mediterranean, anti-inflammatory, low-AGE, phytoestrogen-supportive or ketogenic diets—embedded in rehabilitation. Track adherence, HbA1c, lipid fractions, inflammatory mediators, and patient-reported outcomes.

(E) Focused micronutrient add-on trials (women-centric)

Test vitamin D, manganese, and selected B-vitamins (e.g., B1/B3) where observational signals suggest benefit, using short randomized add-on designs to determine effect sizes and feasibility.

(F) Integrative biomarker panels for stratification

Assemble compact panels combining inflammatory (IL-1β, IL-6, TNF-α, HMGB1), metabolic (HbA1c, HOMA-IR, lipid fractions, AGEs), hormonal (estradiol, SHBG, thyroid function) and vascular markers (NO metabolites, ADMA, ICAM-1/VCAM-1) to classify FS subtypes by systemic dysfunction rather than symptoms alone.

7.2. Long-Term, Exploratory Programs (24–60+ Months)

(G) Estrogen deficiency/resistance and receptor-level interference

Undertake tissue and liquid-biopsy studies to assess estrogen receptor density, nuclear localization, phosphorylation status, and downstream signaling (ERK, PI3K/Akt). Determine whether receptor dysfunction causally links to fibroblast activation, immune dysregulation, and impaired matrix repair.

(H) Systems mapping of the vascular–immune–fibrotic axis

Combine vascular imaging/surrogates, NO/ADMA biology, cytokine profiling, and shoulder imaging (US/MRI) to model causal pathways from endothelial dysfunction to fibrosis and pain sensitization.

(I) Chronobiology and sleep as disease modifiers

Run mechanistic trials aligning sleep/wake timing and light exposure with endocrine outputs (estrogen, GH, thyroid, cortisol) to test whether circadian restoration modifies immuno-metabolic signatures and clinical trajectories.

(J) Gut microbiota and the gut–vascular–joint axis

Integrate microbiome sequencing and intestinal permeability assays with metabolomics (including LPS-related and methylarginine pathways) to delineate diet–microbiome–endothelium crosstalk that impairs estrogen and NO signaling.

(K) Multi-omics and precision medicine frameworks

Deploy metabolomic, transcriptomic, and epigenetic profiling to define FS endotypes, enabling adaptive trials that match interventions (dietary, circadian, endothelial support, hormone modulation when appropriate) to molecular phenotypes.

(L) Scalable interventional platforms and implementation science

Progress from efficacy to effectiveness via pragmatic, multi-arm platforms in real-world PT/orthopedic settings; include cost-effectiveness, equity, and adoption metrics to support health-system uptake.

Therefore, FS should no longer be approached as an isolated orthopedic disease but as a systemic disorder in which vascular dysfunction, hormonal imbalance, metabolic stress, and lifestyle exposures converge. A staged research agenda—pairing near-term, pragmatic studies with ambitious, systems-level programs—can deliver stratified, precision-based therapies that target the underlying immuno–endocrine–vascular networks rather than the symptomatic shoulder alone.

To provide a more visual and practice-oriented synthesis of the evidence reviewed, Table 4 summarizes the key clinical signals, underlying mechanistic drivers, and proposed interventions in FS. By distinguishing between established findings supported by clinical studies and emerging hypotheses drawn from experimental or mechanistic research, this table offers a concise framework that bridges basic science and clinical management. Its purpose is to guide clinicians and researchers toward integrative strategies that combine endocrine, metabolic, vascular, and lifestyle perspectives, facilitating translation of complex concepts into practical applications.

Table 4. Established Evidence vs. Emerging Hypotheses in Frozen Shoulder (FS).

Domain	Established Evidence (Human-Focused)	Emerging Hypotheses (Mechanistic/Early Clinical)	Notes/Level of Evidence
Epidemiology & clinical course	Female predominance; peak in peri-menopause/postmenopause; painful capsular stiffness with staged course.	Sex-specific vulnerability linked to estrogen deficiency/resistance; phenotypes differing by metabolic status.	High-quality observational data; sex-hormone linkage under active study.
Histopathology & cytokines	Capsular fibrosis; myofibroblast proliferation; ↑ TGF-β, IL-1β, TNF-α; neoangiogenesis; mast cells.	Alarmins (HMGB1, IL-33, S100A8/9) drive nerve ingrowth and persistent fibrosis.	Multiple biopsy series; alarmin data growing (moderate).
Metabolic biomarkers (glycemia, lipids)	Higher HbA1c and total cholesterol in FS vs. controls (meta-analyses).	AGE–RAGE axis as fibrosis driver; glycation impairs cholesterol traffic → dyslipidemia → hormonal disruption.	Human meta-analyses (strong); mechanistic links plausible (moderate).
Thyroid dysfunction	Hypothyroidism (overt/subclinical) associated with FS; MR studies suggest causal link.	Autoimmune thyroiditis primes chronic inflammatory milieu, amplifying capsular fibrosis.	Systematic reviews & MR (strong); immune amplification (moderate).

Table 4. *Cont.*

Domain	Established Evidence (Human-Focused)	Emerging Hypotheses (Mechanistic/Early Clinical)	Notes/Level of Evidence
Estrogen axis (deficiency/resistance)	Postmenopausal status correlates with worse pain/stiffness; ERs in capsule; estrogen is anti-inflammatory/antifibrotic (indirect clinical support).	Estrogen resistance from LGI/oxidative stress/EDCs; receptor-level interference in capsule tissue.	Human indirect + robust mechanistic data (moderate).
Endothelial dysfunction & NO biology	Endothelial impairment associates with chronic pain states; lifestyle improves endothelial function.	Local microvascular injury in capsule (↓NO/eNOS, ↑ADMA, oxidized LDL) fuels fibrosis & pain.	Human vascular data (moderate); capsule-specific vascular biology emerging (limited–moderate).
Microbiome & gut barrier	Diets high in ultra-processed foods associate with inflammation; gut barrier compromise in chronic pain cohorts.	Dysbiosis → LPS/ADMA → endothelial & ER signaling disruption; gut–joint axis in FS.	Human associative data (moderate); FS-specific data limited.
Psychoneuroimmunology & sleep	Stress, poor sleep linked to worse pain/function; psychoeducation/exercise benefit shoulder pain.	Circadian misalignment → HPA/SNS activation → ER dysfunction and fibrosis.	Human outcomes (moderate); circadian-ER link mechanistic (moderate).
Exposome/EDCs	Population exposure to BPA/phthalates/parabens widespread; endocrine effects documented in humans.	Xenoestrogens cause ER misactivation/desensitization in capsule, promoting fibrosis.	Human exposure strong; FS-targeted evidence limited (emerging).
Adipose tissue dysfunction	Central adiposity associates with systemic inflammation and shoulder pain risk.	Leptin resistance downregulates ERα; adipokines drive fibroblast activation in capsule.	Human association (moderate); cellular mechanisms strong.
Therapeutics—standard care	Exercise therapy, manual therapy, education; injections/hydrodistension as per guidelines.	Stratified care by immunometabolic/endocrine phenotype to personalize response.	High clinical evidence for core PT; precision phenotyping emerging.
Therapeutics—metabolic & endocrine	Diet/exercise improve pain in shoulder disorders; omega-3s analgesic in inflammatory joint pain.	Low-AGE/anti-inflammatory/phytoestrogen diets; circadian therapy; endocrine optimization (thyroid/estrogen) in selected patients.	Mixed clinical evidence (moderate); targeted trials needed.

Note: FS = Frozen Shoulder; ER = Estrogen Receptor; MR = Mendelian randomization; LGI = Low-grade inflammation; AGE = Advanced glycation end-product; RAGE = Receptor for AGE; NO/eNOS = Nitric Oxide/endothelial Nitric Oxide Synthase; ADMA = Asymmetric dimethylarginine; LPS = lipopolysaccharides; HPA = hypothalamic-pituitary-adrenal; SNS = sympathetic nervous system; EDCs = endocrine-disrupting chemicals; PT = physiotherapy.

8. Clinical Implications

The emerging model of FS as a systemic, hormonally modulated inflammatory–fibrotic condition reframes this disorder far beyond a localized joint pathology. In particular, receptor-level dysfunction of estrogen—exacerbated by menopause, metabolic syndrome, thyroid imbalance, endothelial dysfunction, or chronic environmental burden—may explain the greater pain severity, poor responsiveness to rehabilitation, and increased recurrence observed in many patients.

Accordingly, treatment strategies should not remain confined to orthopedic interventions but integrate metabolic, endocrine, vascular, and lifestyle dimensions. Key implications include:

1. Hormonal, metabolic, and vascular evaluation. Routine assessment of sex hormones (estradiol, progesterone, testosterone), thyroid function, cortisol rhythms, HbA1c, lipid profile, inflammatory mediators (e.g., IL-6, TNF-α), and vascular health (NO metabolites, ADMA, ICAM-1/VCAM-1) should be considered, particularly in women over 40 or in patients with metabolic risk factors.
2. Lifestyle assessment and modification. Screening for sleep quality, circadian rhythm disruption, stress levels, physical activity, and dietary habits must become part of FS evaluation. Personalized interventions may include stress reduction strategies (e.g., mindfulness, CBT), structured physical activity programs, and dietary approaches such as anti-inflammatory, low-AGE, or phytoestrogen-rich diets to support estrogen signaling, endothelial health, and systemic metabolic balance.
3. Targeting environmental and metabolic disruptors. Reducing exposure to endocrine-disrupting chemicals (e.g., BPA, phthalates, heavy metals) and addressing insulin and leptin resistance are essential for restoring endocrine sensitivity. Equally important is supporting mitochondrial function and reducing oxidative stress through antioxidant therapies, which may help normalize estrogen receptor activity and endothelial nitric oxide signaling.
4. Gut–vascular–immune axis modulation. Given growing evidence of the role of dysbiosis and intestinal permeability in systemic inflammation, therapeutic approaches including prebiotics, probiotics, and microbiome-targeted nutrition could be explored as adjunctive strategies to mitigate endothelial dysfunction, reduce ADMA levels, and restore immune tolerance.
5. Interdisciplinary management. Optimal care requires collaboration between orthopedic specialists, endocrinologists, physiotherapists, and nutritionists. Selected patients may benefit from hormonal support (e.g., bioidentical hormone therapy), correction of subclinical hypothyroidism, or integrative metabolic therapies following individualized risk–benefit evaluation.
6. Patient education. Empowering patients with knowledge about how nutrition, sleep, stress, hormonal balance, and environmental exposures influence their condition can foster adherence to lifestyle changes, strengthen self-management, and improve long-term outcomes.

Ultimately, this broader perspective reframes FS as an endocrine–metabolic–vascular musculoskeletal disorder, highlighting the need for integrative and personalized interventions that combine rehabilitation with hormonal, nutritional, vascular, and lifestyle strategies—going far beyond intra-articular corticosteroids or manual therapy alone. In order to enhance clinical applicability, Table 5 presents a structured overview of recommended assessments and potential interventions for FS, categorized by mechanistic domain and graded according to available evidence or expert consensus. This table is designed to serve as a practical tool for clinicians, highlighting how evaluation of hormonal, metabolic, vascular, and lifestyle factors can be integrated into standard FS management. By aligning clinical assessment with targeted interventions, it emphasizes the need for an interdisciplinary and personalized approach that extends beyond conventional orthopedic care.

Table 5. Clinical assessment and interventions in Frozen Shoulder (FS) with level of evidence/consensus.

Domain	Clinical Assessments (Recommended)	Interventions (Examples)	Human Clinical Evidence	Experimental/Mechanistic Support
Hormonal—Estrogen/Female axis	Serum estradiol, progesterone, SHBG; menopausal status; vasomotor and sleep symptom scales. (ER polymorphisms for research).	Lifestyle + nutrition to support estrogen balance; phytoestrogens (e.g., soy isoflavones) when appropriate; consider HRT in selected patients per guidelines; vitamin D repletion.	Observational links between menopausal status and FS severity; small trials on phytoestrogens and musculoskeletal symptoms; indirect evidence from shoulder pain cohorts.	Strong evidence of estrogen anti-inflammatory/antifibrotic actions; ER signaling modulates TGF-β/NF-κB; animal & cellular models.
Thyroid axis	TSH, free T4/T3; thyroid autoantibodies (TPOAb/TgAb) if suspected; hypothyroid symptom checklist.	Treat overt/subclinical hypothyroidism per endocrine guidelines; monitor FS outcomes after euthyroid restoration.	Epidemiology, meta-analyses, and Mendelian randomization support association between hypothyroidism and FS.	Thyroid hormones regulate collagen turnover, MMP/TIMP balance, and mitochondrial function in connective tissue.
Metabolic—Glucose/Insulin & Lipids	HbA1c, fasting glucose/insulin, HOMA-IR; lipid profile (LDL-C, HDL-C, TG); body composition/waist circumference.	Anti-inflammatory or low-AGE diet; Mediterranean or low-glycemic patterns; weight optimization; structured exercise; omega-3 supplementation as appropriate.	Meta-analyses show elevated HbA1c and cholesterol in FS; clinical trials in shoulder pain show benefit of diet/exercise on pain/function.	AGE-RAGE activation drives fibrosis; hyperglycemia and dyslipidemia impair ECM and endothelial health (cell/animal studies).
Vascular, Endothelial & NO biology	CRP/IL-6 (systemic context); ADMA (research); endothelial function (flow-mediated dilation) in studies; ICAM-1/VCAM-1 (research).	Mediterranean-style diet; homocysteine lowering (B-vitamins) when deficient; antioxidant/mitochondrial support; aerobic exercise.	Emerging human data linking endothelial dysfunction with shoulder pain states; diet/exercise improve endothelial function.	Mechanistic evidence for NO/eNOS impairment, oxidized LDL, and AGE-RAGE in fibrosis and pain sensitization.
Lifestyle & Circadian health	Sleep quality (PSQI), actigraphy if available; chronotype; stress scales; physical activity (IPAQ/accelerometry); dietary quality (MEDAS).	Sleep/circadian hygiene (reduce light-at-night, regular schedule); stress reduction (mindfulness/CBT); graded activity programs; anti-inflammatory nutrition.	Multiple RCTs in musculoskeletal pain show benefit of exercise and psychoeducation; FS RCTs support multimodal rehab; early trials on circadian interventions.	Psychoneuroimmunology models show stress-immune-pain links; animal/experimental data on circadian disruption and inflammation.
Orthopedic/Physiotherapy core care	Pain (NPRS/VAS), SPADI/DASH, ROM (goniometry), strength; functional goals; imaging when indicated.	Progressive exercise therapy, manual therapy, joint mobilization; education & pacing; consider hydrodistension or injections per guidelines.	Strong evidence base for exercise/manual therapy in FS and shoulder disorders; guideline-endorsed multimodal care.	Biomechanical & neurophysiological models support tissue adaptation and central desensitization with rehab.

Note: FS = Frozen Shoulder; SHBG = Sex Hormone–Binding Globulin; ER = Estrogen Receptor; HRT = Hormone Replacement Therapy; TSH = Thyroid-Stimulating Hormone; TPOAb/TgAb = Thyroid Peroxidase/Thyroglobulin Antibodies; HbA1c = Glycated Hemoglobin; HOMA-IR = Homeostatic Model Assessment of Insulin Resistance; LDL-C/HDL-C/TG = Low-/High-Density Lipoprotein Cholesterol/Triglycerides; AGE = Advanced Glycation End-product; RAGE = Receptor for AGE; NO/eNOS = Nitric Oxide/endothelial Nitric Oxide Synthase; CRP = C-reactive Protein; ICAM-1/VCAM-1 = Intercellular/Vascular Cell Adhesion Molecule-1; PSQI = Pittsburgh Sleep Quality Index; IPAQ = International Physical Activity Questionnaire; NPRS/VAS = Numeric Pain Rating Scale/Visual Analog Scale; SPADI/DASH = Shoulder Pain and Disability Index/Disabilities of the Arm, Shoulder and Hand.

9. Limitations

Because this is a narrative–scoping review, we did not track database-wise record counts or include a PRISMA flow diagram. While this limits replicability at the level of numeric yields, it is consistent with the goals and conventions of narrative synthesis. We mitigated this by (i) pre-specifying mechanistic domains and eligibility logic, (ii) documenting sources and date limits, and (iii) separating clinical and experimental evidence in text and tables. A future systematic review could extend our framework with comprehensive retrieval and quantitative flow reporting.

10. Conclusions

Emerging evidence suggests that FS may extend beyond a purely local capsular disorder toward a systemic, immunometabolic–vascular condition. Across the literature reviewed, dysfunction of the estrogen axis—via deficiency, resistance, or receptor-level interference—appears to act as a key amplifier of fibrosis, nociception, and impaired tissue repair, particularly in women. This hormonal vulnerability often coexists with hyperglycemia and AGEs, dyslipidemia, adipose and thyroid dysfunction, endothelial injury, gut dysbiosis, circadian and sleep disruption, psychosocial stress, and broader exposome burdens. Together, these factors sustain low-grade inflammation and fibro-inflammatory signaling that characterize the FS phenotype of pain and stiffness. Clinically, this points to the need to look beyond strictly orthopedic approaches and incorporate metabolic and hormonal profiling (estradiol, thyroid function, cortisol rhythms, HbA1c, lipid fractions, inflammatory markers) together with endothelial health surrogates, alongside rehabilitation. Integrative strategies such as anti-inflammatory and estrogen-supportive nutrition, sleep and circadian hygiene, stress-reduction approaches, and risk-adapted endocrine support in selected cases, combined with patient education, may improve outcomes and adherence. Future research should prioritize longitudinal endocrine monitoring linked to pain and function, compact diet-first and circadian/sleep interventions embedded in rehabilitation, and pilot studies of endothelial and microvascular markers. Longer-range work should address estrogen-resistance mechanisms in joint-relevant tissues, map the vascular–immune–fibrotic axis with multi-omic tools, and develop precision endotypes that enable phenotype-matched interventions. By reframing FS within a broader neuro–endocrine–immune–metabolic–vascular model, new opportunities may arise for more effective, personalized, and preventive care—particularly for peri- and postmenopausal women who remain disproportionately affected.

Supplementary Materials: The following supporting information can be downloaded at: https://www.mdpi.com/article/10.3390/jcm14207315/s1, Table S1: Search strategy, databases, eligibility criteria, and sources by mechanistic domain.

Funding: This research received no external funding.

Data Availability Statement: No new data were created or analyzed in this study.

Conflicts of Interest: The author declares no conflicts of interest.

References

1. Sophie, A.; Franck, K.; Sebastian, P.; Joe, C.-H.C.; Patrick, S.; Pierre, H.; Alexandre, L. Frozen Shoulder Is Ill-Defined. How Can It Be Described Better? *EFORT Open Rev.* **2020**, *5*, 145–155. [CrossRef]
2. Brindisino, F.; Turgut, E.; Struyf, F. Frozen Shoulder: Exploration of Terminology and Classification. *Front. Rehabil. Sci.* **2024**, *5*, 1498263. [CrossRef] [PubMed]
3. Brindisino, F.; Silvestri, E.; Gallo, C.; Venturin, D.; Di Giacomo, G.; Peebles, A.M.; Provencher, M.T.; Innocenti, T. Depression and Anxiety Are Associated With Worse Subjective and Functional Baseline Scores in Patients With Frozen Shoulder Contracture Syndrome: A Systematic Review. *Arthrosc. Sports Med. Rehabil.* **2022**, *4*, e1219–e1234. [CrossRef]
4. Lewis, J. Frozen Shoulder Contracture Syndrome—Aetiology, Diagnosis and Management. *Man. Ther.* **2015**, *20*, 2–9. [CrossRef]
5. de la Serna, D.; Navarro-Ledesma, S.; Alayón, F.; López, E.; Pruimboom, L. A Comprehensive View of Frozen Shoulder: A Mystery Syndrome. *Front. Med.* **2021**, *8*, 663703. [CrossRef]
6. Sarasua, S.M.; Floyd, S.; Bridges, W.C.; Pill, S.G. The Epidemiology and Etiology of Adhesive Capsulitis in the U.S. Medicare Population. *BMC Musculoskelet. Disord.* **2021**, *22*, 828. [CrossRef]
7. Whelton, C.; Peach, C.A. Review of Diabetic Frozen Shoulder. *Eur. J. Orthop. Surg. Traumatol.* **2018**, *28*, 363–371. [CrossRef]
8. Navarro-Ledesma, S.; Hamed-Hamed, D.; Pruimboom, L. A New Perspective of Frozen Shoulder Pathology; the Interplay between the Brain and the Immune System. *Front. Physiol.* **2024**, *15*, 1248612. [CrossRef] [PubMed]
9. Chen, B.; Zhu, Z.H.; Li, Q.; Zuo, Z.C.; Zhou, K.L. Causal Associations of Hypothyroidism with Frozen Shoulder: A Two-Sample Bidirectional Mendelian Randomization Study. *BMC Musculoskelet. Disord.* **2024**, *25*, 693. [CrossRef]

10. Kean Ann Phua, S.; Si Ning Loh, R.; Tan, B.Y.; Wei Loong Ho, S. Does Concomitant Thyroid Disorder Lead to Worse Outcomes in Frozen Shoulder? A Systematic Review. *J. Shoulder Elb. Surg.* **2025**, *34*, 1322–1330. [CrossRef] [PubMed]
11. Date, A.; Rahman, L. Frozen Shoulder: Overview of Clinical Presentation and Review of the Current Evidence Base for Management Strategies. *Future Sci. OA* **2020**, *6*, FSO647. [CrossRef]
12. Le, H.V.; Lee, S.J.; Nazarian, A.; Rodriguez, E.K. Adhesive Capsulitis of the Shoulder: Review of Pathophysiology and Current Clinical Treatments. *Shoulder Elb.* **2017**, *9*, 75–84. [CrossRef]
13. Page, M.J.; Green, S.; Kramer, S.; Johnston, R.V.; Mcbain, B.; Chau, M.; Buchbinder, R. Manual Therapy and Exercise for Adhesive Capsulitis (Frozen Shoulder). *Cochrane Database Syst. Rev.* **2014**, *2014*. [CrossRef]
14. Navarro-Ledesma, S. Frozen Shoulder as a Metabolic and Immune Disorder: Potential Roles of Leptin Resistance, JAK-STAT Dysregulation, and Fibrosis. *J. Clin. Med.* **2025**, *14*, 1780. [CrossRef]
15. Sharma, R.; Kumari, S.; Thakur, R.; Ranjan, R. Prevalence of Frozen Shoulder in Post-Menopausal Women: A Cross-Sectional Study. *J. Pharm. Negat. Results* **2022**, *13*, 1124–1130. Available online: https://www.pnrjournal.com/index.php/home/article/view/10667 (accessed on 14 October 2025).
16. Xu, J.-W.; Gong, J.; Chang, X.-M.; Luo, J.-Y.; Dong, L.; Hao, Z.-M.; Jia, A.; Xu, G.-P. Estrogen Reduces CCL 4-Induced Liver Fibrosis in Rats. *World J. Gastroenterol.* **2002**, *8*, 883. [CrossRef] [PubMed]
17. Iorga, A.; Umar, S.; Ruffenach, G.; Aryan, L.; Li, J.; Sharma, S.; Motayagheni, N.; Nadadur, R.D.; Bopassa, J.C.; Eghbali, M. Estrogen Rescues Heart Failure through Estrogen Receptor Beta Activation. *Biol. Sex. Differ.* **2018**, *9*, 48. [CrossRef] [PubMed]
18. Ren, L.; Li, F.; Di, Z.; Xiong, Y.; Zhang, S.; Ma, Q.; Bian, X.; Lang, Z.; Ye, Q.; Wang, Y. Estradiol Ameliorates Acute Kidney Ischemia-Reperfusion Injury by Inhibiting the TGF-BRI-SMAD Pathway. *Front. Immunol.* **2022**, *13*, 822604. [CrossRef] [PubMed]
19. Brun, S.P. Idiopathic Frozen Shoulder. *Aust. J. Gen. Pr.* **2019**, *48*, 757–761. [CrossRef]
20. Cho, C.H.; Song, K.S.; Kim, B.S.; Kim, D.H.; Lho, Y.M. Biological Aspect of Pathophysiology for Frozen Shoulder. *Biomed. Res. Int.* **2018**, *2018*, 7274517. [CrossRef]
21. Akbar, M.; McLean, M.; Garcia-Melchor, E.; Crowe, L.A.N.; McMillan, P.; Fazzi, U.G.; Martin, D.; Arthur, A.; Reilly, J.H.; McInnes, I.B.; et al. Fibroblast Activation and Inflammation in Frozen Shoulder. *PLoS ONE* **2019**, *14*, e0215301. [CrossRef]
22. Ng, M.T.H.; Borst, R.; Gacaferi, H.; Davidson, S.; Ackerman, J.E.; Johnson, P.A.; Machado, C.C.; Reekie, I.; Attar, M.; Windell, D.; et al. A Single Cell Atlas of Frozen Shoulder Capsule Identifies Features Associated with Inflammatory Fibrosis Resolution. *Nat. Commun.* **2024**, *15*, 1394. [CrossRef]
23. Struyf, F.; Mertens, M.G.C.A.M.; Navarro-Ledesma, S. Causes of Shoulder Dysfunction in Diabetic Patients: A Review of Literature. *Int. J. Environ. Res. Public Health* **2022**, *19*, 6228. [CrossRef]
24. Hwang, K.R.; Murrell, G.A.C.; Millar, N.L.; Bonar, F.; Lam, P.; Walton, J.R. Advanced Glycation End Products in Idiopathic Frozen Shoulders. *J. Shoulder Elb. Surg.* **2016**, *25*, 981–988. [CrossRef]
25. Kraal, T.; Lübbers, J.; van den Bekerom, M.P.J.; Alessie, J.; van Kooyk, Y.; Eygendaal, D.; Koorevaar, R.C.T. The Puzzling Pathophysiology of Frozen Shoulders—A Scoping Review. *J. Exp. Orthop.* **2020**, *7*, 91. [CrossRef]
26. Bunker, T.D.; Reilly, J.; Baird, K.S.; Hamblen, D.L. Expression of Growth Factors, Cytokines and Matrix Metalloproteinases in Frozen Shoulder. *J. Bone Jt. Surg.—Ser. B* **2000**, *82*, 768–773. [CrossRef]
27. Lho, Y.M.; Ha, E.; Cho, C.H.; Song, K.S.; Min, B.W.; Bae, K.C.; Lee, K.J.; Hwang, I.; Park, H. Bin Inflammatory Cytokines Are Overexpressed in the Subacromial Bursa of Frozen Shoulder. *J. Shoulder Elb. Surg.* **2013**, *22*, 666–672. [CrossRef] [PubMed]
28. Cher, J.Z.B.; Akbar, M.; Kitson, S.; Crowe, L.A.N.; Garcia-Melchor, E.; Hannah, S.C.; McLean, M.; Fazzi, U.G.; Kerr, S.C.; Murrell, G.A.C.; et al. Alarmins in Frozen Shoulder: A Molecular Association Between Inflammation and Pain. *Am. J. Sports Med.* **2018**, *46*, 671–678. [CrossRef] [PubMed]
29. Navarro-Ledesma, S.; Hamed-Hamed, D.; Gonzalez-Muñoz, A.; Pruimboom, L. Impact of Physical Therapy Techniques and Common Interventions on Sleep Quality in Patients with Chronic Pain: A Systematic Review. *Sleep Med. Rev.* **2024**, *76*, 101937. [CrossRef]
30. Brincisino, F.; Rizzo, V.; Dejaco, B.; Andriesse, A.; Verardo, A.; Turolla, A. Association between Pain, Stiffness, Mood, Catastrophizing, and Perceived Social Support, in Subjects with Frozen Shoulder: A Cross-Sectional Study. *Shoulder Elb.* 2025; *ahead of print*. [CrossRef]
31. Wang, Z.; Li, X.; Liu, X.; Yang, Y.; Yan, Y.; Cui, D.; Meng, C.; Ali, M.I.; Zhang, J.; Yao, Z.; et al. Mechanistic Insights into the Anti-Fibrotic Effects of Estrogen via the PI3K-Akt Pathway in Frozen Shoulder. *J. Steroid Biochem. Mol. Biol.* **2025**, *249*, 106701. [CrossRef] [PubMed]
32. Tanriverdi, F.; Silveira, G.; Maccoll, G.S.; Bouloux, P.M.G. The hypothalamic-pituitary-gonadal axis: Immune function and autoimmunity. *J. Endocrinol.* **2003**, *176*, 293–304. [CrossRef]
33. Athnaiel, O.; Cantillo, S.; Paredes, S.; Knezevic, N.N. The Role of Sex Hormones in Pain-Related Conditions. *Int. J. Mol. Sci.* **2023**, *24*, 1866. [CrossRef]
34. Vegeto, E.; Benedusi, V.; Maggi, A. Estrogen Anti-Inflammatory Activity in Brain: A Therapeutic Opportunity for Menopause and Neurodegenerative Diseases. *Front. Neuroendocr.* **2008**, *29*, 507–519. [CrossRef]

35. Ansar Ahmed, S.; Penhale, W.J.; Talal, N. Sex Hormones, Immune Responses, and Autoimmune Diseases Mechanisms of Sex Hormone Action. *Am. J. Pathol.* **1985**, *121*, 531.
36. Maurer, A.J.; Lissounov, A.; Knezevic, I.; Candido, K.D.; Knezevic, N.N. Pain and Sex Hormones: A Review of Current Understanding. *Pain. Manag.* **2016**, *6*, 258–296. [CrossRef]
37. Aloisi, A.M. Gonadal Hormones and Sex Differences in Pain Reactivity. *Clin. J. Pain.* **2003**, *19*, 168–174. [CrossRef]
38. Arjmand, S.; Ilaghi, M.; Sisakht, A.K.; Guldager, M.B.; Wegener, G.; Landau, A.M.; Gjedde, A. Regulation of Mitochondrial Dysfunction by Estrogens and Estrogen Receptors in Alzheimer's Disease: A Focused Review. *Basic. Clin. Pharmacol. Toxicol.* **2024**, *135*, 115–132. [CrossRef] [PubMed]
39. Young, E.; Korszun, A. Sex, Trauma, Stress Hormones and Depression. *Mol. Psychiatry* **2010**, *15*, 23–28. [CrossRef] [PubMed]
40. Handa, R.J.; Mani, S.K.; Uht, R.M. Estrogen Receptors and the Regulation of Neural Stress Responses. *Neuroendocrinology* **2012**, *96*, 111–118. [CrossRef]
41. Rebecca, M. Modulation of Pain by Estrogens. *Pain* **2007**, *132*, S3–S12. [CrossRef] [PubMed]
42. Harding, A.T.; Heaton, N.S. The Impact of Estrogens and Their Receptors on Immunity and Inflammation during Infection. *Cancers* **2022**, *14*, 909. [CrossRef] [PubMed]
43. Chen, Z.; Lan, H.Q.; Liao, Z.H.; Huang, J.W.; Jian, X.T.; Hu, J.; Liao, H. Regulatory T Cells-Centered Regulatory Networks of Skeletal Muscle Inflammation and Regeneration. *Cell Biosci* **2022**, *12*, 112. [CrossRef] [PubMed]
44. Enright, S.; Werstuck, G.H. Investigating the Effects of Sex Hormones on Macrophage Polarization. *Int. J. Mol. Sci.* **2024**, *25*, 951. [CrossRef] [PubMed]
45. Mao, H.; Zhao, X.; Sun, S.C. NF-KB in Inflammation and Cancer. *Cell Mol. Immunol.* **2025**, *22*, 811–839. [CrossRef]
46. Carr, M.C. The Emergence of the Metabolic Syndrome with Menopause. *J. Clin. Endocrinol. Metab.* **2003**, *88*, 2404–2411. [CrossRef]
47. D'Eon, T.M.; Souza, S.C.; Aronovitz, M.; Obin, M.S.; Fried, S.K.; Greenberg, A.S. Estrogen Regulation of Adiposity and Fuel Partitioning: Evidence of Genomic and Non-Genomic Regulation of Lipogenic and Oxidative Pathways. *J. Biol. Chem.* **2005**, *280*, 35983–35991. [CrossRef]
48. Barros, R.P.A.; Gustafsson, J.Å. Estrogen Receptors and the Metabolic Network. *Cell Metab.* **2011**, *14*, 289–299. [CrossRef]
49. Rettberg, J.R.; Yao, J.; Brinton, R.D. Estrogen: A Master Regulator of Bioenergetic Systems in the Brain and Body. *Front. Neuroendocr.* **2014**, *35*, 8–30. [CrossRef]
50. Ryan, V.; Brown, H.; Minns Lowe, C.J.; Lewis, J.S. The Pathophysiology Associated with Primary (Idiopathic) Frozen Shoulder: A Systematic Review. *BMC Musculoskelet. Disord.* **2016**, *17*, 340. [CrossRef]
51. Konarski, W.; Poboży, T.; Hordowicz, M.; Poboży, K.; Domańska, J. Current Concepts of Natural Course and in Management of Frozen Shoulder: A Clinical Overview. *Orthop. Rev.* **2020**, *12*, 186–190. [CrossRef]
52. Ryu, J.D.; Kirpalani, P.A.; Kim, J.M.; Nam, K.H.; Han, C.W.; Han, S.H. Expression of Vascular Endothelial Growth Factor and Angiogenesis in the Diabetic Frozen Shoulder. *J. Shoulder Elb. Surg.* **2006**, *15*, 679–685. [CrossRef]
53. Miller, W.L.; Auchus, R.J. The Molecular Biology, Biochemistry, and Physiology of Human Steroidogenesis and Its Disorders. *Endocr. Rev.* **2011**, *32*, 81–151. [CrossRef]
54. Simons, K.; Ikonen, E. How Cells Handle Cholesterol. *Science* **2000**, *290*, 1721–1726. [CrossRef]
55. Stocco, D.M. The Role of the StAR Protein in Steroidogenesis: Challenges for the Future. *J. Endocrinol.* **2000**, *164*, 247–253. [CrossRef] [PubMed]
56. Miller, W.L. Steroid Hormone Synthesis in Mitochondria. *Mol. Cell Endocrinol.* **2013**, *379*, 62–73. [CrossRef] [PubMed]
57. Labrie, F. All Sex Steroids Are Made Intracellularly in Peripheral Tissues by the Mechanisms of Intracrinology after Menopause. *J. Steroid Biochem. Mol. Biol.* **2015**, *145*, 133–138. [CrossRef]
58. Hamed-Hamed, D.; Rodríguez-Pérez, C.; Pruimboom, L.; Navarro-Ledesma, S. Influence of the Metabolic and Inflammatory Profile in Patients with Frozen Shoulder—Systematic Review and Meta-Analysis. *BMC Musculoskelet. Disord.* **2025**, *26*, 475.
59. Hamed Hamed, D.; Rodríguez-Pérez, C.; Pruimboom, L.; Navarro-Ledesma, S. Relationship Between Metabolic Profile, Pain, and Functionality in Patients with Frozen Shoulder: A Cross-Sectional Study. *Healthcare* **2024**, *12*, 2444. [CrossRef] [PubMed]
60. Lopes-Virella, M.F.; Klein, R.L.; Lyons, T.J.; Stevenson, H.C.; Witztum, J.L. Glycosylation of Low-Density Lipoprotein Enhances Cholesteryl Ester Synthesis in Human Monocyte-Derived Macrophages. *Diabetes* **1988**, *37*, 550–557. [CrossRef]
61. Payne, A.H.; Hales, D.B. Overview of Steroidogenic Enzymes in the Pathway from Cholesterol to Active Steroid Hormones. *Endocr. Rev.* **2004**, *25*, 947–970. [CrossRef]
62. Miller, Y.I.; Choi, S.H.; Wiesner, P.; Fang, L.; Harkewicz, R.; Hartvigsen, K.; Boullier, A.; Gonen, A.; Diehl, C.J.; Que, X.; et al. Oxidation-Specific Epitopes Are Danger-Associated Molecular Patterns Recognized by Pattern Recognition Receptors of Innate Immunity. *Circ. Res.* **2011**, *108*, 235–248. [CrossRef] [PubMed]
63. Seneviratne, A.N.; Sivagurunathan, B.; Monaco, C. Toll-like Receptors and Macrophage Activation in Atherosclerosis. *Clin. Chim. Acta* **2012**, *413*, 3–14. [CrossRef] [PubMed]
64. Wynn, T.A.; Ramalingam, T.R. Mechanisms of Fibrosis: Therapeutic Translation for Fibrotic Disease. *Nat. Med.* **2012**, *18*, 1028–1040. [CrossRef] [PubMed]

65. Schieber, M.; Chandel, N.S. ROS Function in Redox Signaling and Oxidative Stress. *Curr. Biol.* **2014**, *24*, R453–R462. [CrossRef]
66. Lubis, A.M.T.; Lubis, V.K. Matrix Metalloproteinase, Tissue Inhibitor of Metalloproteinase and Transforming Growth Factor-Beta 1 in Frozen Shoulder, and Their Changes as Response to Intensive Stretching and Supervised Neglect Exercise. *J. Orthop. Sci.* **2013**, *18*, 519–527. [CrossRef]
67. Simpson, E.R. Sources of Estrogen and Their Importance. *J. Steroid Biochem. Mol. Biol.* **2003**, *86*, 225–230. [CrossRef]
68. Nilsson, S.; Gustafsson, J.Å. Estrogen Receptors: Therapies Targeted to Receptor Subtypes. *Clin. Pharmacol. Ther.* **2011**, *89*, 44–55. [CrossRef]
69. Au, A.; Feher, A.; McPhee, L.; Jessa, A.; Oh, S.; Einstein, G. Estrogens, Inflammation and Cognition. *Front. Neuroendocr.* **2016**, *40*, 87–100. [CrossRef]
70. Chakraborty, B.; Byemerwa, J.; Krebs, T.; Lim, F.; Chang, C.Y.; McDonnell, D.P. Estrogen Receptor Signaling in the Immune System. *Endocr. Rev.* **2023**, *44*, 117–141. [CrossRef]
71. Mauvais-Jarvis, F. Estrogen and Androgen Receptors: Regulators of Fuel Homeostasis and Emerging Targets for Diabetes and Obesity. *Trends Endocrinol. Metab.* **2011**, *22*, 24–33. [CrossRef]
72. Hotamisligil, G.S. Inflammation, Metaflammation and Immunometabolic Disorders. *Nature* **2017**, *542*, 177–185. [CrossRef]
73. Mauvais-Jarvis, F.; Manson, J.A.E.; Stevenson, J.C.; Fonseca, V.A. Menopausal Hormone Therapy and Type 2 Diabetes Prevention: Evidence, Mechanisms, and Clinical Implications. *Endocr. Rev.* **2017**, *38*, 173–188. [CrossRef]
74. Zore, T.; Palafox, M.; Reue, K. Sex Differences in Obesity, Lipid Metabolism, and Inflammation—A Role for the Sex Chromosomes? *Mol. Metab.* **2018**, *15*, 35–44. [CrossRef]
75. Nilsen, J.; Diaz Brinton, R. Impact of Progestins on Estrogen-Induced Neuroprotection: Synergy by Progesterone and 19-Norprogesterone and Antagonism by Medroxyprogesterone Acetate. *Endocrinology* **2002**, *143*, 205–212. [CrossRef] [PubMed]
76. Bao, A.M.; Liu, R.Y.; van Someren, E.J.W.; Hofman, M.A.; Cao, Y.X.; Zhou, J.N. Diurnal Rhythm of Free Estradiol during the Menstrual Cycle. *Eur. J. Endocrinol.* **2003**, *148*, 227–232. [CrossRef]
77. Lok, R.; Qian, J.; Chellappa, S.L. Sex Differences in Sleep, Circadian Rhythms, and Metabolism: Implications for Precision Medicine. *Sleep Med. Rev.* **2024**, *75*, 101926. [CrossRef] [PubMed]
78. Bailey, M.; Silver, R. Sex Differences in Circadian Timing Systems: Implications for Disease. *Front. Neuroendocr.* **2014**, *35*, 111–139. [CrossRef] [PubMed]
79. Gamble, K.L.; Resuehr, D.; Johnson, C.H. Shift Work and Circadian Dysregulation of Reproduction. *Front. Endocrinol.* **2013**, *4*, 92. [CrossRef]
80. Logan, R.W.; McClung, C.A. Rhythms of Life: Circadian Disruption and Brain Disorders across the Lifespan. *Nat. Rev. Neurosci.* **2019**, *20*, 49–65. [CrossRef]
81. Hale, G.E.; Zhao, X.; Hughes, C.L.; Burger, H.G.; Robertson, D.M.; Fraser, I.S. Endocrine Features of Menstrual Cycles in Middle and Late Reproductive Age and the Menopausal Transition Classified According to the Staging of Reproductive Aging Workshop (STRAW) Staging System. *J. Clin. Endocrinol. Metab.* **2007**, *92*, 3060–3067. [CrossRef]
82. Asadipooya, K.; Uy, E.M. Advanced Glycation End Products (AGEs), Receptor for AGEs, Diabetes, and Bone: Review of the Literature. *J. Endocr. Soc.* **2019**, *3*, 1799–1818. [CrossRef]
83. Rhee, S.Y.; Kim, Y.S. The Role of Advanced Glycation End Products in Diabetic Vascular Complications. *Diabetes Metab. J.* **2018**, *42*, 188–195. [CrossRef]
84. Yano, T.; Hagiwara, Y.; Ando, A.; Kanazawa, K.; Koide, M.; Sekiguchi, T.; Itaya, N.; Onoki, T.; Suzuki, K.; Tsuchiya, M.; et al. RAGE-Dependent NF-KB Inflammation Processes in the Capsule of Frozen Shoulders. *J. Shoulder Elb. Surg.* **2020**, *29*, 1884–1891. [CrossRef]
85. Guo, Q.; Jin, Y.; Chen, X.; Ye, X.; Shen, X.; Lin, M.; Zeng, C.; Zhou, T.; Zhang, J. NF-KB in Biology and Targeted Therapy: New Insights and Translational Implications. *Signal Transduct. Target Ther.* **2024**, *9*, 53. [CrossRef] [PubMed]
86. Xu, L.; Wang, Y.R.; Li, P.C.; Feng, B. Advanced Glycation End Products Increase Lipids Accumulation in Macrophages through Upregulation of Receptor of Advanced Glycation End Products: Increasing Uptake, Esterification and Decreasing Efflux of Cholesterol. *Lipids Health Dis.* **2016**, *15*, 161. [CrossRef]
87. Miller, W.L.; Bose, H.S. Early Steps in Steroidogenesis: Intracellular Cholesterol Trafficking. *J. Lipid Res.* **2011**, *52*, 2111–2135. [CrossRef] [PubMed]
88. Jiang, H.; Zhou, Y.; Nabavi, S.M.; Sahebkar, A.; Little, P.J.; Xu, S.; Weng, J.; Ge, J. Mechanisms of Oxidized LDL-Mediated Endothelial Dysfunction and Its Consequences for the Development of Atherosclerosis. *Front. Cardiovasc Med.* **2022**, *9*, 925923. [CrossRef] [PubMed]
89. Kilic, G.; Alvarez-Mercado, A.I.; Zarrouki, B.; Opland, D.; Liew, C.W.; Alonso, L.C.; Myers, M.G.; Jonas, J.C.; Poitout, V.; Kulkarni, R.N.; et al. The Islet Estrogen Receptor-α Is Induced by Hyperglycemia and Protects against Oxidative Stress-Induced Insulin-Deficient Diabetes. *PLoS ONE* **2014**, *9*, e87941. [CrossRef]
90. Chakrabarti, S.; Davidge, S.T. High Glucose-Induced Oxidative Stress Alters Estrogen Effects on ERα and ERβ in Human Endothelial Cells: Reversal by AMPK Activator. *J. Steroid Biochem. Mol. Biol.* **2009**, *117*, 99–106. [CrossRef]

91. Hu, J.; Zhang, Z.; Shen, W.J.; Azhar, S. Cellular Cholesterol Delivery, Intracellular Processing and Utilization for Biosynthesis of Steroid Hormones. *Nutr. Metab.* **2010**, *7*, 47. [CrossRef]
92. Pérez-Montilla, J.J.; Guzmán-García, R.; Pruimboom, L.; Navarro-Ledesma, S. Does Leptin and Insulin Levels Influence Pain and Disability in Subjects With Frozen Shoulder? A Cross-Sectional Study. *Eur. J. Pain.* **2025**, *29*, e70007. [CrossRef]
93. Savage, D.B.; Petersen, K.F.; Shulman, G.I. Disordered Lipid Metabolism and the Pathogenesis of Insulin Resistance. *Physiol. Rev.* **2007**, *87*, 507–520. [CrossRef]
94. Vona, R.; Gambardella, L.; Cittadini, C.; Straface, E.; Pietraforte, D. Biomarkers of Oxidative Stress in Metabolic Syndrome and Associated Diseases. *Oxid Med. Cell Longev.* **2019**, *2019*, 8267234. [CrossRef] [PubMed]
95. He, S.; Nelson, E.R. 27-Hydroxycholesterol, an Endogenous Selective Estrogen Receptor Modulator. *Maturitas* **2017**, *104*, 29–35. [CrossRef]
96. Ouchi, N.; Parker, J.L.; Lugus, J.J.; Walsh, K. Adipokines in Inflammation and Metabolic Disease. *Nat. Rev. Immunol.* **2011**, *11*, 85–97. [CrossRef] [PubMed]
97. Austin, D.C.; Gans, I.; Park, M.J.; Carey, J.L.; Kelly, J.D. The Association of Metabolic Syndrome Markers with Adhesive Capsulitis. *J. Shoulder Elb. Surg.* **2014**, *23*, 1043–1051. [CrossRef]
98. Raut, P.K.; Choi, D.Y.; Kim, S.H.; Hong, J.T.; Kwon, T.K.; Jeong, J.H.; Park, P.-H. Estrogen Receptor Signaling Mediates Leptin-Induced Growth of Breast Cancer Cells via Autophagy Induction. *Oncotarget* **2017**, *8*, 109417. [CrossRef]
99. Kirichenko, T.V.; Markina, Y.V.; Bogatyreva, A.I.; Tolstik, T.V.; Varaeva, Y.R.; Starodubova, A.V. The Role of Adipokines in Inflammatory Mechanisms of Obesity. *Int. J. Mol. Sci.* **2022**, *23*, 14982. [CrossRef]
100. Dama, A.; Baggio, C.; Boscaro, C.; Albiero, M.; Cignarella, A. Estrogen Receptor Functions and Pathways at the Vascular Immune Interface. *Int. J. Mol. Sci.* **2021**, *22*, 4254. [CrossRef] [PubMed]
101. Da Silva, R.P.; Zampieri, T.T.; Pedroso, J.A.B.; Nagaishi, V.S.; Ramos-Lobo, A.M.; Furigo, I.C.; Câmara, N.O.; Frazão, R.; Donato, J. Leptin Resistance Is Not the Primary Cause of Weight Gain Associated with Reduced Sex Hormone Levels in Female Mice. *Endocrinology* **2014**, *155*, 4226–4236. [CrossRef]
102. Zheng, J.; Du, M.; Ye, W.; Xie, J.; Zhang, P.; Huang, C.; Lin, H. Editorial: Molecular Mechanisms and Therapeutic Strategies in Inflammation. *Front. Immunol.* **2025**, *16*. [CrossRef]
103. Hetemäki, N.; Robciuc, A.; Vihma, V.; Haanpää, M.; Hämäläinen, E.; Tikkanen, M.J.; Mikkola, T.S.; Savolainen-Peltonen, H. Adipose Tissue Sex Steroids in Postmenopausal Women With and Without Menopausal Hormone Therapy. *J. Clin. Endocrinol. Metab.* **2025**, *110*, 511–522. [CrossRef] [PubMed]
104. Yuxin, L.; Chen, L.; Xiaoxia, L.; Yue, L.; Junjie, L.; Youzhu, L.; Huiliang, Z.; Qicai, L. Research Progress on the Relationship between Obesity-Inflammation-Aromatase Axis and Male Infertility. *Oxid Med. Cell Longev.* **2021**, *2021*, 6612796. [CrossRef] [PubMed]
105. Mair, K.M.; Gaw, R.; MacLean, M.R. Obesity, Estrogens and Adipose Tissue Dysfunction—Implications for Pulmonary Arterial Hypertension. *Pulm. Circ.* **2020**, *10*, 2045894020952019. [CrossRef]
106. Hsieh, C.-C.; Hernández-Ledesma, B.; Kuryłowicz, A. Estrogens in Adipose Tissue Physiology and Obesity-Related Dysfunction. *Biomedicines* **2023**, *11*, 690. [CrossRef]
107. Blüher, M. Importance of Estrogen Receptors in Adipose Tissue Function. *Mol. Metab.* **2013**, *2*, 130–132. [CrossRef]
108. Eaton, S.A.; Sethi, J.K. Immunometabolic Links between Estrogen, Adipose Tissue and Female Reproductive Metabolism. *Biology* **2019**, *8*, 8. [CrossRef] [PubMed]
109. Steiner, B.M.; Berry, D.C. The Regulation of Adipose Tissue Health by Estrogens. *Front. Endocrinol.* **2022**, *13*, 889923. [CrossRef]
110. Liu, W.; Yu, M.; Xie, D.; Wang, L.; Ye, C.; Zhu, Q.; Liu, F.; Yang, L. Melatonin-Stimulated MSC-Derived Exosomes Improve Diabetic Wound Healing through Regulating Macrophage M1 and M2 Polarization by Targeting the PTEN/AKT Pathway. *Stem Cell Res. Ther.* **2020**, *11*, 259. [CrossRef]
111. Bianchi, M.E. DAMPs, PAMPs and Alarmins: All We Need to Know about Danger. *J. Leukoc. Biol.* **2007**, *81*, 1–5. [CrossRef]
112. Moosmann, B.; Behl, C. The Antioxidant Neuroprotective Effects of Estrogens and Phenolic Compounds Are Independent from Their Estrogenic Properties. *Proc. Natl. Acad. Sci. USA* **1999**, *96*, 8867–8872. [CrossRef]
113. Chen, Q.; Zhang, W.; Sadana, N.; Chen, X. Estrogen Receptors in Pain Modulation: Cellular Signaling. *Biol. Sex Differ.* **2021**, *12*, 22. [CrossRef]
114. Longo, U.G.; Mazzola, A.; Carotti, S.; Francesconi, M.; Catapano, S.; Magrì, F.; Perrone, G.; Morini, S.; De Salvatore, S.; Denaro, V. The Role of Estrogen and Progesterone Receptors in the Rotator Cuff Disease: A Retrospective Cohort Study. *BMC Musculoskelet. Disord.* **2021**, *22*, 891. [CrossRef]
115. Xu, J.; Wang, F.; Li, Y.; Huang, Y.; Li, P.; Zhang, Y.; Xu, G.; Sun, K. Estrogen Inhibits TGF-B1-Stimulated Cardiac Fibroblast Differentiation and Collagen Synthesis by Promoting Cdc42. *Mol. Med. Rep.* **2024**, *30*, 123. [CrossRef]
116. Batty, M.J.; Chabrier, G.; Sheridan, A.; Gage, M.C. Metabolic Hormones Modulate Macrophage Inflammatory Responses. *Cancers* **2021**, *13*, 4661. [CrossRef] [PubMed]

117. Belbool, A.; Ashworth, J.; Fadel, A.; Mcloughlin, J.; Mahmoud, A.; El Mohtadi, M. Estrogen Induces the Alternative Activation of Macrophages through Binding to Estrogen Receptor-Alpha. *Exp. Mol. Pathol.* **2025**, *143*, 104971. [CrossRef] [PubMed]
118. Mafu, T.S.; September, A.V.; Shamley, D. The Potential Role of Angiogenesis in the Development of Shoulder Pain, Shoulder Dysfunction, and Lymphedema after Breast Cancer Treatment. *Cancer Manag. Res.* **2018**, *10*, 81–90. [CrossRef]
119. Kumar, M.; Sarma, D.K.; Shubham, S.; Kumawat, M.; Verma, V.; Prakash, A.; Tiwari, R. Environmental Endocrine-Disrupting Chemical Exposure: Role in Non-Communicable Diseases. *Front. Public Health* **2020**, *8*, 553850. [CrossRef] [PubMed]
120. Gupta, R.; Kumar, P.; Fahmi, N.; Garg, B.; Dutta, S.; Sachar, S.; Matharu, A.S.; Vimaleswaran, K.S. Endocrine Disruption and Obesity: A Current Review on Environmental Obesogens. *Curr. Res. Green Sustain. Chem.* **2020**, *3*, 100009. [CrossRef]
121. La Merrill, M.A.; Vandenberg, L.N.; Smith, M.T.; Goodson, W.; Browne, P.; Patisaul, H.B.; Guyton, K.Z.; Kortenkamp, A.; Cogliano, V.J.; Woodruff, T.J.; et al. Consensus on the Key Characteristics of Endocrine-Disrupting Chemicals as a Basis for Hazard Identification. *Nat. Rev. Endocrinol.* **2020**, *16*, 45–57. [CrossRef]
122. Heindel, J.J.; Blumberg, B. Environmental Obesogens: Mechanisms and Controversies. *Annu. Rev. Pharmacol. Toxicol.* **2019**, *59*, 89–106. [CrossRef] [PubMed]
123. Thambirajah, A.A.; Wade, M.G.; Verreault, J.; Buisine, N.; Alves, V.A.; Langlois, V.S.; Helbing, C.C. Disruption by Stealth—Interference of Endocrine Disrupting Chemicals on Hormonal Crosstalk with Thyroid Axis Function in Humans and Other Animals. *Environ. Res.* **2022**, *203*, 111906. [CrossRef]
124. Tamai, K.; Hamada, J.; Nagase, Y.; Morishige, M.; Naito, M.; Asai, H.; Tanaka, S. Frozen Shoulder. An Overview of Pathology and Biology with Hopes to Novel Drug Therapies. *Mod. Rheumatol.* **2024**, *34*, 439–443. [CrossRef] [PubMed]
125. Cutolo, M.; Capellino, S.; Sulli, A.; Serioli, B.; Secchi, M.E.; Villaggio, B.; Straub, R.H. Estrogens and autoimmune diseases. *Ann. N Y Acad. Sci.* **2006**, *1089*, 538–547. [CrossRef] [PubMed]
126. Pruimboom, L.; Alayon Rocio, F.; Navarro-Ledesma, S. Psychoneuroimmunology in the Daily Clinic Is Only Possible Within a Contextual Frame. In *PsychoNeuroImmunology: Integration of Psychology, Neurology, and Immunology*; Springer Nature: Berlin/Heidelberg, Germany, 2025; Volume 1, pp. 515–563.
127. Furman, D.; Campisi, J.; Verdin, E.; Carrera-Bastos, P.; Targ, S.; Franceschi, C.; Ferrucci, L.; Gilroy, D.W.; Fasano, A.; Miller, G.W.; et al. Chronic Inflammation in the Etiology of Disease across the Life Span. *Nat. Med.* **2019**, *25*, 1822–1832. [CrossRef]
128. De Punder, K.; Pruimboom, L. Stress Induces Endotoxemia and Low-Grade Inflammation by Increasing Barrier Permeability. *Front. Immunol.* **2015**, *6*, 223. [CrossRef]
129. Bosma-Den Boer, M.M.; Van Wetten, M.L.; Pruimboom, L. Chronic Inflammatory Diseases Are Stimulated by Current Lifestyle: How Diet, Stress Levels and Medication Prevent Our Body from Recovering. *Nutr. Metab.* **2012**, *9*, 32. [CrossRef] [PubMed]
130. Libby, P. Inflammation in Atherosclerosis—No Longer a Theory. *Clin. Chem.* **2021**, *67*, 131–142. [CrossRef]
131. Dai, M.; Mei, B.; Zheng, F.; Ballestar, E. Sex Hormones and Epigenetic Dysregulation in Autoimmune Disease. *Curr. Opin. Immunol.* **2025**, *95*, 102595. [CrossRef]
132. Tristan Asensi, M.; Napoletano, A.; Sofi, F.; Dinu, M. Low-Grade Inflammation and Ultra-Processed Foods Consumption: A Review. *Nutrients* **2023**, *15*, 1546. [CrossRef]
133. Lane, M.M.; Davis, J.A.; Beattie, S.; Gómez-Donoso, C.; Loughman, A.; O'Neil, A.; Jacka, F.; Berk, M.; Page, R.; Marx, W.; et al. Ultraprocessed Food and Chronic Noncommunicable Diseases: A Systematic Review and Meta-Analysis of 43 Observational Studies. *Obes. Rev.* **2021**, *22*, e13146. [CrossRef]
134. Ludwig, D.S. The Glycemic Index Physiological Mechanisms Relating to Obesity, Diabetes, and Cardiovascular Disease. *Jama* **2002**, *287*, 2414–2423. [CrossRef]
135. Simopoulos, A.P. The Importance of the Omega-6/Omega-3 Fatty Acid Ratio in Cardiovascular Disease and Other Chronic Diseases. *Exp. Biol. Med.* **2008**, *233*, 674–688. [CrossRef] [PubMed]
136. Valdes, A.M.; Walter, J.; Segal, E.; Spector, T.D. Role of the Gut Microbiota in Nutrition and Health. *BMJ* **2018**, *361*, 36–44. [CrossRef]
137. Liu, Z.; Xiao, T.; Liu, H. Leptin Signaling and Its Central Role in Energy Homeostasis. *Front. Neurosci.* **2023**, *17*, 1238528. [CrossRef] [PubMed]
138. Casanova, A.; Wevers, A.; Navarro-Ledesma, S.; Pruimboom, L. Mitochondria: It Is All about Energy. *Front. Physiol.* **2023**, *14*, 1114231. [CrossRef] [PubMed]
139. Bajbouj, K.; Shafarin, J.; Taneera, J.; Hamad, M. Estrogen Signaling Induces Mitochondrial Dysfunction-Associated Autophagy and Senescence in Breast Cancer Cells. *Biology* **2020**, *9*, 68. [CrossRef]
140. Vianello, E.; Beltrami, A.P.; Aleksova, A.; Janjusevic, M.; Fluca, A.L.; Corsi Romanelli, M.M.; La Sala, L.; Dozio, E. The Advanced Glycation End-Products (AGE)–Receptor for AGE System (RAGE): An Inflammatory Pathway Linking Obesity and Cardiovascular Diseases. *Int. J. Mol. Sci.* **2025**, *26*, 3707. [CrossRef]
141. Palmisano, B.T.; Zhu, L.; Stafford, J.M. Role of Estrogens in the Regulation of Liver Lipid Metabolism. In *Advances in Experimental Medicine and Biology*; Springer: New York, NY, USA, 2017; Volume 1043, pp. 227–256.
142. Xiao, Z.; Liu, H. The Estrogen Receptor and Metabolism. *Women's Health* **2024**, *20*, 17455057241227362. [CrossRef]

143. Mahboobifard, F.; Pourgholami, M.H.; Jorjani, M.; Dargahi, L.; Amiri, M.; Sadeghi, S.; Tehrani, F.R. Estrogen as a Key Regulator of Energy Homeostasis and Metabolic Health. *Biomed. Pharmacother.* **2022**, *156*, 113808. [CrossRef]
144. Safe, S.; Kim, K. Non-Classical Genomic Estrogen Receptor (ER)/Specificity Protein and ER/Activating Protein-1 Signaling Pathways. *J. Mol. Endocrinol.* **2008**, *41*, 263–275. [CrossRef]
145. Oakley, R.H.; Cidlowski, J.A. The Biology of the Glucocorticoid Receptor: New Signaling Mechanisms in Health and Disease. *J. Allergy Clin. Immunol.* **2013**, *132*, 1033–1044. [CrossRef]
146. Eckschlager, T.; Plch, J.; Stiborova, M.; Hrabeta, J. Histone Deacetylase Inhibitors as Anticancer Drugs. *Int. J. Mol. Sci.* **2017**, *18*, 1414. [CrossRef]
147. Bulun, S.E.; Simpson, E.R. Regulation of Aromatase Expression in Human Tissues. *Breast Cancer Res. Treat.* **1994**, *30*, 19–29. [CrossRef]
148. Fattahi, R.; Chamkhorami, F.M.; Taghipour, N.; Keshel, S.H. The Effect of Extracellular Matrix Remodeling on Material-Based Strategies for Bone Regeneration: Review Article. *Tissue Cell* **2022**, *76*, 101748. [CrossRef]
149. Zomer, H.D.; Cooke, P.S. Targeting Estrogen Signaling and Biosynthesis for Aged Skin Repair. *Front. Physiol.* **2023**, *14*, 1281071. [CrossRef]
150. Jung, U.J.; Choi, M.S. Obesity and Its Metabolic Complications: The Role of Adipokines and the Relationship between Obesity, Inflammation, Insulin Resistance, Dyslipidemia and Nonalcoholic Fatty Liver Disease. *Int. J. Mol. Sci.* **2014**, *15*, 6184–6223. [CrossRef]
151. Dong, W.; Peng, Q.; Liu, Z.; Xie, Z.; Guo, X.; Li, Y.; Chen, C. Estrogen Plays an Important Role by Influencing the NLRP3 Inflammasome. *Biomed. Pharmacother.* **2023**, *167*, 115554. [CrossRef] [PubMed]
152. Tan, C.K.; Chong, H.C.; Tan, E.H.P.; Tan, N.S. Getting "Smad" about Obesity and Diabetes. *Nutr. Diabetes* **2012**, *2*, e29. [CrossRef] [PubMed]
153. Atasoy-Zeybek, A.; Showel, K.K.; Nagelli, C.V.; Westendorf, J.J.; Evans, C.H. The Intersection of Aging and Estrogen in Osteoarthritis. *npj Women's Health* **2025**, *3*, 15. [CrossRef] [PubMed]
154. Bottalico, L.N.; Weljie, A.M. Cross-Species Physiological Interactions of Endocrine Disrupting Chemicals with the Circadian Clock. *Gen. Comp. Endocrinol.* **2021**, *301*, 113650. [CrossRef] [PubMed]
155. Bansal, A.; Henao-Mejia, J.; Simmons, R.A. Immune System: An Emerging Player in Mediating Effects of Endocrine Disruptors on Metabolic Health. *Endocrinology* **2018**, *159*, 32–45. [CrossRef] [PubMed]
156. Koop, S.; Oster, H. Eat, Sleep, Repeat—Endocrine Regulation of Behavioural Circadian Rhythms. *FEBS J.* **2022**, *289*, 6543–6558. [CrossRef]
157. Alvord, V.M.; Kantra, E.J.; Pendergast, J.S. Estrogens and the Circadian System. *Semin. Cell Dev. Biol.* **2022**, *126*, 56–65. [CrossRef]
158. Guzmán-García, R.; Pérez-Montalbán, M.; Pruimboom, L.; Navarro-Ledesma, S. Impact of a Multimodal Intervention Combining Manual Therapy, Exercise, Reduced Methylxanthine Intake, and Nocturnal Light Avoidance on Inflammatory and Metabolic Profiles, Pain, Functionality, and Sleep Quality in Patients with Frozen Shoulder: A Single-Blind Randomized Controlled Trial. *J. Clin. Med.* **2025**, *14*, 4539. [CrossRef]
159. Beroukhim, G.; Esencan, E.; Seifer, D.B. Impact of Sleep Patterns upon female neuroendocrinology and Reproductive Outcomes: A Comprehensive Review. *Reprod. Biol. Endocrinol.* **2022**, *20*, 16. [CrossRef]
160. Kim, T.W.; Jeong, J.H.; Hong, S.C. The Impact of Sleep and Circadian Disturbance on Hormones and Metabolism. *Int. J. Endocrinol.* **2015**, *2015*, 591729. [CrossRef]
161. Zhou, P.; Li, H.; Li, H.; Chen, Y.; Lv, Y. A Possible Important Regulatory Role of Estrogen in Obstructive Sleep Apnea Hypoventilation Syndrome. *Front. Med.* **2025**, *12*, 1369393. [CrossRef]
162. Carter, E. Examining the Effects of Cortisol on Insulin. *Endocrinol. Diabetes Res.* **2024**, *10*, 5.
163. Unluhizarci, K.; Karaca, Z.; Kelestimur, F. Role of Insulin and Insulin Resistance in Androgen Excess Disorders. *World J. Diabetes* **2021**, *12*, 616–629. [CrossRef] [PubMed]
164. González-González, A.; Mediavilla, M.D.; Sánchez-Barceló, E.J. Melatonin: A Molecule for Reducing Breast Cancer Risk. *Molecules* **2018**, *23*, 336. [CrossRef]
165. Huang, W.; Zheng, J.; Wang, M.; Du, L.Y.; Bai, L.; Tang, H. The Potential Therapeutic Role of Melatonin in Organ Fibrosis: A Comprehensive Review. *Front. Med.* **2024**, *11*, 1502368. [CrossRef] [PubMed]
166. Chang, A.M.; Aeschbach, D.; Duffy, J.F.; Czeisler, C.A. Evening Use of Light-Emitting EReaders Negatively Affects Sleep, Circadian Timing, and next-Morning Alertness. *Proc. Natl. Acad. Sci. USA* **2015**, *112*, 1232–1237. [CrossRef] [PubMed]
167. Irwin, M.R. Sleep and Inflammation: Partners in Sickness and in Health. *Nat. Rev. Immunol.* **2019**, *19*, 702–715. [CrossRef]
168. Schiefer, M.; Teixeira, P.F.S.; Fontenelle, C.; Carminatti, T.; Santos, D.A.; Righi, L.D.; Conceição, F.L. Prevalence of Hypothyroidism in Patients with Frozen Shoulder. *J. Shoulder Elb. Surg.* **2017**, *26*, 49–55. [CrossRef]
169. Tran, M.; Stovitz, S.D. Prevalence of Diabetes Mellitus and Thyroid Disease in Patients Diagnosed with Adhesive Capsulitis (Frozen Shoulder). *Ann. Sports Med. Res.* **2021**, *8*, 1178.

170. Chuang, S.H.; Chen, Y.P.; Huang, S.W.; Kuo, Y.J. Association between Adhesive Capsulitis and Thyroid Disease: A Meta-Analysis. *J. Shoulder Elb. Surg.* **2023**, *32*, 1314–1322. [CrossRef] [PubMed]
171. Alonso-Merino, E.; Orozco, R.M.; Ruíz-Llorente, L.; Martínez-Iglesias, O.A.; Velasco-Martín, J.P.; Montero-Pedrazuela, A.; Fanjul-Rodríguez, L.; Contreras-Jurado, C.; Regadera, J.; Aranda, A. Thyroid Hormones Inhibit TGF-β Signaling and Attenuate Fibrotic Responses. *Proc. Natl. Acad. Sci. USA* **2016**, *113*, E3451–E3460. [CrossRef]
172. El Amrousy, D.; El-Afify, D.; Salah, S. Insulin Resistance, Leptin and Adiponectin in Lean and Hypothyroid Children and Adolescents with Obesity. *BMC Pediatr.* **2022**, *22*, 245. [CrossRef]
173. Trotta, M.C.; Esposito, D.; Carotenuto, R.; di Fraia, R.; Selvaggio, L.D.; Allosso, F.; Russo, M.; Accardo, G.; Alfano, R.; D'Amico, M.; et al. Thyroid Dysfunction in Hashimoto's Thyroiditis: A Pilot Study on the Putative Role of MiR-29a and TGFβ1. *Endocrine* **2024**, *86*, 1090–1096. [CrossRef]
174. Brown, E.D.L.; Obeng-Gyasi, B.; Hall, J.E.; Shekhar, S. The Thyroid Hormone Axis and Female Reproduction. *Int. J. Mol. Sci.* **2023**, *24*, 9815. [CrossRef]
175. Kjaergaard, A.D.; Marouli, E.; Papadopoulou, A.; Deloukas, P.; Kuś, A.; Sterenborg, R.; Teumer, A.; Burgess, S.; Åsvold, B.O.; Chasman, D.I.; et al. Thyroid Function, Sex Hormones and Sexual Function: A Mendelian Randomization Study. *Eur. J. Epidemiol.* **2021**, *36*, 335–344. [CrossRef]
176. Sutkowska, E.; Kisiel, M.; Zubkiewicz-Kucharska, A. When Should the Treatment of Obesity in Thyroid Disease Begin? *Biomedicines* **2025**, *13*, 157. [CrossRef]
177. Song, C.H.; Kim, N.; Kim, D.H.; Lee, H.N.; Surh, Y.J. 17-β Estradiol Exerts Anti-Inflammatory Effects through Activation of Nrf2 in Mouse Embryonic Fibroblasts. *PLoS ONE* **2019**, *14*, e0221650. [CrossRef]
178. Deng, Z.; Fan, T.; Xiao, C.; Tian, H.; Zheng, Y.; Li, C.; He, J. TGF-β Signaling in Health, Disease, and Therapeutics. *Signal Transduct. Target Ther.* **2024**, *9*, 61. [CrossRef] [PubMed]
179. Strehlow, K.; Rotter, S.; Wassmann, S.; Adam, O.; Grohé, C.; Laufs, K.; Böhm, M.; Nickenig, G. Modulation of Antioxidant Enzyme Expression and Function by Estrogen. *Circ. Res.* **2003**, *93*, 170–177. [CrossRef]
180. Sun, J.X.; Xu, X.H.; Jin, L. Effects of Metabolism on Macrophage Polarization Under Different Disease Backgrounds. *Front. Immunol.* **2022**, *13*, 880286. [CrossRef]
181. Pérez, S.; Rius-Pérez, S. Macrophage Polarization and Reprogramming in Acute Inflammation: A Redox Perspective. *Antioxidants* **2022**, *11*, 1394. [CrossRef] [PubMed]
182. Russart, K.L.G.; Nelson, R.J. Light at Night as an Environmental Endocrine Disruptor. *Physiol. Behav.* **2018**, *190*, 82–89. [CrossRef]
183. Ott, C.; Jacobs, K.; Haucke, E.; Navarrete Santos, A.; Grune, T.; Simm, A. Role of Advanced Glycation End Products in Cellular Signaling. *Redox Biol.* **2014**, *2*, 411–429. [CrossRef] [PubMed]
184. Schmidt, S.; Monk, J.M.; Robinson, L.E.; Mourtzakis, M. The Integrative Role of Leptin, Oestrogen and the Insulin Family in Obesity-Associated Breast Cancer: Potential Effects of Exercise. *Obes. Rev.* **2015**, *16*, 473–487. [CrossRef] [PubMed]
185. Reid, I.R.; Baldock, P.A.; Cornish, J. Effects of Leptin on the Skeleton. *Endocr. Rev.* **2018**, *39*, 938–959. [CrossRef]
186. Baser, K.H.C.; Haskologlu, I.C.; Erdag, E. Molecular Links Between Circadian Rhythm Disruption, Melatonin, and Neurodegenerative Diseases: An Updated Review. *Molecules* **2025**, *30*, 1888. [CrossRef]
187. Hardeland, R. Melatonin and Inflammation—Story of a Double-Edged Blade. *J. Pineal Res.* **2018**, *65*, e12525. [CrossRef]
188. Huang, X.; Pan, C.H.; Yin, F.; Peng, J.; Yang, L. The Role of Estrogen in Mitochondrial Disease. *Cell Mol. Neurobiol.* **2025**, *45*, 68. [CrossRef]
189. Sánchez-Robalino, A.; Sinchi-Sinchi, H.; Ramírez, A. Effectiveness of Pain Neuroscience Education in Physical Therapy: A Systematic Review and Meta-Analysis. *Brain Sci.* **2025**, *15*, 658. [CrossRef]
190. Watson, J.A.; Ryan, C.G.; Cooper, L.; Ellington, D.; Whittle, R.; Lavender, M.; Dixon, J.; Atkinson, G.; Cooper, K.; Martin, D.J. Pain Neuroscience Education for Adults With Chronic Musculoskeletal Pain: A Mixed-Methods Systematic Review and Meta-Analysis. *J. Pain.* **2019**, *20*, e1–e1140. [CrossRef] [PubMed]
191. Cuenca-Martínez, F.; Suso-Martí, L.; Calatayud, J.; Ferrer-Sargues, F.J.; Muñoz-Alarcos, V.; Alba-Quesada, P.; Biviá-Roig, G. Pain Neuroscience Education in Patients with Chronic Musculoskeletal Pain: An Umbrella Review. *Front. Neurosci.* **2023**, *17*, 1272068. [CrossRef] [PubMed]
192. Ray, A.; Maharana, K.C.; Meenakshi, S.; Singh, S. Endothelial Dysfunction and Its Relation in Different Disorders: Recent Update. *Health Sci. Rev.* **2023**, *7*, 100084. [CrossRef]
193. Pacinella, G.; Ciaccio, A.M.; Tuttolomondo, A. Endothelial Dysfunction and Chronic Inflammation: The Cornerstones of Vascular Alterations in Age-Related Diseases. *Int. J. Mol. Sci.* **2022**, *23*, 15722. [CrossRef]
194. Li, J.; Liu, F.; Liang, F.; Yang, Y.; Lu, X.; Gu, D. Air Pollution Exposure and Vascular Endothelial Function: A Systematic Review and Meta-Analysis. *Environ. Sci. Pollut. Res.* **2023**, *30*, 28525–28549. [CrossRef]
195. de Bont, J.; Jaganathan, S.; Dahlquist, M.; Persson, Å.; Stafoggia, M.; Ljungman, P. Ambient Air Pollution and Cardiovascular Diseases: An Umbrella Review of Systematic Reviews and Meta-Analyses. *J. Intern. Med.* **2022**, *291*, 779–800. [CrossRef] [PubMed]
196. Förstermann, U.; Sessa, W.C. Nitric Oxide Synthases: Regulation and Function. *Eur. Heart J.* **2012**, *33*, 829–837. [CrossRef]

197. Böger, R.H. The Emerging Role of Asymmetric Dimethylarginine as a Novel Cardiovascular Risk Factor. *Cardiovasc. Res.* **2003**, *59*, 824–833. [CrossRef]
198. Radi, R. Peroxynitrite, a Stealthy Biological Oxidant. *J. Biol. Chem.* **2013**, *288*, 26464–26472. [CrossRef]
199. Förstermann, U.; Xia, N.; Li, H. Roles of Vascular Oxidative Stress and Nitric Oxide in the Pathogenesis of Atherosclerosis. *Circ. Res.* **2017**, *120*, 713–735. [CrossRef]
200. Thaiss, C.A.; Zmora, N.; Levy, M.; Elinav, E. The Microbiome and Innate Immunity. *Nature* **2016**, *535*, 65–74. [CrossRef] [PubMed]
201. Fan, Y.; Pedersen, O. Gut Microbiota in Human Metabolic Health and Disease. *Nat. Rev. Microbiol.* **2021**, *19*, 55–71. [CrossRef] [PubMed]
202. Tilg, H.; Zmora, N.; Adolph, T.E.; Elinav, E. The Intestinal Microbiota Fuelling Metabolic Inflammation. *Nat. Rev. Immunol.* **2020**, *20*, 40–54. [CrossRef]
203. Cani, P.D.; Amar, J.; Iglesias, M.A.; Poggi, M.; Knauf, C.; Bastelica, D.; Neyrinck, A.M.; Fava, F.; Tuohy, K.M.; Chabo, C.; et al. Metabolic Endotoxemia Initiates Obesity and Insulin Resistance. *Diabetes* **2007**, *56*, 1761–1772. [CrossRef]
204. Böger, R.H.; Maas, R.; Schulze, F.; Schwedhelm, E. Asymmetric Dimethylarginine (ADMA) as a Prospective Marker of Cardiovascular Disease and Mortality-An Update on Patient Populations with a Wide Range of Cardiovascular Risk. *Pharmacol. Res.* **2009**, *60*, 481–487. [CrossRef] [PubMed]
205. Monnier, V.M.; Mustata, G.T.; Biemel, K.L.; Reihl, O.; Lederer, M.O.; Zhenyu, D.; Sell, D.R. Cross-Linking of the Extracellular Matrix by the Maillard Reaction in Aging and Diabetes: An Update on "a Puzzle Nearing Resolution". In *Annals of the New York Academy of Sciences*; New York Academy of Sciences: New York, NY, USA, 2005; Volume 1043, pp. 533–544.
206. Taguchi, K.; Fukami, K. RAGE Signaling Regulates the Progression of Diabetic Complications. *Front. Pharmacol.* **2023**, *14*, 1128872. [CrossRef] [PubMed]
207. Ungvari, Z.; Tarantini, S.; Kiss, T.; Wren, J.D.; Giles, C.B.; Griffin, C.T.; Murfee, W.L.; Pacher, P.; Csiszar, A. Endothelial Dysfunction and Angiogenesis Impairment in the Ageing Vasculature. *Nat. Rev. Cardiol.* **2018**, *15*, 555–565. [CrossRef] [PubMed]

Journal of *Clinical Medicine*

MDPI

Review

Injury Characteristics and Physical Therapy Management Strategies for Circus Artists: A Scoping Review

Jessica Straub [1,*], Dhinu J. Jayaseelan [2], Clara Honigberg [2] and David A. Scalzitti [2]

[1] Alliance Physical Therapy, Baltimore, MD 21211, USA
[2] Program in Physical Therapy, The George Washington University, Washington, DC 20006, USA; scalzitt@gwu.edu (D.A.S.)
* Correspondence: jlstraub4@gmail.com

Abstract: Background: Circus arts are gaining popularity across the globe and lifespan. Despite growing participation rates, there is limited high-quality evidence describing the physical therapy evaluation and management of injury within this population. The purpose of this scoping review was to identify and summarize evidence related to the injury characteristics and management of circus artists. Methods: With a research librarian, computerized searches were developed and performed using online databases (PubMed, CINAHL, Scopus, SPORTDiscus and Cochrane), gray literature and non-medical databases. Two authors independently voted on article inclusion with a third author blinded to previous voting used in case of conflict. Concept mapping identified five primary themes related to circus injuries and physical therapy treatment. Data was extracted from each article based on content relevant to the classification. Results: In total, 1095 titles were retrieved from electronic searches, of which 49 studies were included. Overall, 20 studies related to injury characteristics, 10 to risk factors, 9 to each psychosocial variables and interventions, and 8 to screening. Acrobats with required ground elements were the most commonly injured discipline, particularly at the shoulder, ankle and spine. Intrinsic and extrinsic risk factors were identified and numerous psychosocial and lifestyle contributing factors were reported. Literature guiding treatment is limited. Conclusions: This scoping review mapped and synthesized evidence related to the evaluation and management of circus artist injuries. While injury patterns and characteristics are generally understood, the treatment of this population is poorly described. Clear gaps in screening, injury prevention strategies, and interventions for this group were identified.

Keywords: performing arts; physical therapy; rehabilitation

1. Introduction

Circus arts are practiced globally in a variety of contexts, with expertise ranging from professional companies to recreational participants. In the United States participation in the circus arts has grown substantially, with more than 78% of the circus organizations founded after 2000 [1]. Of these circus organizations, 74.4% offer adult recreational classes. The circus arts are highly demanding athletic activities that require similar strength, balance, flexibility, and motor coordination to gymnastics [2], and activity that carries substantial injury risk [3]. Coupled with these sport-specific demands, there is often a high work load and short recovery time due to frequent performance schedules [4]. Even for professionals, performance and training may require considerable travel, and access to appropriate care may not be perceived to be available [5]. Respecting these variables, it becomes apparent that circus artist athletes are unique and their sport complex, and physical therapy management requires a deep understanding of the population.

Unfortunately, despite the need for high-quality evidence guiding management, available evidence includes inconsistent injury definitions for circus arts, making it difficult to compare and contrast trends. In 2020 Greenspan et al. [6] created an International Olympic Committee (IOC) consensus statement on reporting injury. The consensus statement comes after a 2017 systematic review including literature through March 2016, reporting substantial variance and a need for consistent reporting of musculoskeletal circus injuries [7]. The review noted a relatively low injury rate among professionals, ranging from 7.37 to 9.27/1000 artist exposures, mostly affecting the spine and ankle. Although not captured in the previous review, it should also be noted that circus artists may suffer from substantial emotional distress [8] which may elevate their risk of injury [9]. In addition to the substantial psychosocial demands, evaluation and management of injury is likely made challenging by the wide-ranging task-specific demands of circus arts. Greenspan [10] separated ground and aerial activity due to the differences in physical demands. Subgroups consisted of aerial acrobatics with ground elements, aerial acrobatics, ground acrobatics with human propulsion, ground acrobatics with balance/control, manipulation, and character. More research is needed to precisely describe injury patterns of this specialized group of athletes.

In addition to understanding injury patterns among circus artists, it seems appropriate to investigate factors that may elevate risk and develop instruments to identify potential risk prior to injury. Without validated pre-participation screening instruments, tools used in other similar sports (e.g., gymnastics) could be useful. In fact, perhaps due to sport-specific similarities, some gymnasts transition to careers in circus arts [11]. However, while the evaluation and management of gymnastics injuries has been well described [12–15], the management of circus artist injuries is not. In fact, there has not been a single randomized controlled trial with circus artist participants. Clinical reasoning and treatment decision making should be guided by high-quality evidence, but none appears available for circus artists. In order to create baseline knowledge to guide clinicians, an extensive evaluation of available evidence describing the treatment of the injured circus artist is required.

Despite the rapid increase in circus arts participation at the professional and recreational level and subsequent injury risk, there is limited evidence describing circus arts, particularly the contemporary injury patterns and treatment approaches. Synthesized evidence can help to inform clinical practice and identify literature gaps to guide future research, but such evidence does not exist for this unique population. This scoping review aims to identify and report on the injury characteristics and management strategies for circus artists.

2. Materials and Methods

This scoping review was pre-registered on the Open Science Framework (OSF) website 8 March 2024, and is freely available online. Reporting followed guidance of the Preferred Reporting Items for Systematic Reviews and Meta-Analyses extension for scoping reviews (PRISMA-ScR).

2.1. Data Sources and Searches

A comprehensive and systematic computerized search of the electronic databases PubMed, Scopus, CINAHL, the Cochrane library, and SPORTDiscus was conducted to identify articles relevant to the clinical question. All articles from database inception through 3 September 2024 were considered for inclusion. With the assistance of a research librarian, key search terms and various combinations of synonyms related to the concepts of injury characteristics and management of circus artists were entered into each database.

Specific search strategies are presented in the Supplementary Materials. The reference lists of eligible articles were manually examined for key review articles and additional relevant studies. Finally, clinical trial registries, Google, and the Open Grey database were scanned for pertinent work not captured otherwise.

A basic example search string is as follows, with relevant truncation, adjustments, Boolean operators, and MeSH terms used depending on the database: ("circus artist*" OR circus OR aerialist* OR acrobat*) AND (("Wounds and Injuries" [Mesh] OR "Epidemiologic Methods" [Mesh]) OR (injury AND (prevention OR assessment OR screening)) OR ("Psychiatry and Psychology Category" [Mesh] OR psychosocial) AND ("Physical Therapy Modalities" [Mesh] OR "physical therapy" OR physiotherapy OR rehabilitation OR recovery OR "conservative management")).

2.2. Eligibility Criteria

Studies were considered in this review if they related to the clinical question and had a full-text report published in the English language in a peer-reviewed journal. The clinical question was categorized into thematic areas after concept mapping was completed by the research team (Figure 1). For inclusion, the population of interest was circus artists and the study aim was related to any of the following: injury trends or characteristics, risk factors, screening or injury prevention instruments, physical therapy management or psychosocial variables. Studies were excluded if they were published in abstract form only or protocols, were not in the English language or reasonably translated to English, not related to circus artists, primarily related to gymnasts or dancers, or if they were not within the scope of injury characteristics or management.

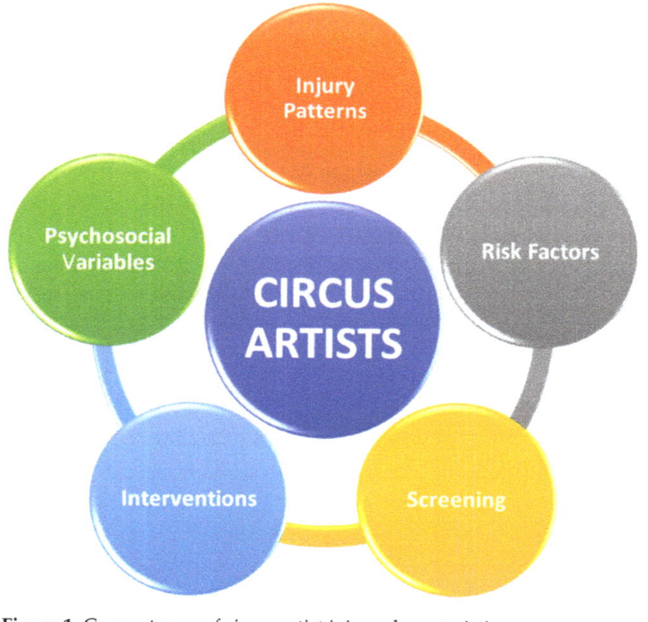

Figure 1. Concept map of circus artist injury characteristics.

2.3. Study Selection

Prior to screening, all individuals involved in screening used 10 titles for a reliability exercise. Each individual independently voted for inclusion or exclusion, and upon completion, the authors met to discuss results, appropriateness for decision making, and create a consensus for future screening principles. After the electronic search was completed and duplicates removed, two reviewers independently screened the titles and abstracts for eligibility using the web-based literature review manager Covidence, with criteria determined a priori. After the preliminary search of the above databases, any article that included circus artists and injury characteristics or management was retained for further analysis. In cases where details of the study methods were unclear, the study's corresponding author was contacted for additional information. Amongst those articles in which disagreement occurred, a third author blinded to previous voting made the final decision for inclusion. Full-text articles were procured through institutional access, interlibrary loan, or requesting copies from the corresponding authors. After full-text articles were obtained, two reviewers independently evaluated the study for appropriateness. If consensus regarding inclusion was not achieved, a third author blinded to previous voting was consulted for a final vote to include or exclude the article.

2.4. Data Extraction and Reporting

Upon final full-text article inclusion, data from studies were extracted to standardized forms. Grouping of data was subclassified into the 5 thematic areas. In cases where studies were pertinent to multiple concepts (e.g., injury patterns and risk factors), data was extracted and reported for each rather than one. Data was extracted by an author and independently cross-checked for accuracy and consistency by a separate author. An assessment of available evidence, and strength of evidence, was synthesized qualitatively.

2.5. Quality Assessment

The purpose of this scoping review was not to determine individual study quality as much as the overall quality of evidence related to a given topic. No formal assessment of study quality was performed for this project.

3. Results

In total 1094 titles were retrieved from the searches. After the removal of duplicates, 817 studies were screened, of which 49 studies were retained for final inclusion in this scoping review (Figure 2). The study design and primary themes of the studies are presented in Figure 3. The highest proportion of studies were related to injury characteristics (n = 20) followed almost equivalently by studies related to interventions, psychosocial variables, risk factors and screening methods for circus artists. Nine studies were tagged with multiple classifications. Less consistent than the number of studies evaluating a given topic was the sample size associated with the topic. Of the 10,272 unique participants included in all retained studies related to circus artists, 5397 (50.26%) participants were included in the 20 studies examining injury characteristics as compared to only 57 (0.55%) participants in the 9 studies describing management of injury (Figure 4).

3.1. Injury Patterns

The type of studies related to injury patterns is presented in Figure 3. Of the 20 studies, there were 2 systematic reviews [7,16], 7 cohort studies [2,4,10,17–20], 1 longitudinal study [21], 2 cross-sectional studies [22,23], 2 descriptive epidemiological studies [24,25], 1 retrospective descriptive epidemiology study [26], 1 case series [27], 1 narrative review [28], and 2 case reports [29,30]. Sample size ranged from 1 to 1376 participants with a diverse level of performer expertise (e.g., professional versus pre-professional, adolescents versus adult circus performers). There was notable variation in injury reporting, particularly as it related to the athlete characteristics, type and impact of injuries. Specific data from individual studies is presented in Table 1.

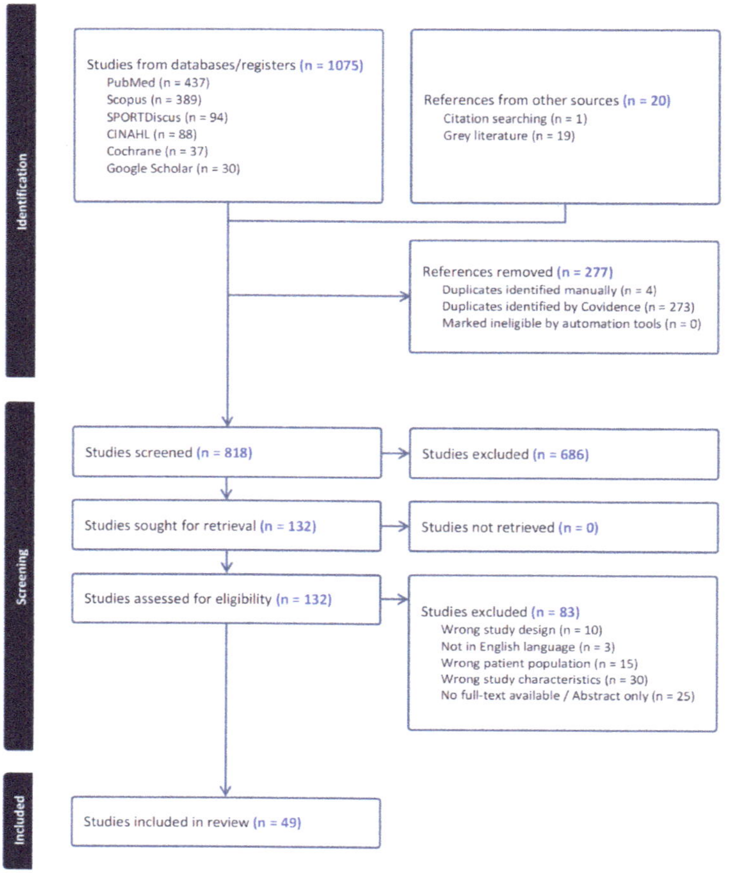

Figure 2. PRISMA flow diagram.

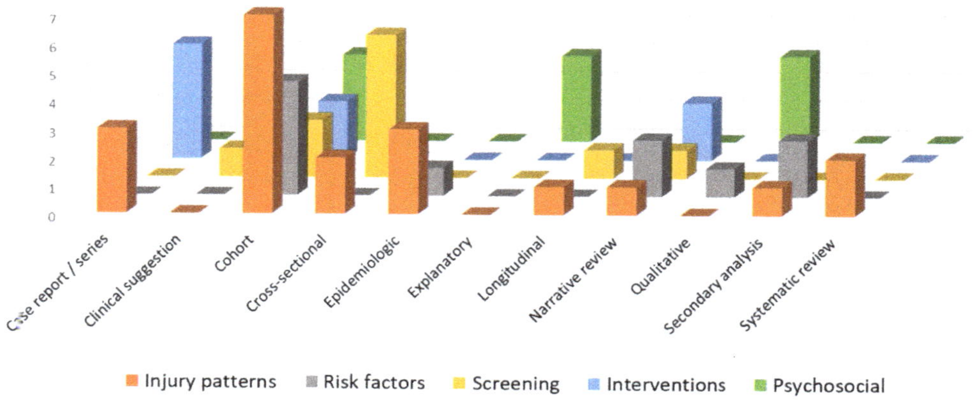

Figure 3. Study design type frequency by characteristic.

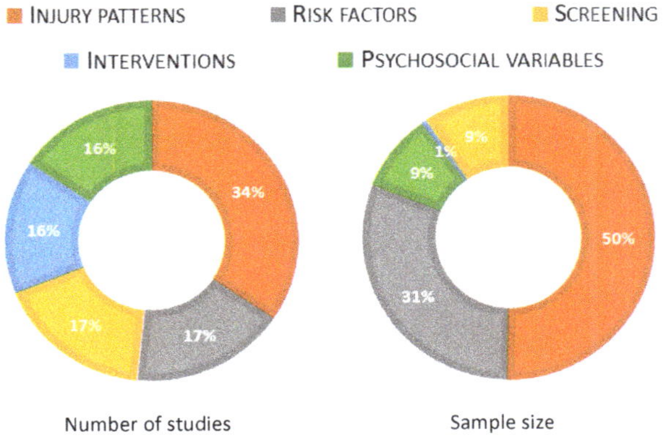

Figure 4. Proportion of included studies (**left**) and sample size (**right**) by injury characteristic.

Table 1. Studies reporting on injury patterns in circus artists.

Study	Study Design	Sample Size	Participant Characteristics	Mechanism of Injury	Injury Characteristics
Al-Kashmiri [29]	Case report	n = 1	26 y/o male	Overuse	Fibular stress fracture
Asselin [27]	Case series	n = 9	8 performers, 1 staff member Age range: 19–34 years 8 females, 1 male	Traumatic; fall while performing hair hanging during a 'human chandelier' maneuver	Fractures of the face, cervical, thoracic and lumbar spine, humerus, radius, wrist and hand, ribs, sacrum, femur, tibia, fibula, and ankle; concussions; lacerations of the knee, liver and scalp; pulmonary contusion; pneumothorax
Greenspan [17]	Prospective cohort	n = 21	Adolescents: Mean age: 14.7 (1.3) years 12 females Mean circus experience: 5.1 years Primary discipline: 35.9% aerial, 21.4% ground, 42.9% mixed Adults: Mean age: 30.7 (3.1) years 5 females, 4 males Mean circus experience: 10.5 years Primary discipline: 30% aerial, 40% ground, 20% mixed, 10% Chinese pole	Overuse (44% of adolescent injuries, 55% of adult injuries); Traumatic (56% of adolescent injuries, 45% of adult injuries)	Tissues involved (most to least frequent): joint, muscle/tendon, nerve, bone, central nervous system, integument. Body region involved (reported as lower extremity, upper extremity, spine): adolescents—44%, 33%, 22%; adults—32%, 45%, 24% Injury rate per 1000 session exposures was 3 for adolescents and 13 for adults Time-loss injury rates were 1.3 and 7.2, respectively Time-loss injury frequency: 44% adolescents, 55% adults
Greenspan [10]	Prospective cohort	n = 201	Mean age: 31.4 (8.9) years 16 adolescents, 185 adults 172 females, 29 males Mean circus experience: 7.0 (4.2) years 130 pre-professionals, 71 professionals	Acute–sudden (32%), repetitive–sudden (12%), repetitive–gradual (54%), unknown (1%)	Most common tissue involved: muscle/tendon injuries (52%) Most common body region involved: shoulder 22%, lumbosacral region 13%, elbow 10%, all others < 10% Injury rates per 1000 sessions: 3.8 overall, 2.42 adolescents, 4.0 adults, 3.5 female, 5.7 male, 5.9 aerialists with ground elements, 4.3 aerial, 3.7 ground (balance and control)
Greenspan [2]	Cohort	n = 24	Mean age: 21.4 (8.3) years 20 females, 4 males Mean circus experience: 7.3 (4.4) years	Overuse: 55.3% Traumatic: 44.7%	Most common tissue involved: joint (46.8%), muscle/tendon (25.5%), nerve (14.9%) all others < 10% Most common body region involved: shoulder 21.3%, wrist/hand 17.0%, hip/thigh and ankle/foot 12.8% each, upper trunk 10.6%, all others < 10% Injury rate per 1000 session exposures was 5 overall, 2.3 for aerialists, 7.0 for the ground group, 3.8 for the mixed group Time-loss injury frequency: 53.2%

Table 1. *Cont.*

Study	Study Design	Sample Size	Participant Characteristics	Mechanism of Injury	Injury Characteristics
Hakim [18]	Cohort	n = 31	Mean age: 22.5 (2) years 14 females, 17 males	Not specified	Most common body region involved: lower limb (44%; ankle 68%, knee 27%, tibia 5%), upper limb (32%; 50% shoulder, 25% wrist, elbow 19%, forearm 6%), trunk (16%), neck (8%)
Hamilton [31]	Secondary analysis of prospective injury data	n = 1281	Circus artists	Not specified	64% incurred at least 2 medical attention injuries 23.1% incurred at least 2 time-loss injuries
Kraan [16]	Systematic review	n = 67, 1 trapeze artist	Mean age of total sample: 27.1 years Male trapeze artist age not specified	Overuse	Posterior circumflex humeral artery pathology
Long [22]	Cross-sectional	n = 30	Mean age: 16.6 years	Not specified	13.3% reported losing at least one day of participation to injury. Fear of losing playing/practice time cited as most common reason to not report injury (42.9%)
Munro [19]	Prospective cohort	n = 63	Mean age: 22 years 33 females, 30 males	Not specified	Most common body region involved: spine 35%, ankle 26%, shoulder 12%, all others < 10% Injury activity frequency: acrobatics/tumbling (23%), handstands (12%), adagio (11%), Chinese pole (10%), others < 10%
Orlando [20]	Cohort	n = 584	208 females, 378 males Mean age: females, 25.3 (9.4) years; males: 30.3 (9.4) Type of performer: females—sudden load (71.4%), non-sudden load (16.5%), musician (12.1%); males—sudden load (66.7%), non-sudden load (18.0%), musician (15.3%)	Not specified	Rate ratio estimates for medical attention injuries = 1.5, TL-1 = 1.3, TL-15 = 1.1
Rossini [23]	Cross-sectional	n = 31	Mean age: 21.1 (2.6) years 18 females, 13 males Mean circus experience: 8.0 (4.3) years	Not specified	Lumbar multifidi asymmetry in prone was greater in artists reporting LBP in the past 4 weeks or 3 months
Russell [28]	Narrative review	Not applicable	Dancers, circus performs, theatre performers, and film/television performers	Traumatic	Notes concussions may be classified under 'head and neck' category of injury reporting
Shrier [25]	Descriptive epidemiological	n = 962	Professional artists Mean age: not reported 303 females, 659 males	Not specified	89.4% incurred an injury requiring medical attention, 74.2% incurred at least 1 TL-1 injury, 50.8% incurred at least 1 TL-15 injury Injury risk per 1000 performances: 5.1 medical attention, 2.5 TL-1, 0.86 TL-15
Shrier [24]	Descriptive epidemiological	n = 1376	Professional artists Mean age: not reported 534 females, 842 males Primary discipline: 80.5% acrobats, 11.8% non-acrobats, 7.8% musicians	Not specified	Types of injury (most to least frequent): muscle/tendon, other, joint and ligament, contusions/lacerations, fractures and bone, nerve Body region involved (most to least frequent): lower extremity, upper extremity, spine, head and neck, trunk, other Injury rates per 1000 performances: overall 9.7, acrobats 11.2, non-acrobats 6.8, musicians: 4.3 4.4% injuries classified as TL-15

Table 1. *Cont.*

Study	Study Design	Sample Size	Participant Characteristics	Mechanism of Injury	Injury Characteristics
Stubbe [4]	Prospective cohort	n = 44	Mean age: 22.0 (2.8) years 21 females, 23 males	Not specified	Most common body region involved: shoulder 27.7%, lower back 15.8%, wrist 14.1%, all others < 10% Mean duration of injury: 6.9 days Injury incidence rate of 3.3 injuries/1000 h
Stuckey [21]	Longitudinal	n = 334	Mean age: 19.2 (2.1) years 134 females, 200 males	Not specified	Overall injury rate per 1000 training hours = 1.89; rate of injuries lasting more than 4 weeks per 1000 training hours = 0.94 Clinical incidence of injury/student/year = 1.78, which decreased over time with experience
Wanke [26]	Retrospective descriptive epidemio-logic	n = 169	Age range: 11–22 years 99 females, 70 males	Traumatic	Most common tissue involved: joint (48.8%), bone (23.8%), ligament (14.9%) all others < 10% Most common body region involved: lower extremity (37%), cervical spine (28.3%), upper extremities (19.6%), thoracic spine (17.2%), lumbar spine (10.9%) Injury risk per 1000 h = 0.3
Wojciuk [30]	Case report	n = 1	64 y/o female 8-year history of an acrobat	Overuse	Bilateral upper limb arterial stenosis
Wolfenden [7]	Systematic review	n = 4795, 8 studies included	High school through professional circus artists	Floor acrobatics/tumbling most common mechanism (23–50.3%) followed by handstands (12%), adagio (11%) and Chinese pole (10%)	Most common type of injury: soft tissue Most common body region involved: spine and ankle Injury rate per 1000 exposures ranged from 7.4 to 9.3

Of the 20 studies, 9 did not specifically report the mechanism of injury. There were five studies reporting overuse conditions to be most prominent, five reporting traumatic injuries to be most prominent, and one study noting that trauma occurred more frequently in adolescents while overuse was more common in adults. One study used the recently developed circus-specific extension of the International Olympic Committee injury recording guidelines [10], while two studies used and adapted version of the International Association of Dance Medicine and Science (IADMS) Standard Consensus Initiative guidelines [2,17]. Outside of these studies, reporting differed across author groups.

Grouping of participant discipline for injuries varied between studies. Greenspan [2] described circus athletes in the following groups: aerial acrobatics with ground elements, aerial acrobatics, ground acrobatics with human propulsion, ground acrobatics with balance/control, manipulation, and character. A separate study used acrobat, non-acrobat, and musician to broadly classify circus artists [24]. The authors used the terms acrobat to describe a performer that required gymnastics, diving, martial arts, and aerial movements, non-acrobat to describe dancers, jugglers, swimmers, clowns, and characters in a show that do not perform gymnastic or martial arts or aerial movements, and musician to describe people that play music. Alternatively, Orlando et al. [20] utilized the terms sudden load, non-sudden load, and musicians to categorize circus injury.

The types of injuries encountered were more consistent across studies than the way injuries were reported. Injury rates ranged from 1.89 to 9.7; however, studies varied rates based on hours or exposures. Acrobats who performed ground elements were the most commonly injured discipline. Although most injuries likely led to some time away from their sport, time lost (TL) injuries were explicitly detailed in 7/20 (35%) studies. When considering the type of tissue injured, three studies reported joint injuries to be most common while three studies noted muscle/tendon injuries to be most common. While all body regions were prone to injury, the most commonly injured sites are shown in Figure 5.

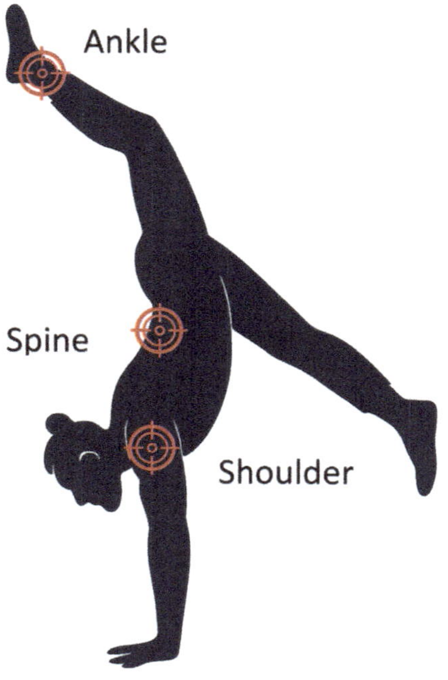

Figure 5. Most frequently reported circus injury sites.

3.2. Risk Factors

Of the 49 studies included, 10 studies [9,10,17,20,25,28,31–34] were related to risk factors (Figure 3) with a total of 4459 participants analyzed. Extracted data from individual studies is presented in Table 2.

Table 2. Risk factors for circus artist injuries.

Study	Study Design	Sample Size	Participant Characteristics	Reported Risk Characteristics
Bolling [32]	Qualitative	n = 82	Professional coaches, physiotherapists, athletic trainers and performance medicine therapists, and artists Participant demographics not reported	Injury risk reported to increase with higher workload. Busy daily schedule, more cues, fewer rotations and backups, less rest/recovery time, higher mental load, fatigue, improper technique, and external factors (weather, area, and touring conditions) increased risk
Faltus [33]	Narrative review	Not applicable	Circus artists	Risk increases with higher volume and frequency of circus performances, lack of a true "off season", certain cultural considerations (e.g., language barriers and pain ideologies), certain psychological considerations (e.g., emotional, social and cognitive loads)

Table 2. *Cont.*

Study	Study Design	Sample Size	Participant Characteristics	Reported Risk Characteristics
Greenspan [17]	Prospective cohort	n = 21	Adolescents: Mean age: 14.7 (1.3) years 12 females Mean circus experience: 5.1 years Primary discipline: 35.9% aerial, 21.4% ground, 42.9% mixed Adults: Mean age: 30.7 (3.1) years 5 females, 4 males Mean circus experience: 10.5 years Primary discipline: 30% aerial, 40% ground, 20% mixed, 10% Chinese pole	Higher age predictive of injury risk
Greenspan [10]	Prospective cohort	n = 201	Mean age: 31.4 (8.9) years 16 adolescents, 185 adults 172 females, 29 males Mean circus experience: 7.0 (4.2) years 130 pre-professionals, 71 professionals	Extrinsic risk factors: Discipline (aerial with ground elements), pre-professional (less experience) Intrinsic risk factors: Age (adults more than adolescents), female sex, disordered eating history
Hamilton [34]	Secondary analysis	n = 1281	Circus artists	Injury risk dependent on injury definition Sudden-load artists and age > 20 years had increased risk across injury classifications. Female sex and age > 30 years had increased risk for medical attention injuries. European artists more likely to sustain time-loss injuries than North American artists.
Hamilton [31]	Secondary analysis	n = 1281	Circus artists	Previous injury not identified to be a casual risk factor.
Orlando [20]	Cohort	n = 584	208 females, 378 males Mean age: females, 25.3 (9.4) years; males: 30.3 (9.4) Type of performer: females—sudden load (71.4%), non-sudden load (16.5%), musician (12.1%); males—sudden load (66.7%), non-sudden load (18.0%), musician (15.3%)	Injury risk is higher among sudden load and non-sudden load artists for medical attention and time loss injuries after breaks (2 days post activity)
Russell [28]	Narrative review	Not applicable	Dancers, circus artists, theatre, film and television performers	Suggests while circus artists sustain concussions, determining risk is limited by barriers in reporting and injury pattern definition.
Shrier [9]	Retrospective cohort	n = 47	Professional circus artists 17 females, 30 males	Prior injury, emotional exhaustion, self-efficacy, and fatigue were associated with an increased in injury risk. Conflicts or pressure not associated with increased injury risk. Low self-efficacy had the strongest relationship.
Shrier [25]	Descriptive epidemio-logical	n = 962	Professional artists Mean age: not reported 303 females, 659 males	Observed injury risk was not consistent with theoretical injury risk in circus performers.

Risk factors were analyzed in extrinsic and intrinsic categories. Extrinsic risk factors were broadly related to performance demands and environment (high performance workload and frequency with a lack of rest [20,32,33]). Pre-professional artists had higher injury rates (4.08/1000 sessions) compared to professional artists (3.49/1000) and those requiring sudden-load discipline demands also were at higher risk than other disciplines (5.93/1000 to 4.26/1000) [10,20]. Qualitative data identified poor touring conditions and weather as a risk factor for injury [32]. Intrinsic risk factors included older age [10,17,34], female sex [10,34], disordered eating [10], and psychological factors (e.g., self-efficacy, emotional exhaustion, higher mental load) [9,32,33]. There were conflicting results related to previous injury being a risk factor for a future injury [9,20,31], which is consistent with Shrier et al. [25], who reported that observed injury risk was not consistent with theoretical injury risk.

3.3. Screening

Of the 49 studies included, 10 studies [23,35–43] were related to screening tools or principles in circus artists (Figure 3) reporting on a total of 913 participants, with individual study data presented in Table 3. Studies included participants across the expertise spectrum, from professionals with Cirque du Soleil through pre-professionals/amateurs, although participant skill was unspecified in three studies. Two screening-related studies were narrative reviews which suggested screening for physical performance, hypermobility, training and lifestyle [36] or using a movement system impairment classification [41]. Four of the studies [35,39,40,43] completed physical performance testing relevant to participant screening. Circus artists were found to have generally more than normal mobility although findings were not discipline-specific. Not all physical testing may provide consistent results; specifically, the Harvard step test, 60 s jump test, and dynamic balance test did not have good reliability in circus athlete testing [35]. Four studies [23,37,38,42] screened mental health, mood, lifestyle and perceptions of health. Studies found self-reported outcomes were feasibly completed and students had different baseline measures compared to professionals. Instruments identified different mood levels at different time points (e.g., beginning versus end of a semester) although surveys can be perceived as burdensome if distributed too frequently [42].

Table 3. Studies reporting on screening tools or principles in circus artists.

Study	Study Design	Sample Size	Participant Characteristics	Instrument/ Process Description	Outcome(s)
Burnstein [35]	Cohort	n = 238	Professional circus performers 76 females, 162 males Mean age: 28.7 (6.4) years	Physical capacity assessment which included dynamic balance, modified Harvard step test, grip strength, vertical jump test, pull-up test, and 60 s jump test; data collected at baseline, 6, 12, and 18 months	Acceptable test–retest reliability over long periods of time for handgrip, vertical jump, and pull-up assessments; Harvard step test and 60 s jump test had poor reliability with comparison of baseline but acceptable reliability otherwise; Dynamic balance test never reached a level of acceptability at any time point; unclear if same tester was used

Table 3. *Cont.*

Study	Study Design	Sample Size	Participant Characteristics	Instrument/ Process Description	Outcome(s)
Callahan [36]	Narrative review	Not applicable	Dancers and circus artists	Suggested subjective screening: artist identity and participation level, injury management, habitual postures, fatigue, sleep, nutrition, menstrual history, support systems, other activities and participation; Suggested physical screening: The Beighton Score, Brighton criteria, 5-point screening questionnaire, The Lower Limb Assessment Score, The Upper Limb Hypermobility Assessment Tool, assessment of strength, functional movements, closed and open chain activities	Not applicable
Decker [37]	Longitudinal	n = 92	Circus students 32 females, 60 males Mean age: 20.9 (2.4) years	Modified Consensus Sleep Diary, ratings of fatigue, wakefulness and perceived exertion; measures taken for 7 consecutive days at 4 different time points	Significant fluctuations in fatigue, wakefulness, and perceived exertion over time points with increased challenge to achieve adequate sleep noted at end of year. Significant correlation between wakefulness and other sleep parameters (duration, latency, and quality). Sleep quality and perceived exertion related to fatigue. No significant differences between disciplines, sex, or year in program.
Donohue [38]	Cross-sectional	n = 109	Professional circus artists (n = 88) and circus students (n = 21) 42 females, 67 males Mean age: 28.5 (7.3) years	Sport Interference Checklist Student Athlete Relationship Instrument; Patient-Reported Outcomes Measurement Information System (anxiety, depression, satisfaction with social roles and activities, social isolation, emotional support, informational support, fatigue, sleep disturbance); Social Skill in Work Environment; satisfaction with overall circus performance	Mental health: Students scored higher for anxiety and professionals demonstrated lower levels of depression. Social health: Professionals scored higher on informational and emotional support and social skills, and lower on social isolation than students. Physical health: Students reported higher fatigue. Performance: Professionals reported less interferences than students. Professionals reported higher overall satisfaction with performance, social roles and responsibilities than students.

Table 3. *Cont.*

Study	Study Design	Sample Size	Participant Characteristics	Instrument/ Process Description	Outcome(s)
Greenspan [39]	Cross-sectional	n = 201	Professional (n = 71) and pre-professional (n = 130) 172 females, 29 males Age range: 13–69 years	Physical examination battery of upper and lower extremity flexibility, strength, and balance and cardiorespiratory measures to determine normative data	Mobility: Females had more lumbar mobility, shoulder and hip (except for external rotation) passive range of motion, hamstring and straddle flexibility, males had more pectoralis minor flexibility; Younger participants generally had more mobility than older counterparts; Strength: Males demonstrated more upper body strength, females had greater hip abduction strength; Professionals demonstrated more lower abdominal and upper body strength; Professionals had lower recovery heart rates than pre-professionals; Findings were not discipline-specific.
Huberman [40]	Cross-sectional	n = 189	Professional and amateur acrobats 157 females, 30 males Mean age = 31.9 years Acrobatic subgroup: aerial (n = 40), ground (n = 21), both (n = 128)	Shoulder range of motion and strength, grip strength	Males and females demonstrated significantly more shoulder range of motion, except for flexion, than established norms Acrobats had greater shoulder strength than the general population, while males had significantly less grip strength than the general population. No significant strength or range of motion differences across age groups.
Rossini [23]	Cross-sectional	n = 33	Circus artist students 19 females, 14 males Mean age: 21.2 (2.5) years Discipline: floor acrobatics (n = 11), aerial acrobatics (n = 15), balancing (n = 6), juggling (n = 1)	Self-reported training, injury and low back pain history; Oswestry Disability Index, Athlete Disability Index, Pain Catastrophizing Scale	Positive correlation between athlete and Oswestry disability indices. Athlete disability index positively correlated with pain intensity and pain catastrophizing. No significant correlations between pain duration and assessment tools.
Scherb [41]	Clinical suggestion	Not applicable	Circus artists with low back pain	Movement system impairment classification	Suggestion based on expert opinion to match the movement needs of circus artists
Shrier [42]	Prospective longitudinal	n = 36	Professional circus artists 16 females, 21 males Median age = 32.4	State-Trait Anxiety Inventory, Ways of Coping, Profile of Mood States, Likert scales to assess anxiety, sleep, confidence, fatigue, well-being; assessed at baseline, daily, weekly for 4 weeks	Monitoring psychological states were generally successful regarding time to complete, distribution, acceptability, and comprehension of questionnaires. Respondents believed questionnaires could be burdensome to complete at expected rate.

Table 3. *Cont.*

Study	Study Design	Sample Size	Participant Characteristics	Instrument/ Process Description	Outcome(s)
Smith [43]	Cross-sectional	n = 15	Pre-professional circus artists 15 females Mean age: 13.6 (2.3) years	Isokinetic testing of knee and ankle, trunk strength, lumbar range of motion, lower extremity flexibility; Modified SafeDance IV survey report	Acrobats generally demonstrated more than normal range of motion. Significant peak torque correlations noted between the ankle and hip/knee. Although the ankle was most commonly injured, and often hypermobile, most injuries were not related to acrobatic participation.

3.4. Interventions

Of the 49 studies included, 9 were related to the physical therapy management of circus artists (Figure 3) with a total of 57 participants included [33,36,41,44–49]. Intervention-specific data is presented in Table 4. Narrative review and suggestion topics were related to making interventions patient-specific, using a movement systems-based approach, and using an interdisciplinary management strategy. Cohort design studies reported on the use of telehealth to treat atraumatic shoulder instability or feasibility of a calf muscle strengthening program. Case reports detailed the management of traumatic soft tissue tears or symptoms associated with hypermobility. No randomized controlled trials or comparative studies examining the effects of interventions for the circus artist were found in this scoping review. Of the five studies including the management of patients, as compared to suggestions, reviews, or feasibility studies, each reported clinically significant improvement in pain and/or functional outcomes. However, only three of the five studies (26 patients) reported on long-term follow-up [47–49].

Table 4. Studies related to the physical therapy management of circus artists.

Study	Study Design	Sample Size	Participant Characteristics	Intervention	Frequency/ Duration	Comparison	Outcome(s)
Callahan [36]	Narrative review	Not applicable	Hypermobility in aesthetic performing artists	Suggested patient-specific utilization of interventions such as bracing, education (self-management, pain science, fatigue), posture and movement retraining, strength and proprioceptive training	Not applicable	Not applicable	Not applicable
Chimenti [44]	Case report	n = 1	16 y/o female Clinical diagnosis: lumbar extension-rotation syndrome	1. Education regarding movement impairments 2. Home exercises and taping to minimize lumbar extension–rotation/ improve abdominal and gluteal recruitment and hip flexor flexibility	16 visits over 16 weeks	Not applicable	Assessed at baseline, at each phase of intervention, and discharge; Clinically significant improvement in pain and function
Faltus [33]	Narrative review	Not applicable	Circus performance artist and acrobat	Suggested use of trans-disciplinary approach for management of the population	Not applicable	Not applicable	Not applicable

Table 4. *Cont.*

Study	Study Design	Sample Size	Participant Characteristics	Intervention	Frequency/ Duration	Comparison	Outcome(s)
Fecteau [45]	Case report	n = 1	15 y/o female Clinical diagnosis: transitional vertebrae and lumbar retrolisthesis	1. Manual therapy for lumbar hypomobility 2. Therapeutic exercise for hip strengthening 3. Neuromuscular re-education for lumbopelvic stability 4. Sport-specific training	16 visits over 8 weeks	Not applicable	Assessed at baseline, 5th and 10th visit; Clinically significant improvement in pain; No functional measure or self-reported questionnaire reported
Gandertcn [46]	Cohort	n = 29	13 females, 16 males Active touring professional circus performers	Feasibility study for calf muscle training Maximal set of calf raises with proper form, each limb, once daily each workday	47 exercise sessions over 9 weeks	Not applicable	Feasibility and endurance assessed at study completion; injury questionnaire administered weekly; High adherence and substantial improvement noted in calf endurance
Gandertcn [47]	Cohort	n = 24	Mean age: 23.82 (2.88) 16 females, 8 males, student circus performers Clinical diagnosis: atraumatic shoulder instability	Telehealth delivery mode Phasic exercise progression emphasizing scapular control and strengthening in increasing ranges of motion towards circus specific training	12 visits over 12 weeks	Not applicable	Assessed at baseline, 6 and 12 weeks, 6 and 9 months; Statistically and clinically significant improvement in function, strength and kinesiophobia
Roubea [48]	Case report	n = 1	16 y/o female acrobat Clinical diagnosis: partial tear right UCL	Phasic progression consisting primarily of 1. Manual therapy for pain relief 2. Progressive wrist, elbow and scapular strengthening, core stability progressing to closed chain activities, plyometric and sport-specific exercise	10 visits over 8 weeks	Not applicable Not applicable	Assessed at baseline, weeks 3, 6, 10 and 3 months; Clinically significant improvements in pain and function
Scherb [41]	Clinical sugges-tion	Not applicable	Not applicable	Suggestion to use movement system impairment classification in management of circus athletes	Not applicable	Not applicable	Not applicable
Teo [49]	Case report	n = 1	42 y/o male rigger Clinical diagnosis: flexor carpi ulnaris tear	1. Wrist splinting × 6 weeks 2. Intermittent mobilization at 4 weeks 3. Progressive forearm strengthening and loading activities at 6 weeks	Not reported	Not applicable	Return to normal activity at 3 months, pain and grip assessed at 6 months; Clinically significant improvement in pain and grip strength

3.5. Psychosocial Variables

Of the 49 studies included, 9 studies were related to psychosocial variables (Figure 3) [5,8,9,11,50–54]. A total of 961 unique circus artists were included with relevant study results presented in Table 5. There was a nearly equal range of expertise, as three studies included professional or retired circus artists [5,9,11], three studies included pre-professional circus artists [50,51,54], and three studies included professional and pre-professional circus artists [8,52,53]. Eight of the studies reported on participants' mental health or emotional perceptions of their body, career, or lifestyle. Four of these studies reported on stress and negative emotions, two studies reported on fatigue, three studies reported on anxiety and fear, one study reported on depression, and one study reported on overall mental health. Overall, results indicated high levels of fatigue, negative emotions, increased anxiety, and low self-efficacy.

Table 5. Studies reporting on psychosocial variables in circus artists.

Study	Study Design	Sample Size	Participant Characteristics	Instrument(s) Used	Outcomes
Cayrol [5]	Qualitative	n = 10	Professional circus artists 5 females, 5 males Mean age: 33 (range 27–42) years Mean performance experience: 12 years At least one injury reported	Semi-structured, individual interviews (virtual or in-person)	4 themes of perceptions and beliefs of injury identified: 1. The injured artists—circus training and performance viewed as their whole life, not a job; injury has negative effect on mood and emotion. 2. Professionalism—work and the performance should take precedence over personal issues or injuries. 3. Circus life—work perceived as challenging, lack of a fixed address limited injury management, injuries often self-managed or treated by other artists. 4. Artists' experience of healthcare—personalized and specialized healthcare is required but not typically available.
Decker [37]	Prospective cohort	n = 92	Professional circus students 32 females, 60 males Mean age: 20.4 (2.4) years	Circus Daily Challenges Questionnaire; Scales perceiving coping, state anxiety, sleep and distress	Highest scores of challenge level, state anxiety, and fatigue at end of year Schedule demands overall highest challenge item. Technical development, artistic expression, physical prep, and sleep 2nd highest challenge item. Sleep, artistic expression, and fear of injury were most frequently reported over the year. Increase in challenge level was associated with an increase in anxiety state and fatigue.
Shrier [9]	Retrospective cohort	n = 47	Professional circus artists 17 females, 30 males	The Recovery-Stress Questionnaire	High measures of fatigue, emotional exhaustion, injury, and low self-efficacy were associated with a 2–3× increase in risk for injury. High levels of social stress or a low level of either success or personal accomplishment may be a predictor of injury.
Stubbe [51]	Prospective cohort	n = 98 total; circus artists n = 25	Performing arts students 74 females, 24 males Mean age: 19.9 (2) years	Oslo Sports Trauma Research Centre Questionnaire; Stress (0–100, 100 = more stressed); Sleep quality (1–10, 10 = good sleep); Subjective mental health (higher score = worse), loneliness and mental health Inventory	Higher prevalence of mental health problems during 3-month COVID-19 lockdown. Average stress 40.38 pre-COVID-19 and 37.66 during lockdown. Average sleep quality 6.44 sleep quality pre-COVID, 6.87 during lockdown. Subjective mental health: 27.6% in March, 32.7% in April, 35.7% in May. Loneliness: 75.5% of people dealt with severe loneliness during lockdown.
van Rens [52]	Explanatory research	n = 248	Expertise included amateurs, students, professionals, retired professionals 188 females, 54 males, 6 other/prefer not to say Mean age: 30.7 (8.4) years Mean circus experience: 7.3 (6.7) years	Sensation seeking, Emotional regulation, and Agency Scale; Ten Item Personality Inventory; Accidents and Close Calls in Sport Inventory; Perceived risk of Activities	No significant difference between circus categories for sensation. Aerial acrobats experienced more emotional regulation, agency, conscientiousness and agreeableness than object manipulators. Floor acrobats reported more near misses and accidents than both aerialists and object manipulators. Object manipulators had significantly lower perceived risk than aerial and floor acrobatics.

Table 5. *Cont.*

Study	Study Design	Sample Size	Participant Characteristics	Instrument(s) Used	Outcomes
van Rens [11]	Qualitative	n = 8	Professional circus artists who were formerly gymnasts 4 female, 4 male Mean age: 30.9 (4.4) years Mean circus experience: 5.8 years	Semi-structured individual interview	3 phases were identified in transitioning from gymnastics to professional circus: (1) realizing, (2) adaptation, (3) thriving. Realizing phase included hard work, motivation to accomplish the transition, social support, optimism. Adaptation phase included general stress, loss of competence, social adjustment, taking calculated risks, physical recovery. Thriving phase included freedom, personal development, social connectedness. Career transition process included an emergence of a circus artist identity.
van Rens [8]	Explanatory research	n = 500	Expertise included amateurs, students, professionals, retired professionals 415 females, 62 males, 23 transgender/gender-diverse Mean age: 31.1 (8.2) years Mean circus experience: 7.6 (5.9) years	Depression Anxiety Stress Scale-21; The Flourishing Scale; State Trait Assessment of Resilience	Circus artists experience lower levels of mental health than other populations despite higher levels of psychological resilience. Circus artists had higher levels of depression, anxiety, and stress, and lower flourishing than other populations, with object manipulators reporting worse scores than other disciplines. Higher state/trait resilience associated with higher psychological well-being. Transgender and gender-diverse individuals had higher depression scores.
van Rens [53]	Explanatory research	n = 500	Expertise included amateurs, students, professionals, retired professionals 415 females, 62 males, 23 transgender/gender-diverse Mean age: 31.1 (8.2) years Mean circus experience: 7.6 (5.9) years	Circus Addiction Inventory; Eating Attitudes Test short form; State Trait Assessment of Resilience	Exercise addiction positively related to being at risk of eating disorders and negatively related to experience. Males scored lower on the circus addiction inventory than female or transgender/gender-diverse peers. Aerial acrobatics were more likely to be at risk for eating disorders than floor artists and had higher addiction scores compared to equilibrium and floor acrobatics.
Walby [54]	Qualitative	n = 31	Circus aerialists 19 females, 12 males Age range: 22–37 years	Semi-structured individual interview	Primary emergent themes included training with pain, body image, performance, aerialism and risk, injury and the erosion of body capital, and aging out. Recognizing the circus performance span is brief, artists often push their bodies through pain and risk boundaries.

4. Discussion

This scoping review sought to describe injury characteristics and management strategies for circus artists. Circus arts participation is becoming more popular across the lifespan, and research is helping to identify injury trends and those at risk for injury. However, based on the results of this review, there appears to be substantial variation in reporting, few appropriate screening instruments for injury risk mitigation, and minimal evidence guiding the treatment of circus artist injuries.

Based on the results of this scoping review, the largest proportion of retained articles were related to the injury patterns and trends of circus artists. In a 2017 systematic review of circus artist injuries, Wolfenden and Angioi identified eight studies reporting on 4795 participants (1281 of which were duplicated from two studies) [7]. This scoping review found 11 new studies on injury patterns since that publication, suggesting a growing scholarly interest in the topic. Despite reporting variability, this review identified acrobats performing ground elements to be the most commonly injured discipline, the shoulder, ankle and spine to be common regions of injury, joint and muscle/tendon tissues to be commonly injured, and traumatic and overuse injuries to be equally common. Physical therapists are well-positioned to manage the gamut of circus injuries, but knowing the task-specific demands and mechanism of injury can allow for comprehensive and individualized care.

Variability and inconsistency across studies can make synthesis of findings difficult. Although a circus-specific reporting extension of the IOC consensus statement was published in 2022 [6], knowledge translation can take time, and only one study implemented the reporting methodology [10]. The lack of standardized surveillance, in part due to heterogeneity among study design and injury definitions, should be rectified for future prospective protocols across circus disciplines. Additionally, the potential for underreporting should be considered. In a recent systematic review, between 20 and 91% of workers failed to report their injury to their supervisors or worker's compensation, with a variety of socioeconomic and employment characteristics, psychosocial variables, and healthcare providers often cited as contributing factors [55]. Circus artists may have pessimistic views of healthcare for their conditions and substantial internal and external pressure to push through injuries [5]. The quantitative results of this review related to injury patterns should be considered in context of possible underestimation.

This review identified intrinsic (personal) and extrinsic (environmental) risk factors that impact injury. Intrinsic risk factors identified were chronological age, history of eating disorder, and sex at birth, while extrinsic risk factors were type of performer, level of performer, and rest time between performances [17]. Greenspan [10,17] and Hamilton [34] found chronological age and age over 30 were associated with increased risk of injury. This contrasts with injury trends in gymnastics, where adolescents face a higher risk. The discrepancy may stem from differences in participation patterns, as adults are more likely to engage in circus arts, whereas gymnastics is predominantly practiced by younger individuals [56]. Individuals with an eating disorder averaged increased injury rates than individuals without an eating disorder [10], which is consistent with previous work in high school athletes [57]. This may be related to body image and esthetic expectations of circus performers [54] and possible exercise addiction [53] with implications for injury for sudden-load disciplines. Three of the studies noted discipline type as a risk factor. Greenspan [17] identified aerial with ground elements to have higher instances of injury per 1000 exposures, whereas Hamilton identified sudden load to have higher rate of time loss injuries [34]. Although higher workload and less rest between practice or performance were identified as risk factors for circus injuries [32,33], so too was being a pre-professional or less experienced artist [10]. Given the highly specialized and intricate physical demands of circus artists, good technique and appropriate rest are important factors in reducing injury risk. If clinicians are aware of common risk factors for injury in circus artists, they can create and implement screening and prevention strategies and create physical therapy plans of care that minimize risk of reinjury.

This review identified various screening tools and processes utilized for circus artists. Professional circus artists made up 68% of the studies included and pre-professional circus artists made up 32% of the studies. There was variation in assessment timing, which was collected at a single time point [35] or serially [23] at different points during a circus artists' career. Callahan et al. [36] emphasized the importance of posture and movement retraining, education on when to use a mid versus full range of motion, and strength training to manage hypermobility. Although the authors did not suggest a specific strength training program, high-load strength training was superior in the short term to low-load training for individuals with hypermobile shoulders [58]. Long-term effectiveness was not different and the study did not include elite-level athletes, which limits generalizability to this population. Various testing modes including functional tests, manual muscle tests, dynamometers, and isokinetic testing were used to assess muscle performance [36,39,40,43]. The authors found that female circus artists tend to have greater passive range of motion compared to males, and professionals had greater muscle performance compared to pre-professionals. This may be a contributing factor associated with the greater injury risk of female athletes and pre-professionals.

Despite the substantial amount of evidence detailing injury patterns in the circus athlete population, there is a relative dearth of literature guiding the physical therapy management of this unique group. While some task-specific movements mimic those required in other well-researched sports (e.g., gymnastics, dance, cheerleading), the management of this group compared to its similar activities is nearly non-existent. The treatment of only 57 unique participants was identified with this review, approximately 0.5% of the total population assessed. Available evidence is limited to small cohorts, case studies, or suggestions, preventing the assessment of treatment effectiveness. From the limited evidence, clinicians can imply that circus artists who have substantial and unique physical and psychological demands require multimodal and tailored rehabilitation programs. One could postulate that the limited data describing circus athlete management parallels the psychosocial findings of this review, identifying a lack of willingness of circus artists to report injuries or perceived challenges with obtaining appropriate sport-specific care [5]. Recognizing that circus artists may be required to travel for performances, it may be difficult to establish continuous care. While telehealth options may be appropriate [46,47], classic in-person physical therapy care may be challenging and should be reconceptualized for this population. The discrepancy between rising circus performance popularity and injury research compared to intervention studies highlights the need for additional high-quality research.

This review found that circus artists and circus students reported high rates of mental health issues, including depression, anxiety, sleep deprivation, and stress. While none of the psychological studies included a control group of non-circus participants, 88.8% of the studies on psychological variables found emergence of negative emotions surrounding their craft [5,8,9,50–54]. Circus artists' livelihood is dependent on how they are able to physically perform both during training and performances. Shrier [9] reported that high fatigue, emotional exhaustion, injury, and low self-efficacy put an individual at a 2–3× increased risk for injury. High stress and/or anxiety was reported in 55.5% of the psychological studies for circus artists [8,9,11,50,51]. Being impeded from doing one's job can result in a mass of negative emotions, whereas having a more positive disposition has been found to improve long-term recovery and survival [59]. While circus artists experience many negative emotions, they also report a high amount of resiliency and motivation in their craft [8,11]. Poor sleep quality and high fatigue levels were another major theme reported among circus artists [9,50,51]. Previous research has suggested that a lack of sleep may put an individual at a greater risk of injury [60]. If an artist is stressed or anxious, this may lead to poor sleep, which in turn may predispose them to a higher likelihood of injury, which will begin a perpetuating cycle. This cycle has been previously discussed in the context of elite athletes [61]. Poor sleep hygiene also imposes a delay in injury recovery [62,63]. While impaired sleep and anxiety were not compared to one another in the included studies, these characteristics were reported in as high in 100% of the population in studies that reported data on those variables [9,37,51]. Evaluating negative psychosocial and lifestyle variables involved in an individual's healthcare experience is essential, and physical therapists should recognize the prevalence of these problems in circus athletes.

While this review is novel and carries important clinical and research implications, there are limitations. The literature search included numerous databases and gray literature, and was created collaboratively by authors with systematic review experience and a research librarian. However, it is possible that potentially relevant work was not retained by the search itself or during the screening process. Specific clinical guidance offered from this report is limited, in large part due to limited evidence and variable reporting. However, the synthesis of key concepts related to the management of circus artists identified important information and opportunities for investigation. While not required for scoping reviews, if quality assessment was formally completed for the included studies, additional information could be provided regarding the topic.

While this review identified and synthesized key aspects of injury patterns and management strategies, a number of evidence gaps were recognized. The average age range across studies varied from 11 to 34 years old. According to the 2022 Circus Census Report, circus performers ranged in age from 6 to 55 and beyond [1]. Additional data on participants aged 6–11 and adults over 34 would help create a more comprehensive understanding of the entire circus artist community. Although the synthesized results of this review help understand injury patterns, it is clear that screening tools and management strategies are limited. Developing and validating sport- and discipline-specific physical and holistic screening instruments can allow clinicians to identify pre-participation injury risk and implement preventative programs to minimize or mitigate the risk. Finally, it is clear that although much is known about how circus artists get injured, and what their injury experience entails, the management of circus injuries is absent. Studies evaluating and describing the effectiveness of intervention strategies are needed. Specifically, comparative studies including multiple treatment options or patient populations would be useful.

5. Conclusions

The purpose of this review was to describe the evidence related to the injury characteristics and management strategies for circus artists. This review found injury trends and characteristics are well-researched but variably reported. Acrobats, particularly those incorporating ground elements, are most often injured, with shoulder, ankle, and spine injuries commonly reported. Although some risk factors are known and can predict who may develop injury, few sport-specific screening tools are available or used for this unique population. Further proactive assessment of psychological variables and screening instruments for this population appear warranted. Importantly, the physical therapy management of circus injuries is limited to few studies of low-level evidence and should be a point of emphasis in this scholarly area. While a growing population globally, the evidence related to physical therapy evaluation and management of circus artists would benefit from consistent reporting and high-quality prospective and comparative studies.

Supplementary Materials: The following supporting information can be downloaded at https://www.mdpi.com/article/10.3390/jcm14175948/s1: Supplementary: Circus artist scoping review search strings.

Author Contributions: Conceptualization, J.S. and D.J.J.; methodology, J.S., D.J.J., C.H. and D.A.S.; software, D.J.J.; validation, J.S., D.J.J., C.H. and D.A.S.; formal analysis, J.S., D.J.J., C.H. and D.A.S.; investigation, J.S., D.J.J. and C.H.; resources, D.J.J.; data curation, D.J.J.; writing—original draft preparation, J.S., D.J.J. and C.H.; writing—review and editing, J.S., D.J.J., C.H. and D.A.S.; visualization, D.J.J.; supervision, D.J.J.; project administration, J.S. and D.J.J. All authors have read and agreed to the published version of the manuscript.

Funding: This research received no external funding.

Institutional Review Board Statement: This study was deemed exempt for formal institutional review due to the study design using previously published data.

Informed Consent Statement: Not applicable.

Data Availability Statement: All relevant data are provided within the manuscript and in the Supplementary Materials.

Conflicts of Interest: The authors declare no conflicts of interest.

References

1. American Circus Educators, C.C.T. Circus Consensus 2022. Available online: https://www.americancircuseducators.org/wp-content/uploads/2022/10/ACE-AYCO-Survey-Final-Report.pdf (accessed on 1 July 2025).
2. Greenspan, S. Injury Patterns in Subgroups of Circus Artists by Circus Discipline: A Pilot Study. *Orthop. Phys. Ther. Pract.* **2022**, *34*, 162–170.
3. Campbell, R.A.; Bradshaw, E.J.; Ball, N.B.; Pease, D.L.; Spratford, W. Injury epidemiology and risk factors in competitive artistic gymnasts: A systematic review. *Br. J. Sports Med.* **2019**, *53*, 1056–1069. [CrossRef]
4. Stubbe, J.H.; Richardson, A.; van Rijn, R.M. Prospective cohort study on injuries and health problems among circus arts students. *BMJ Open Sport Exerc. Med.* **2018**, *4*, e000327. [CrossRef]
5. Cayrol, T.; Godfrey, E.; Draper-Rodi, J.; Bearne, L. Exploring Professional Circus Artists' Experience of Performance-Related Injury and Management: A Qualitative Study. *Med. Probl. Perform. Art.* **2019**, *34*, 14–24. [CrossRef]
6. Greenspan, S.; Munro, D.; Nicholas, J.; Stubbe, J.; Stuckey, M.I.; Van Rijn, R.M. Circus-specific extension of the International Olympic Committee 2020 consensus statement: Methods for recording and reporting of epidemiological data on injury and illness in sport. *BMJ Open Sport Exerc. Med.* **2022**, *8*, e001394. [CrossRef] [PubMed]
7. Wolfenden, H.E.; Angioi, M. Musculoskeletal Injury Profile of Circus Artists: A Systematic Review of the Literature. *Med. Probl. Perform. Art.* **2017**, *32*, 51–59. [CrossRef] [PubMed]
8. van Rens, F.E.C.A.; Heritage, B. Mental health of circus artists: Psychological resilience, circus factors, and demographics predict depression, anxiety, stress, and flourishing. *Psychol. Sport Exerc.* **2021**, *53*, 101850. [CrossRef]
9. Shrier, I.; Hallé, M. Psychological predictors of injuries in circus artists: An exploratory study. *Br. J. Sports Med.* **2011**, *45*, 433–436. [CrossRef]
10. Greenspan, S.; Stuckey, M.I. Untangling risk factors including discipline-specific exposure for injuries in preprofessional and professional circus artists in the USA. *BMJ Open Sport Exerc. Med.* **2023**, *9*, e001551. [CrossRef]
11. van Rens, F.E.C.A.; Filho, E. Realizing, Adapting, and Thriving in Career Transitions From Gymnastics to Contemporary Circus Arts. *J. Clin. Sport Psychol.* **2020**, *14*, 127–148. [CrossRef]
12. Desai, N.; Vance, D.D.; Rosenwasser, M.P.; Ahmad, C.S. Artistic Gymnastics Injuries; Epidemiology, Evaluation, and Treatment. *J. Am. Acad. Orthop. Surg.* **2019**, *27*, 459–467. [CrossRef]
13. Sweeney, E.A.; Howell, D.R.; James, D.A.; Potter, M.N.; Provance, A.J. Returning to Sport After Gymnastics Injuries. *Curr. Sports Med. Rep.* **2018**, *17*, 376–390. [CrossRef]
14. Hart, E.; Meehan, W.P., 3rd; Bae, D.S.; d'Hemecourt, P.; Stracciolini, A. The Young Injured Gymnast: A Literature Review and Discussion. *Curr. Sports Med. Rep.* **2018**, *17*, 366–375. [CrossRef] [PubMed]
15. Thomas, R.E.; Thomas, B.C. A systematic review of injuries in gymnastics. *Physician Sportsmed.* **2019**, *47*, 96–121. [CrossRef] [PubMed]
16. Kraan, R.B.; Beers, L.; van de Pol, D.; Daams, J.G.; Maas, M.; Kuijer, P.P. A systematic review on posterior circumflex humeral artery pathology: Sports and professions at risk and associated risk factors. *J. Sports Med. Phys. Fit.* **2019**, *59*, 1058–1067. [CrossRef] [PubMed]
17. Greenspan, S. Injury Frequency and Characteristics in Adolescent and Adult Circus Artists: A Pilot Prospective Cohort Study. *Med. Probl. Perform. Art.* **2021**, *36*, 103–107. [CrossRef]
18. Hakim, H.; Puel, F.; Bertucci, W. Injury assessment in circus student-artists population; preliminary study. *Sci. Sports* **2020**, *35*, 154–160. [CrossRef]
19. Munro, D. Injury patterns and rates amongst students at the national institute of circus arts: An observational study. *Med. Probl. Perform. Art.* **2014**, *29*, 235–240. [CrossRef]
20. Orlando, C.; Levitan, E.B.; Mittleman, M.A.; Steele, R.J.; Shrier, I. The effect of rest days on injury rates. *Scand. J. Med. Sci. Sports* **2011** *21*, 64. [CrossRef]
21. Stuckey, M.I.; Bruinooge, B.; Aubertin, P.; Kriellaars, D. Clinical Burden of Injuries in Students at a Professional Circus College: A 7.5-Year Longitudinal Study. *Med. Probl. Perform. Art.* **2022**, *37*, 98–105. [CrossRef]
22. Long, A.S.; Ambegaonkar, J.P.; Fahringer, P.M. Injury reporting rates and injury concealment patterns differ between high-school cirque performers and basketball players. *Med. Probl. Perform. Art.* **2011**, *26*, 200–205. [CrossRef] [PubMed]
23. Rossini, B.; Anstruther, M.; Fortin, M. Comparing assessment methods of low back pain related disability in student circus artists: A cross-sectional study. *J. Back Musculoskelet. Rehabil.* **2024**, *37*, 1141–1150. [CrossRef] [PubMed]

24. Shrier, I.; Meeuwisse, W.H.; Matheson, G.O.; Wingfield, K.; Steele, R.J.; Prince, F.; Hanley, J.; Montanaro, M. Injury patterns and injury rates in the circus arts: An analysis of 5 years of data from Cirque du Soleil. *Am. J. Sports Med.* **2009**, *37*, 1143–1149. [CrossRef]
25. Shrier, I.; Mattiello, R.; Caron, M.; Verhagen, E.; Steele, R.J. Observed Injury Rates Did Not Follow Theoretically Predicted Injury Risk Patterns in Professional Human Circus Artists. *Clin. J. Sport Med.* **2022**, *32*, e627–e634. [CrossRef]
26. Wanke, E.M.; McCormack, M.; Koch, F.; Wanke, A.; Groneberg, D.A. Acute injuries in student circus artists with regard to gender specific differences. *Asian J. Sports Med.* **2012**, *3*, 153–160. [CrossRef]
27. Asselin, N.; Proano, L.; Williams, K.; Partridge, R. Circus disaster: Case report, response, and review of injuries. *Am. J. Disaster Med.* **2016**, *11*, 137–141. [CrossRef]
28. Russell, J.A.; McIntyre, L.; Stewart, L.; Wang, T. Concussions in Dancers and Other Performing Artists. *Phys. Med. Rehabil. Clin. N. Am.* **2021**, *32*, 155–168. [CrossRef]
29. Al-Kashmiri, A.; Delaney, J.S. Case report: Fatigue fracture of the proximal fibula with secondary common peroneal nerve injury. *Clin. Orthop. Relat. Res.* **2007**, *463*, 225–228. [CrossRef]
30. Wojciuk, J.; Bury, R.W.; Brack, M.J. Acrobatic vascular disease. *Heart Vessel.* **2006**, *21*, 199–200. [CrossRef]
31. Hamilton, G.M.; Meeuwisse, W.H.; Emery, C.A.; Steele, R.J.; Shrier, I. Past injury as a risk factor: An illustrative example where appearances are deceiving. *Am. J. Epidemiol.* **2011**, *173*, 941–948. [CrossRef]
32. Bolling, C.; Mellette, J.; Pasman, H.R.; van Mechelen, W.; Verhagen, E. From the safety net to the injury prevention web: Applying systems thinking to unravel injury prevention challenges and opportunities in Cirque du Soleil. *BMJ Open Sport Exerc. Med.* **2019**, *5*, e000492. [CrossRef]
33. Faltus, J.; Richard, V. Considerations for the Medical Management of the Circus Performance Artist and Acrobat. *Int. J. Sports Phys. Ther.* **2022**, *17*, 307–316. [CrossRef]
34. Hamilton, G.M.; Meeuwisse, W.H.; Emery, C.A.; Shrier, I. Examining the effect of the injury definition on risk factor analysis in circus artists. *Scand. J. Med. Sci. Sports* **2012**, *22*, 330–334. [CrossRef] [PubMed]
35. Burnstein, B.D.; Steele, R.J.; Shrier, I. Reliability of fitness tests using methods and time periods common in sport and occupational management. *J. Athl. Train.* **2011**, *46*, 505–513. [CrossRef] [PubMed]
36. Callahan, A.; Squires, A.; Greenspan, S. Management of Hypermobility in Aesthetic Performing Artists: A Review. *Orthop. Phys. Ther. Pract.* **2022**, *34*, 134–145.
37. Decker, A.; Aubertin, P.; Kriellaars, D. Sleep and Fatigue of Elite Circus Student-Artists During One Year of Training. *Med. Probl. Perform. Art.* **2019**, *34*, 125–131. [CrossRef]
38. Donohue, B.; Gavrilova, Y.; Galante, M.; Burnstein, B.; Aubertin, P.; Gavrilova, E.; Funk, A.; Light, A.; Benning, S.D. Empirical development of a screening method for mental, social, and physical wellness in amateur and professional circus artists. *Psychol. Aesthet. Creat. Arts* **2020**, *14*, 313–324. [CrossRef]
39. Greenspan, S.J.; Stuckey, M.I. Preparation For Flight: The Physical Profile of Pre-Professional and Professional Circus Artists in the United States. *Int. J. Sports Phys. Ther.* **2024**, *19*, 591–608. [CrossRef]
40. Huberman, C.; Scales, M.; Vallabhajosula, S. Shoulder Range of Motion and Strength Characteristics in Circus Acrobats. *Med. Probl. Perform. Art.* **2020**, *35*, 145–152. [CrossRef]
41. Scherb, E. Low Back Pain in Circus Artists: Using a Movement System Impairment Framework as a Component of Care. *Orthop. Phys. Ther. Pract.* **2022**, *34*, 148–151.
42. Shrier, I.; Raglin, J.S.; Levitan, E.B.; Mittleman, M.A.; Steele, R.J.; Powell, J. Procedures for assessing psychological predictors of injuries in circus artists: A pilot prospective study. *BMC Med. Res. Methodol.* **2014**, *14*, 77. [CrossRef]
43. Smith, D.; Noorbhai, H. Prevalence of muscle imbalance and its potential influence on injury among female acrobatic dancers. *BMJ Open Sport Exerc. Med.* **2022**, *8*, e001322. [CrossRef] [PubMed]
44. Chimenti, R.L.; Van Dillen, L.R.; Khoo-Summers, L. Use of a Patient-Specific Outcome Measure and a Movement Classification System to Guide Nonsurgical Management of a Circus Performer with Low Back Pain: A Case Report. *J. Danc. Med. Sci.* **2017**, *21*, 185–192. [CrossRef] [PubMed]
45. Fecteau, L.; Freitas, N. Management of Transitional Vertebra in An Amateur Level Teenage Circus Acrobat: A Case Report. *Orthop. Phys. Ther. Pract.* **2022**, *34*, 152–156.
46. Ganderton, C.; Henry, M.; Walker, A.; McGinley, P.; Verhagen, E. Implementation of Calf Endurance Training in a Touring Group of Professional Circus Performers: A Feasibility Study. *Med. Probl. Perform. Art.* **2021**, *36*, 54–60. [CrossRef]
47. Ganderton, C.L.; Tirosh, O.; Munro, D.; Meyer, D.; Lenssen, R.; Balster, S.; Watson, L.; Warby, S. Rehabilitation for atraumatic shoulder instability in circus arts performers: Delivery via telehealth. *J. Shoulder Elb. Surg.* **2022**, *31*, e246–e257. [CrossRef]
48. Roubea, I.; Korakakis, V. Rehabilitation following ulnar collateral ligament injury of the elbow in a female acrobatic athlete: A case report. *J. Bodyw. Mov. Ther.* **2024**, *38*, 329–338. [CrossRef]
49. Teo, W.Z.W.; Kaur, R.; Sebastin, S. Traumatic Rupture of the Flexor Carpi Ulnaris Muscle Belly in a Circus Rigger. *J. Hand Surg. Asian Pac. Vol.* **2021**, *26*, 274–279. [CrossRef]

50. Decker, A.; Richard, V.; Cairney, J.; Jefferies, P.; Houser, N.; Aubertin, P.; Kriellaars, D. Assessment of Professional Circus Students' Psychological Characteristics at Four Strategic Timepoints over the Scholastic Year: A Longitudinal Study Using the Stress Process Model. *Med. Probl. Perform. Art.* **2022**, *37*, 249–258. [CrossRef]
51. Stubbe, J.H.; Tiemens, A.; Keizer-Hulsebosch, S.C.; Steemers, S.; van Winden, D.; Buiten, M.; Richardson, A.; van Rijn, R.M. Prevalence of Mental Health Complaints Among Performing Arts Students Is Associated With COVID-19 Preventive Measures. *Front. Psychol.* **2021**, *12*, 676587. [CrossRef]
52. van Rens, F.E.C.A.; Filho, E. Not just clowning around: Investigating psychological mechanisms underlying accidents in a heterogeneous group of contemporary circus artists. *Psychol. Aesthet. Creat. Arts* **2021**, *15*, 377–385. [CrossRef]
53. van Rens, F.E.C.A.; Metse, A.P.; Heritage, B. Exploring the mental health of circus artists: Circus factors, psychological resilience, and demographics predict disordered eating and exercise addictions. *Psychol. Sport Exerc.* **2022**, *59*, 102107. [CrossRef]
54. Walby, K.; Stuart, S. "You Have to Accept the Pain": Body Callusing and Body Capital in Circus Aerialism. *Qual. Sociol. Rev.* **2021**, *17*, 6–23. [CrossRef]
55. Kyung, M.; Lee, S.; Dancu, C.; Hong, O. Underreporting of workers' injuries or illnesses and contributing factors: A systematic review. *BMC Public Health* **2023**, *23*, 558. [CrossRef] [PubMed]
56. Tisano, B.; Zynda, A.J.; Ellis, H.B.; Wilson, P.L. Epidemiology of Pediatric Gymnastics Injuries Reported in US Emergency Departments: Sex- and Age-Based Injury Patterns. *Orthop. J. Sports Med.* **2022**, *10*, 23259671221102478. [CrossRef] [PubMed]
57. Rauh, M.J.; Nichols, J.F.; Barrack, M.T. Relationships among injury and disordered eating, menstrual dysfunction, and low bone mineral density in high school athletes: A prospective study. *J. Athl. Train.* **2010**, *45*, 243–252. [CrossRef]
58. Liaghat, B.; Juul-Kristensen, B.; Faber, D.A.; Christensen, E.O.; Søgaard, K.; Skou, S.T.; Søndergaard, J.; Juhl, C.B. One-year effectiveness of high-load compared with low-load strengthening exercise on self-reported function in patients with hypermobile shoulders: A secondary analysis from a randomised controlled trial. *Br. J. Sports Med.* **2024**, *58*, 373–381. [CrossRef]
59. Lamers, S.M.A.; Bolier, L.; Westerhof, G.J.; Smit, F.; Bohlmeijer, E.T. The impact of emotional well-being on long-term recovery and survival in physical illness: A meta-analysis. *J. Behav. Med.* **2012**, *35*, 538–547. [CrossRef]
60. Grier, T.; Dinkeloo, E.; Reynolds, M.; Jones, B.H. Sleep duration and musculoskeletal injury incidence in physically active men and women: A study of U.S. Army Special Operation Forces soldiers. *Sleep Health* **2020**, *6*, 344–349. [CrossRef]
61. Vitale, J.A.; Mathieu, N.; Sabrina, S.; Michele, L. Editorial: The Reciprocal Relationship Between Sleep and Stress in Elite Athletes. *Front. Psychol.* **2021**, *12*, 797847. [CrossRef]
62. Chennaoui, M.; Vanneau, T.; Trignol, A.; Arnal, P.; Gomez-Merino, D.; Baudot, C.; Perez, J.; Pochettino, S.; Eirale, C.; Chalabi, H. How does sleep help recovery from exercise-induced muscle injuries? *J. Sci. Med. Sport* **2021**, *24*, 982–987. [CrossRef]
63. Copenhaver, E.A.; Diamond, A.B. The Value of Sleep on Athletic Performance, Injury, and Recovery in the Young Athlete. *Pediatr. Ann.* **2017**, *46*, e106–e111. [CrossRef]

Journal of
Clinical Medicine

MDPI

Review

Frozen Shoulder as a Metabolic and Immune Disorder: Potential Roles of Leptin Resistance, JAK-STAT Dysregulation, and Fibrosis

Santiago Navarro-Ledesma

Department of Physiotherapy, Faculty of Health Sciences, Campus of Melilla, University of Granada, Querol Street 5, 52004 Melilla, Spain; snl@ugr.es

Abstract: Frozen shoulder (FS) is a complex and multifactorial condition characterized by persistent inflammation, fibrosis, and metabolic dysregulation. Despite extensive research, the underlying drivers of FS remain poorly understood. Recent findings indicate the coexistence of pro-inflammatory and fibrosis-resolving macrophages within affected tissues, suggesting a dysregulated immune response influenced by metabolic and neuroendocrine factors. This review proposes that leptin resistance, a hallmark of metabolic syndrome and chronic inflammation, may play a central role in FS pathogenesis by impairing macrophage polarization, perpetuating inflammation, and disrupting fibrosis resolution. The JAK-STAT signaling pathway, critically modulated by leptin resistance, may further contribute to immune dysregulation by sustaining inflammatory macrophage activation and interfering with tissue remodeling. Additionally, FS shares pathogenic features with fibrotic diseases driven by TGF-β signaling, mitochondrial dysfunction, and circadian disruption, further linking systemic metabolic dysfunction to localized fibrotic pathology. Beyond immune and metabolic regulation, alterations in gut microbiota, bacterial translocation, and chronic psychosocial stress may further exacerbate systemic inflammation and neuroendocrine imbalances, intensifying JAK-STAT dysregulation and leptin resistance. By examining the intricate interplay between metabolism, immune function, and fibrotic remodeling, this review highlights targeting leptin sensitivity, JAK-STAT modulation, and mitochondrial restoration as novel therapeutic strategies for FS treatment. Future research should explore these interconnections to develop integrative interventions that address both the metabolic and immune dysregulation underlying FS, ultimately improving clinical outcomes.

Keywords: frozen shoulder; metabolism; immunology; psychology; rehabilitation

1. Introduction

Frozen shoulder (FS), also known as adhesive capsulitis, is a musculoskeletal condition characterized by progressive pain and significant limitation in the range of motion of the shoulder joint. Affecting approximately 2% to 5% of the general population, FS is particularly prevalent among individuals between the ages of 40 and 60, with a higher incidence observed in women compared to men [1–3]. The condition can be classified into primary or idiopathic and secondary forms, with the latter often associated with trauma, surgery, or systemic diseases such as diabetes mellitus. FS not only impacts patients' quality of life, but also has considerable socioeconomic implications, including high healthcare costs and significant work-related disability. Studies have shown that up to 50% of individuals with FS experience a reduction in their capacity to perform work-related tasks, leading to decreased productivity and increased absenteeism [4]. The long duration of the disease, which can last from 1 to 3 years or more, further exacerbates these socioeconomic burdens, as patients often require prolonged treatment and rehabilitation [5].

The etiology of FS remains largely unclear, though it is generally accepted to be a multifactorial condition involving both mechanical and biochemical components [6]. Systemic diseases such as diabetes mellitus, cardiovascular disease, and metabolic syndrome have been strongly associated with an increased risk of developing FS [7]. These conditions, characterized by chronic low-grade inflammation and insulin resistance, contribute to altered tissue repair mechanisms, leading to fibrosis and thickening of the joint capsule [4]. In particular, metabolic disturbances, including the dysregulation of adipokines, have been proposed as central to the inflammatory processes driving FS [8,9]. One of the key adipokines involved is leptin, a hormone produced by adipose tissue that plays a significant role in both energy metabolism and immune regulation. Elevated leptin levels and leptin resistance may be linked to the chronic inflammation and fibrosis observed in FS, suggesting a possible metabolic pathway contributing to the disease's progression, and positioning it as a pivotal player in the emerging field of immunometabolism [10]. Leptin receptors are widely expressed throughout the immune system, and their regulatory effects encompass both innate and adaptive immune cells. Leptin is among the adipokines contributing to the chronic inflammatory state associated with obesity, which predisposes individuals not only to type 2 diabetes, metabolic syndrome, and cardiovascular disease, but also to autoimmune and allergic disorders [11].

In this regard, it has been hypothesized that the GABAergic system may play a crucial role in the development of FS, suggesting a potential link between type 1 diabetes, autoimmune endocrine disorders, and FS through shared pathophysiological mechanisms [9]. According to Nataf et al., antibodies against GAD65, which are implicated in both type 1 diabetes and central nervous system disorders, often arise from two synergistic risk factors: immune challenges and psycho-emotional stress. This combination increases the likelihood of T cell priming against GAD65, potentially leading to both type 1 diabetes and central nervous system disorders [12]. Antibody spreading is a known mechanism in autoimmune diseases, and the propagation of GAD65 antibodies has been observed in individuals with type 1 diabetes, although antibody levels were not consistently high enough to predict autoreactivity in infiltrated tissues [13]. Proteomics could be employed to test this hypothesis regarding why type 1 diabetes (DM1) is more closely associated with FS than type 2 diabetes (DM2). Such research aims to identify immune-related proteins, including T lymphocyte markers and the presence of GAD65 or other superantigens, along with their corresponding antibodies. Nonetheless, disturbances in the GABAergic system could contribute to a fear of physical activity, and movement neglect has been identified as a significant risk factor for the development of FS [8].

A study by Kawahara et al. analyzed the proteomic profiles of FS in different regions of the shoulder capsule across various patient groups. Their analysis compared twelve patients with severe primary FS to seven patients with FS and rotator cuff tears, who served as a control group. Significant proteomic differences were found between the two groups, with several proteins highlighted for their clinical relevance [14]. Notably, proteins involved in the PI3K-Akt and PPAR signaling pathways—key components of insulin and leptin metabolism—were more prominent in patients with primary FS [15,16]. This increased signaling activity suggests the heightened involvement of insulin and leptin pathways in the pathophysiology of primary FS, potentially linked to insulin and leptin resistance [16,17]. Conversely, the proteome of patients with rotator cuff damage was more closely related to direct tissue injury rather than metabolic disturbances. These findings were supported by the detection of proteins indicating Staphylococcus aureus infection, antigen processing and presentation, and lysosome/phagosome activity [14]. The involvement of phagosomal and lysosomal activity suggests the presence of damage-associated molecular patterns (DAMPs) and pathogen-associated molecular patterns (PAMPs) [18,19]. In cases of FS following rotator cuff damage, barrier disruption between the blood and capsule may underlie symptomatology. This distinction implies that patients with primary FS may benefit from treatments targeting lifestyle modifications and metabolic interventions to address insulin and leptin resistance, while those with traumatic FS may require more orthopedic-focused approaches. The study also concluded that primary and secondary FS have distinct etiologies and pathophysiologies, necessitating differentiated therapeutic strategies [9,14].

Additionally, Hand et al. identified immune cell infiltration in the shoulder capsules of 22 patients with refractory primary FS. Mast cells were the most prevalent, followed by T lymphocytes, B lymphocytes, and macrophages, indicating a chronic inflammatory state in primary FS. The interaction between mast cells and fibroblasts suggests that inflammation drives fibrosis through mast cell-mediated mechanisms [20]. The presence of T and B lymphocytes, components of the adaptive immune system, raises the possibility of an autoimmune reaction targeting fibrotic tissue in FS, although alternative hypotheses may exist. Latest studies utilizing single-cell RNA sequencing (scRNA-seq) to map the cellular landscape of frozen shoulder tissue identified key cell types and their roles in the resolution of inflammatory fibrosis. The main findings suggest that FS differs from other fibrotic conditions because it is a self-limiting disease, with pro-inflammatory and fibrosis-resolving macrophages (MERTK+ macrophages) coexisting in the affected tissues. These macrophages interact with specific fibroblast subtypes (DKK3+ and POSTN+ fibroblasts) to promote matrix remodeling and inflammation resolution. Moreover, the study found similarities in the gene expression profiles of MERTK+ macrophages in FS and those in synovial tissues from rheumatoid arthritis patients in remission, supporting the hypothesis that these macrophages facilitate the resolution of inflammation. The study suggests that the cellular mechanisms for resolving FS fibrosis may be pre-established during human shoulder development. These findings open avenues for new therapeutic strategies aimed at promoting resolution of fibrosis in chronic inflammatory diseases by targeting the interactions between specific macrophage and fibroblast populations [21].

Despite growing evidence linking metabolic dysfunction with FS pathophysiology, the precise mechanisms remain unclear. The interplay between leptin resistance, JAK-STAT signaling, and immune responses has not been thoroughly investigated in FS, leading to a gap in understanding its systemic nature. This review aims to: (1) explore the link between metabolic dysregulation and immune dysfunction in FS, (2) examine the role of JAK-STAT signaling in chronic inflammation and fibrosis, (3) compare JAK-STAT signaling with other fibrotic pathways such as TGF-β, and (4) propose novel therapeutic strategies targeting metabolic–immune interactions in FS.

2. Scoping the Role of JAK-STAT Signaling and MERTK+ Macrophages in Inflammatory Fibrosis Resolution

The aforementioned discovery aligns with the hypothesis that metabolic signals, potentially mediated by leptin, influence the activity of these immune cells. Leptin's role in energy regulation may extend to regulating the metabolic energy requirements of immune cells, particularly macrophages and fibroblasts, thereby influencing their capacity for fibrosis resolution. Given leptin's dual role in metabolism and immunity, it is plausible that disruptions in leptin signaling—such as those observed in metabolic syndrome and obesity—contribute to prolonged inflammation and delayed fibrosis resolution in FS [22,23]. The cellular energy demands of MERTK+ macrophages and fibroblasts during matrix remodeling may be influenced by leptin sensitivity and overall metabolic health.

Hypothetically, enhancing leptin sensitivity or targeting its downstream signaling pathways could improve the efficiency of these immune cells in resolving fibrosis, providing a potential therapeutic target. Thus, leptin may act as a bridge between metabolic dysfunction and impaired immune responses, perpetuating conditions like FS unless metabolic and immune homeostasis are restored [24]. The role of leptin and metabolic signals becomes even more pronounced when considering the JAK-STAT signaling pathway, as discussed in Sarapultsev et al. [25]. JAK-STAT is a key signaling mechanism in both immune and metabolic regulation, with direct implications for inflammation and cellular stress responses [26]. Dysregulation of this pathway, such as through leptin resistance, can perpetuate chronic inflammation and hinder the resolution of fibrosis, as seen in conditions like FS [10]. This pathway interacts with the immune system at various levels, promoting or dampening inflammatory responses based on metabolic inputs, such as leptin levels and signaling [27].

The presence of leptin resistance in FS patients may impair the proper functioning of the JAK-STAT pathway, leading to prolonged inflammation and delayed resolution of fibrosis [28]. This highlights the need for therapeutic interventions targeting both metabolic dysfunction and immune regulation, such as enhancing leptin sensitivity or directly modulating the JAK-STAT pathway to restore immune and metabolic balance in affected tissues [29]. Future research should focus on the combined role of metabolic regulators, like leptin, and immune-modulating pathways, like JAK-STAT, in promoting tissue repair and fibrosis resolution in frozen shoulder [9]. The JAK-STAT signaling pathway, a critical mediator of immune responses and leptin signaling, may also be implicated in FS pathophysiology. In the context of leptin resistance, dysregulation of the JAK-STAT pathway exacerbates inflammatory responses, activating transcription factors involved in fibrosis and tissue remodeling [30]. This suggests that therapies targeting JAK-STAT signaling could potentially mitigate the chronic inflammation and fibrosis characteristic of FS [31]. In this regard, a key aspect of fibrosis progression is the dysregulation of transcription factors, which are downstream targets of the JAK-STAT pathway [32]. Activation of STAT proteins, such as STAT3, has been implicated in promoting fibroblast proliferation and collagen production, exacerbating fibrotic responses [33]. The continuous stimulation of STAT3 in response to cytokines and growth factors, such as TGF-β, leads to unchecked ECM accumulation, a process that is central to the fibrotic pathology observed in FS [34]. Recent transcriptomic analyses from patients with FS reveal the upregulation of genes involved in immune responses and extracellular matrix modification, such as MMP9 and MMP13, which are closely associated with collagen degradation and fibrosis progression [35]. These findings suggest that metabolic dysregulation, mediated by leptin resistance, may directly influence the cellular processes that perpetuate inflammation and fibrosis in FS.

3. JAK-STAT, TGF-β, and Leptin Signaling in Frozen Shoulder

The TGF-β signaling pathway is well recognized as a central driver of fibrosis across multiple organ systems, including the musculoskeletal system. Elevated TGF-β activity has been implicated in fibroblast proliferation, extracellular matrix (ECM) deposition, and persistent myofibroblast activation, all of which contribute to joint capsule fibrosis and stiffness [36,37]. However, recent evidence suggests that the JAK-STAT pathway may also modulate fibroblast function and ECM production, establishing an important link between immune-mediated inflammation and fibrotic progression [38,39].

Notably, leptin signaling appears to intersect with both JAK-STAT and TGF-β pathways. Leptin promotes TGF-β-induced fibroblast differentiation into myofibroblasts in various fibrotic conditions, including pulmonary and hepatic fibrosis [40,41]. Moreover, studies suggest that STAT3 activation can directly upregulate TGF-β expression, amplifying fibrotic responses [42]. In contrast, leptin resistance may lead to a dysregulated JAK-STAT response, potentially altering its interaction with TGF-β and promoting a sustained fibrotic environment [43].

Both TGF-β and JAK-STAT pathways contribute to fibrosis progression, but through distinct and complementary mechanisms. TGF-β primarily drives fibrosis via SMAD-dependent pathways, promoting fibroblast-to-myofibroblast differentiation, ECM production, and tissue remodeling [36,37]. The JAK-STAT pathway, on the other hand, is primarily involved in immune regulation, but also plays a role in fibroblast activation and ECM remodeling, particularly through STAT3-mediated transcriptional regulation of fibrotic genes [38,39]. The crosstalk between these pathways is evident in various fibrotic conditions, where persistent STAT3 activation has been linked to increased TGF-β expression, reinforcing the fibrotic response [42].

The interplay between leptin resistance, JAK-STAT signaling, and TGF-β in FS remains an area of significant interest. Leptin resistance disrupts homeostatic metabolic signaling, which in turn influences immune and fibrotic pathways, creating a chronic inflammatory state that favors fibrosis progression. The effects of leptin on TGF-β signaling could be direct, through its influence on fibroblast activation, or indirect, by modulating the inflammatory microenvironment that sustains TGF-β activity [40,41]. Given that leptin resistance is closely linked to metabolic dysfunction, obesity, and chronic inflammation, its impact on both JAK-STAT and TGF-β could provide a unifying explanation for the metabolic–immune dysregulation observed in FS [43].

While JAK-STAT and TGF-β function as independent pathways, their interaction in the fibrotic progression of FS remains underexplored. Given the evidence that leptin influences both pathways, further research is warranted to determine whether leptin resistance disrupts this balance and fosters a chronic inflammatory-fibrotic state in FS. Targeting both pathways simultaneously—through JAK-STAT inhibitors, TGF-β modulators, or metabolic interventions aimed at improving leptin sensitivity—could provide a novel therapeutic strategy for FS patients.

4. Chronic Neuroinflammation, Leptin Resistance, and JAK-STAT Signaling

The coexistence of both pro-inflammatory and fibrosis-resolving macrophages (MERTK+) within the fibrotic tissues of frozen shoulder (FS) may be further explained through the lens of neuroinflammation and leptin resistance, particularly regarding the JAK-STAT signaling pathway [21]. Neuroinflammation, a state of chronic inflammation within the central nervous system (CNS), often results from a dysregulated immune response, driven by the JAK-STAT pathway [44]. This pathway is activated by various cytokines that promote both immune and inflammatory responses, playing a crucial role in diseases such as multiple sclerosis and Parkinson's disease [34].

Leptin resistance at the hypothalamic level, which is often present in individuals with metabolic syndrome, can exacerbate neuroinflammation by disrupting the normal regulation of energy balance and immune responses [45]. Leptin normally acts on hypothalamic receptors to regulate appetite and energy expenditure, but when leptin signaling is impaired, a state of chronic low-grade inflammation ensues [46]. This inflammatory state may spill over into peripheral tissues, such as those involved in FS, creating an environment where pro-inflammatory and fibrosis-resolving macrophages coexist [47]. The JAK-STAT pathway plays a central role in both the central and peripheral inflammatory processes, amplifying the inflammatory signals in response to neuroinflammation [34,48].

In FS, this disrupted signaling could manifest as a failure to effectively transition macrophages from a pro-inflammatory to a pro-resolving phenotype, leading to the persistence of fibrosis [38,49]. The involvement of JAK-STAT signaling in neuroinflammation suggests that targeting this pathway could mitigate not only the peripheral fibrotic response, but also the central neuroinflammatory drivers of FS [26,50]. The pathway's role in activating transcription factors associated with fibrosis and inflammation further underscores its importance [51,52]. Future research should explore the potential cross-talk between neuroinflammation, JAK-STAT signaling, and leptin resistance in FS, as this might unveil novel therapeutic strategies aimed at resolving both neuroinflammation and peripheral fibrosis [47]. Furthermore, in FS, the role of leptin may be further complicated by the inhibition of its signaling by SOCS3, which binds to the leptin receptor, particularly at sites necessary for STAT3 activation [53]. This attenuation of leptin signaling may exacerbate both peripheral inflammation and fibrosis because it disrupts the balance of macrophage activation [54]. SOCS3, by inhibiting the JAK-STAT signaling pathway, prevents effective immune resolution and promotes sustained inflammation. Moreover, SOCS3's role extends beyond leptin resistance [55]. It is also implicated in insulin resistance, which contributes to the broader metabolic dysregulation observed in FS patients [7]. In these individuals, overexpression of SOCS3 in both hypothalamic and peripheral tissues reduces the effectiveness of insulin signaling, further fueling systemic inflammation [54]. The link between metabolic disorders and fibrotic diseases, like FS, may thus be mediated, in part, by the SOCS3-induced blockade of both leptin and insulin pathways, perpetuating chronic inflammation and tissue fibrosis.

This insight prompts further investigation into the metabolic regulation of immune cell functions in FS and other chronic fibrotic diseases. It suggests that therapies aimed at improving metabolic health—particularly those enhancing leptin sensitivity—could also facilitate immune resolution processes, opening new avenues for treating FS by targeting both the metabolic and immune aspects of the disease.

The role of chronic psychosocial stress in FS pathophysiology is an emerging area of interest, particularly in its interaction with metabolic and immune dysregulation. Psychological factors such as pain-related fear, anxiety, and depression have been identified as key prognostic markers in FS, influencing functional disability, pain intensity, and recovery duration [56]. Stress-induced activation of the hypothalamic–pituitary–adrenal (HPA) axis and the resultant low-grade systemic inflammation may create a metabolic and immunological context that predisposes individuals to FS [9]. Chronic exposure to stressors not only contributes to increased circulating levels of pro-inflammatory cytokines, but also disrupts the homeostatic regulation of leptin and insulin signaling, further exacerbating immune dysregulation and fibrotic remodeling in FS. In this context, leptin resistance may serve as a metabolic link between chronic psychosocial stress and the inflammatory processes driving FS, as persistent stress is known to impair leptin signaling, fostering behavioral patterns characterized by reduced physical activity and heightened pain perception [8]. These findings suggest that targeting stress-related metabolic dysregulation, alongside immune and fibrotic pathways, could offer a more integrative therapeutic approach to FS management. Future studies should explore the potential of interventions aimed at mitigating stress-induced immune activation and leptin resistance as a novel strategy to improve both clinical outcomes and patient quality of life in FS (See Figure 1).

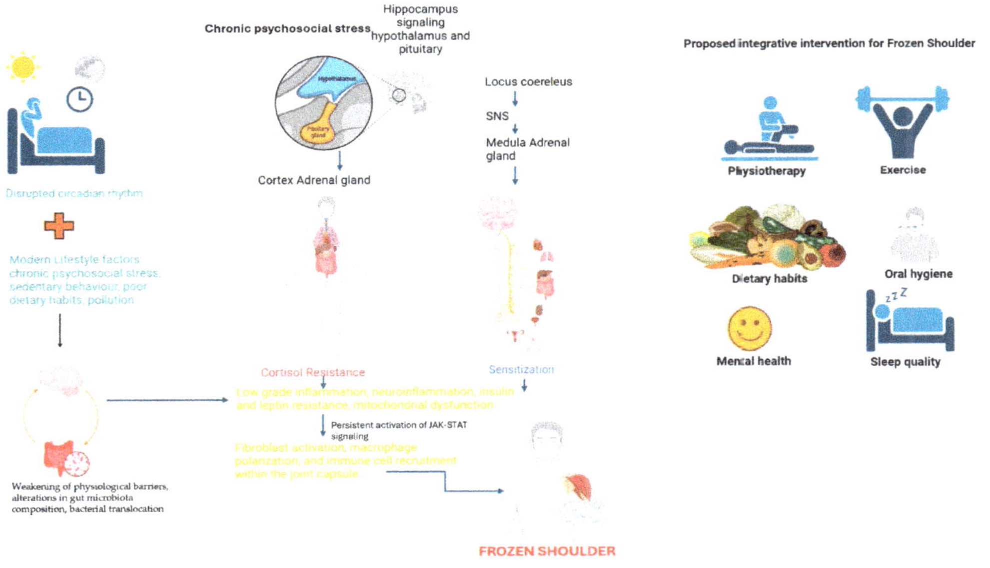

Figure 1. Note. Pathophysiological mechanisms and integrative treatment approaches in frozen shoulder. This figure provides a comprehensive overview of the multifactorial pathophysiology of frozen shoulder (FS) and the proposed integrative treatment strategies. On the left side of the figure, key lifestyle and environmental factors, such as circadian rhythm desynchronization and modern lifestyle influences (chronic psychosocial stress, sedentary behavior, poor dietary habits, and pollution), are depicted as major contributors to systemic dysregulation. When sustained over time, these factors promote low-grade inflammation, neuroinflammation, and a state of insulin and leptin resistance, disrupting normal metabolic and immune homeostasis. This condition fosters the weakening of physiological barriers, alterations in gut microbiota composition, and bacterial translocation, further amplifying systemic inflammation and immune dysregulation. In the central portion of the figure, the interconnected pathways of metabolic, immune, and neuroendocrine dysfunctions are highlighted. Chronic psycho-emotional stress and circadian rhythm disruption lead to persistent activation of the sympathetic nervous system (SNS) and the hypothalamic–pituitary–adrenal (HPA) axis, which, over time, results in cortisol resistance and SNS sensitization. This prolonged neuroendocrine dysfunction fosters low-grade inflammation and neuroinflammation, further impairing insulin and leptin signaling. Leptin resistance, in particular, contributes to a sustained activation of the JAK-STAT signaling pathway, which is known to promote chronic inflammation and fibrotic processes. The dysregulation of this pathway is likely responsible for the coexistence of pro-inflammatory and fibrosis-resolving macrophages in FS, perpetuating a pathological state where fibrosis is initiated but not efficiently resolved. Furthermore, gut microbiota dysbiosis and bacterial translocation contribute to the systemic immune activation, exacerbating the inflammatory environment and fibrosis progression in FS. On the right side of the figure, a multi-targeted, integrative treatment strategy for FS is proposed, addressing both systemic metabolic–immune imbalances and localized tissue pathology. These interventions include physiotherapy, exercise, dietary habits, oral health, mental health, and sleep quality.

5. Low-Grade Infections, Altered Microbiota, and Leptin Resistance

Interestingly, systemic leptin levels are known to decrease in states of malnutrition and starvation, which underscores leptin's role as a mediator between nutritional status and immune function [57]. Leptin deficiency is linked to heightened vulnerability to various infections [58]. Furthermore, certain infections can mimic malnutrition by downregulating leptin levels, contributing to an immune-compromised state [59]. For example, a significant drop in leptin levels during starvation has been associated with increased sensitivity to endotoxins like lipopolysaccharides (LPS) and TNF-α in animal models. However, leptin replacement has been shown to reverse these effects, protecting against fasting-induced immune deficiencies, such as lymphopenia [60,61].

Phagocytosis, a key immune mechanism for eliminating pathogens, is enhanced by leptin, which stimulates macrophage activity and prevents apoptosis in multiple immune cells involved in both innate and adaptive immunity [62]. Numerous studies support the idea that leptin supplementation can reduce infections caused by pathogens such as *Listeria monocytogenes*, *Klebsiella pneumoniae*, *Escherichia coli*, and *Mycobacterium tuberculosis* by boosting macrophage phagocytosis [10,59,63]. Leptin also plays a crucial role in combating sepsis, a severe inflammatory response that can lead to organ failure and death. In leptin-deficient mice, exogenous leptin administration improved survival rates during sepsis by reducing systemic IL-6 levels and controlling inflammation [10,64]. In humans, higher leptin levels have been observed in survivors of sepsis compared to non-survivors, underscoring leptin's protective role in immune responses during infection [59].

Obesity, on the other hand, is associated with elevated leptin levels, which can promote chronic low-grade inflammation by activating both innate and adaptive immune cells [65]. This pro-inflammatory environment contributes to the breakdown of immune tolerance, priming immune cells for a Th1-dominated response [10,66]. This persistent inflammation heightens the risk of developing metabolic diseases such as cardiovascular disease and type 2 diabetes, as well as autoimmune conditions like multiple sclerosis, thyroiditis, rheumatoid arthritis, and inflammatory bowel disease [67].

Chronic inflammation, whether due to infection or autoimmune disease, can lead to leptin resistance, particularly in the hypothalamus [68]. This leptin resistance impairs appetite regulation and energy expenditure, further exacerbating obesity [69]. In obesity, the interaction between hypertrophic adipocytes and immune cells, such as macrophages, leads to an overproduction of pro-inflammatory cytokines and adipokines, like leptin [70]. These molecules perpetuate local and systemic inflammation, contributing to leptin resistance at both the peripheral and central levels [71]. Inflammatory cytokines activate signaling pathways, such as NF-κB, which induce suppressors of cytokine signaling (SOCS3) and protein tyrosine phosphatases (PTP1B), further inhibiting leptin receptor signaling via the JAK/STAT pathway [26,72,73].

Emerging research highlights the role of gut microbiota in regulating systemic metabolism, particularly energy balance, glucose homeostasis, and low-grade inflammation associated with obesity [74–76]. Alterations in the gut microbiota, such as those caused by a high-fat diet, have been linked to a reduction in beneficial bacterial populations, like *Bifidobacterium* spp., *Lactobacillus* spp., and *Roseburia* spp. [77–79]. The interaction between gut microbiota and the immune system is mediated by pattern recognition receptors like Toll-like receptors (TLRs), which detect microbial components such as LPS. Fatty acids can stimulate innate immunity by interacting with the TLR4/CD14 complex, further promoting inflammatory responses [80]. Alterations in the gut microbiota have been implicated in the development of obesity and its related metabolic disorders, with evidence suggesting that modulating the gut microbiota can influence leptin sensitivity and metabolic outcomes [81–83].

Interestingly, the gut microbiota also appears to regulate leptin action, with studies showing that dietary interventions, like prebiotics, can improve leptin sensitivity in obese and diabetic mice [84]. This suggests that gut microbiota modulation may offer a novel therapeutic strategy for restoring leptin sensitivity and addressing metabolic dysregulation in FS.

Additionally, recent findings suggest a possible infectious etiology in frozen shoulder (FS), linked to bacteria that commonly inhabit human skin, such as *Propionibacterium acnes* (*P. acnes*) [85–87]. Although some studies argue against this hypothesis, others have found evidence of infection in FS patients. For instance, markers such as HMGB1, IL-33, S100A8, and S100A9 were elevated in the joint capsules of FS patients, supporting the notion of a low-grade infection contributing to the pathology [88]. *P. acnes*, often dismissed as a contaminant due to its slow growth in anaerobic conditions, has been implicated in post-surgical infections and other conditions, like disk herniation [89–91]. The systemic spread of these bacteria, along with species like *Streptococcus epidermis* and *Corynebacterium propinquum*, could contribute to persistent low-grade infections that play a role in the chronic inflammation observed in FS [92].

Bacterial infiltration can occur through daily activities, such as tooth brushing, leading to microbial dissemination via the bloodstream [93]. These bacteria may enter tissues with low oxygen levels, such as the intervertebral disks and possibly the shoulder joint, particularly in areas with reduced movement [8,94]. Such low-grade infections may be an under-recognized factor in the development of FS and other inflammatory conditions [95].

6. Discussion

This review highlights the complex interplay between leptin resistance, JAK-STAT signaling, metabolic dysregulation, and immune dysfunction in the pathophysiology of frozen shoulder (FS). We summarize evidence suggesting that FS shares common inflammatory and fibrotic pathways with metabolic disorders, particularly in conditions characterized by chronic low-grade inflammation, insulin resistance, and dysregulated adipokine signaling. Leptin, traditionally recognized for its role in energy homeostasis, emerges as a key immunometabolic regulator, influencing fibroblast activation, macrophage polarization, and immune cell recruitment within the joint capsule. Moreover, we discuss how JAK-STAT dysregulation, particularly through leptin resistance and SOCS3 overexpression, may perpetuate chronic inflammation and fibrosis in FS, similar to its role in other fibrotic conditions. Recent findings demonstrate the coexistence of both pro-inflammatory and fibrosis-resolving macrophages (MERTK+) in FS tissue, suggesting that metabolic and immune cross-talk influences the progression and resolution of fibrosis, a concept that aligns with recent transcriptomic and proteomic studies. Additionally, the review explores the potential role of chronic psychosocial stress as a driver of immune–metabolic dysregulation and discusses emerging evidence linking gut microbiota alterations and bacterial translocation to systemic inflammation and immune priming in FS. These insights broaden the traditional understanding of FS as a purely orthopedic condition, instead positioning it as a multisystem disorder influenced by metabolic, inflammatory, and immune dysfunctions.

A recent study reveals the coexistence of both pro-inflammatory macrophages and fibrosis-resolving MERTK+ macrophages within the same affected tissue in FS, raising important questions regarding the underlying metabolic and signaling mechanisms that allow such cellular dynamics [21]. In traditional models of inflammation, pro-inflammatory macrophages (often referred to as M1) dominate the early stages of the immune response, followed by a transition to pro-resolving macrophages (M2) as the inflammation subsides [96]. However, the coexistence of these two distinct macrophage phenotypes in the fibrotic tissue of FS suggests a more complex regulatory environment, which is potentially driven by metabolic and immunological factors [97].

One possible explanation for this paradox may lie in the metabolic state of the tissue, particularly in relation to leptin resistance [98]. Leptin, a key regulator of both metabolism and immune responses, plays a crucial role in macrophage polarization [99]. In the context of leptin resistance, which is commonly observed in metabolic syndromes such as obesity and type 2 diabetes, macrophages may exhibit a dysregulated response [98]. This dysregulation could impair the typical transition from pro-inflammatory to pro-resolving states, allowing both phenotypes to coexist within the same tissue [100]. Specifically, leptin resistance may impair the energetic capacity of macrophages, altering their metabolic flexibility, which is required for the shift toward a fibrosis-resolving phenotype [101]. The inability to efficiently switch from glycolysis (which favors M1 polarization) to oxidative phosphorylation (which supports M2 activity) could result in the persistence of both pro-inflammatory and pro-resolving macrophages in the fibrotic environment of FS [102].

Moreover, the JAK-STAT signaling pathway, which is critically involved in both immune regulation and leptin signaling, may further contribute to this phenomenon [103]. Dysregulation of the JAK-STAT pathway due to leptin resistance can exacerbate chronic inflammation by promoting the persistence of inflammatory macrophages while simultaneously activating downstream signals that encourage tissue remodeling and fibrosis resolution [27]. In the presence of leptin resistance, the failure to adequately suppress the pro-inflammatory arm of the JAK-STAT pathway may lead to an environment where fibrosis-resolving processes are initiated but not fully effective, thereby allowing these seemingly opposing macrophage populations to coexist [51].

Thus, the coexistence of pro-inflammatory and fibrosis-resolving macrophages in FS tissue may be indicative of a metabolic and signaling imbalance, where leptin resistance and JAK-STAT pathway dysregulation prevent the efficient resolution of inflammation while simultaneously promoting fibrosis. This dynamic highlights the need for further research into how metabolic interventions, particularly those targeting leptin sensitivity and JAK-STAT modulation, could restore proper immune balance and improve fibrosis outcomes in FS.

7. Current Treatments and Future Directions

The treatment of FS remains a challenging and complex endeavor due to the multifactorial nature of the disease, involving both metabolic and inflammatory components. Current therapeutic approaches range from non-surgical interventions, such as physical therapy, corticosteroid injections, and manual mobilization, to more invasive procedures, like arthroscopic capsular release and hydrodilation [3]. However, these methods primarily focus on symptom relief and improving shoulder mobility, with limited effectiveness in addressing the underlying inflammatory and fibrotic processes [104].

Conventional Therapies and Their Limitations

Non-surgical approaches, such as corticosteroid injections, have demonstrated effectiveness in reducing pain and improving joint function during the early "freezing" phase of FS. Nonetheless, the long-term impact of corticosteroids remains limited, as they do not target the underlying causes of fibrosis and inflammation [3,104]. Similarly, physical therapy and manual mobilization are beneficial for improving the range of motion, particularly in the later stages of FS, but they also fall short in addressing the root metabolic and inflammatory factors driving disease progression [8,105].

Among non-surgical treatments, corticosteroid injections are widely used to reduce pain and improve joint function during the early "freezing" phase of FS [106]. Despite their short-term efficacy, long-term corticosteroid use does not modify the disease course and is associated with significant risks, including joint deterioration, cartilage degeneration, and systemic metabolic side effects, such as hyperglycemia and insulin resistance, particularly in patients with pre-existing metabolic disorders [107]. Similarly, physical therapy and manual mobilization remain the mainstay of conservative treatment, with benefits in the range of motion improvement, particularly in the later stages of FS [108,109].

However, overly aggressive mobilization may worsen pain and inflammation, potentially prolonging recovery [110].

For patients with persistent symptoms, surgical interventions such as arthroscopic capsular release and hydrodilation are considered. While capsular release is effective in improving mobility, it carries risks such as postoperative stiffness, adhesion reformation, and persistent pain [111]. Hydrodilation, which involves the injection of large fluid volumes into the joint capsule to increase capsular distension, has shown variable success rates and does not target the fibrotic and metabolic dysfunction underlying FS [112].

8. Emerging Therapeutic Approaches

Recent insights into metabolic dysregulation, particularly leptin resistance, suggest that FS should not only be viewed as a mechanical disorder, but also as a metabolic–immunological condition. Given the role of leptin in immune regulation and fibrosis, novel therapeutic strategies targeting leptin sensitivity, JAK-STAT signaling, and microbiome modulation have gained attention [8].

8.1. Targeting Leptin Resistance and Metabolic Dysregulation

Given the potential role leptin may play in FS pathophysiology, therapeutic interventions aimed at improving leptin sensitivity could prove beneficial. Studies have shown that exercise, particularly resistance and aerobic training, can improve leptin sensitivity and reduce systemic inflammation [8,105]. In addition, dietary modifications, such as time-restricted feeding or intermittent fasting, have been found to modulate leptin levels, offering a potential avenue for metabolic correction in FS patients [105]. However, while restoring leptin sensitivity could theoretically ameliorate fibrosis and inflammation, potential risks remain. Excessive leptin modulation could impact systemic metabolism, potentially influencing appetite regulation, insulin sensitivity, and immune function [113]. Further research is required to determine the optimal balance between therapeutic benefits and metabolic stability in FS treatment.

8.2. JAK-STAT Pathway as a Target

Persistent activation of this pathway contributes to the overproduction of pro-inflammatory cytokines, macrophage polarization, and fibroblast activation, leading to excessive extracellular matrix deposition and fibrosis [34,48]. Thus, the JAK-STAT signaling pathway, activated by inflammatory cytokines and impaired leptin signaling, may play a crucial role in both immune regulation and fibrotic progression in FS. Therapies aimed at modulating the JAK-STAT pathway could reduce inflammation and promote tissue repair, making it a promising target for FS treatment [8,105]. However, JAK-STAT inhibitors, which are already in clinical use for autoimmune and inflammatory conditions like rheumatoid arthritis, have shown promise in reducing fibrosis by modulating macrophage activity and fibroblast proliferation [114]. Moreover, their immunosuppressive effects pose significant risks, including increased susceptibility to infections, impaired immune surveillance, and potential long-term metabolic alterations [115]. Future research should aim to determine whether selective JAK-STAT modulation can provide anti-fibrotic benefits while minimizing immune suppression, potentially making it a viable therapeutic option for FS.

8.3. Gut Microbiota Modulation

Recent studies have highlighted the role of the gut microbiota in regulating systemic inflammation and metabolic health, including leptin sensitivity [116]. Alterations in gut microbiota composition, often observed in obesity and metabolic syndrome, can exacerbate leptin resistance and inflammatory processes via bacterial translocation and LPS-mediated activation of the JAK-STAT pathway [117]. Probiotic and prebiotic interventions may offer a novel therapeutic strategy to improve metabolic and immune regulation in FS patients, potentially reducing the chronic inflammation and fibrosis associated with the condition [8,118]. However, the precise role of microbiota-driven inflammation in FS remains to be fully elucidated, warranting further clinical investigation.

9. Future Research Directions

Given the complex interplay of metabolic, inflammatory, and fibrotic processes in FS, future research must explore novel pathways that may provide insight into the underlying mechanisms of this condition. One promising area of investigation involves the relationship between mental health, mitochondrial dysfunction, circadian rhythm disruption, leptin resistance, and the JAK-STAT signaling pathway, which together could play a pivotal role in FS progression.

9.1. Lifestyle Interventions as a Potential Therapeutic Approach in FS

In light of the growing evidence linking chronic psychosocial stress, metabolic dysregulation, and immune dysfunction in FS, lifestyle interventions emerge as a promising avenue for disease management [24]. Modern lifestyle factors, including sedentary behavior, poor dietary habits, and chronic exposure to psychosocial stressors, have been implicated in the disruption of homeostatic regulatory systems, including the hypothalamic–pituitary–adrenal (HPA) axis and the autonomic nervous system [24]. These disruptions, in turn, contribute to chronic low-grade inflammation, gut barrier dysfunction, and neuroimmune activation, which have been proposed as key drivers of immune-mediated musculoskeletal conditions such as FS [119]. From a psychoneuroimmunological perspective, interventions that promote physical activity, circadian alignment, and metabolic flexibility could mitigate the sustained immune activation and metabolic disturbances associated with shoulder pain [120]. Regular exercise has been shown to improve leptin and insulin sensitivity, while also exerting anti-inflammatory effects through modulation of the gut microbiome and systemic cytokine profiles [121]. Additionally, circadian rhythm regulation through light exposure, sleep hygiene, and structured feeding patterns has been proposed as an essential component in restoring immune–metabolic balance, particularly in individuals experiencing stress-related immune dysfunction [122]. Given the interplay between environmental stressors, immune dysregulation, and FS progression, future research should focus on integrative lifestyle-based interventions that address both the physiological and psychosocial dimensions of the disease. These approaches may hold significant potential in improving patient outcomes while reducing reliance on pharmacological therapies that primarily target symptom relief rather than the underlying pathophysiology of FS.

9.2. Mitochondrial Dysfunction and FS Progression

Mitochondrial health is critical for maintaining cellular energy homeostasis and regulating immune responses. Mitochondrial dysfunction, often a result of chronic inflammation and metabolic stress, is associated with decreased ATP production, increased oxidative stress, and impaired tissue repair [123]. In the context of FS, mitochondrial dysfunction may exacerbate the chronic inflammation and fibrosis observed in the joint capsule [8]. As immune cells, such as macrophages, rely on mitochondrial energy production to facilitate their transition from pro-inflammatory (M1) to fibrosis-resolving (M2 or MERTK+), mitochondrial dysfunction could delay this transition, prolonging inflammation and fibrosis [21]. Understanding how mitochondrial impairment influences macrophage function and fibroblast activity in FS could provide valuable insight into the disease's metabolic underpinnings and suggest potential therapeutic targets aimed at restoring mitochondrial function to improve tissue repair.

9.3. Disruption of Circadian Rhythms

Circadian rhythms regulate a wide array of physiological processes, including immune function and energy metabolism. Disruption of these rhythms, whether due to sleep disorders, shift work, or other environmental factors, has been linked to metabolic diseases and chronic inflammation [124]. In shoulder disorders, the dysregulation of circadian rhythms could further impair the already-compromised metabolic pathways, such as leptin signaling, thereby perpetuating the disease state [120]. Leptin levels are known to follow a circadian pattern, and disruptions in these rhythms may worsen leptin resistance, impairing the body's ability to regulate energy balance and immune responses effectively [125,126]. Investigating how circadian rhythm disturbances contribute to metabolic dysregulation and inflammation in FS could open new avenues for chronotherapy-based interventions that realign circadian patterns to improve metabolic outcomes and reduce inflammation [127,128].

9.4. Leptin Resistance and JAK-STAT Pathway

Leptin resistance may play a central role in the chronic inflammation and metabolic disturbances observed in FS [24,129]. The JAK-STAT pathway, activated by inflammatory cytokines and impaired leptin signaling, is a critical mediator of immune responses and fibrosis [38]. In FS, persistent activation of the JAK-STAT pathway due to leptin resistance may promote the sustained activation of pro-inflammatory macrophages and fibroblasts, leading to excessive extracellular matrix deposition and tissue fibrosis [38]. Future research should focus on the precise mechanisms by which leptin resistance amplifies JAK-STAT signaling and how this contributes to the maintenance of a chronic inflammatory state in FS [129]. Targeting the JAK-STAT pathway in conjunction with restoring leptin sensitivity may provide a dual approach to reducing inflammation and fibrosis in FS patients.

10. Conclusions

This review highlights the potential critical role of metabolic–immune dysregulation, particularly leptin resistance and JAK-STAT signaling, in the pathophysiology of FS. The persistence of both pro-inflammatory and fibrosis-resolving (MERTK+) macrophages within FS tissue suggests a disrupted immune resolution process, potentially driven by metabolic impairments. Leptin resistance, a hallmark of metabolic disorders, not only contributes to sustained inflammation, but also disrupts macrophage polarization, delaying fibrosis resolution. This metabolic dysfunction is further amplified by chronic neuroinflammation, mitochondrial dysfunction, and circadian rhythm disruption, which collectively impair the transition from acute to resolving phases of inflammation.

The JAK-STAT pathway, as a central mediator of immune and metabolic responses, likely plays a pivotal role in maintaining this dysfunctional environment.

Given the complexity of FS pathogenesis, effective therapeutic strategies should move beyond symptom management and target the root causes of metabolic and immune dysregulation. Restoring leptin sensitivity, modulating JAK-STAT signaling, improving mitochondrial function, and aligning circadian rhythms emerge as promising avenues for intervention. Additionally, integrative approaches, including exercise, dietary modifications, gut microbiota-targeted therapies, and psychological stress management, may enhance immune resilience and metabolic homeostasis.

Future research should prioritize investigating the mechanistic links between metabolic dysfunction, immune dysregulation, and fibrosis progression in FS. A deeper understanding of how chronic stress, neuroendocrine alterations, and systemic inflammation intersect in FS pathophysiology may open new therapeutic opportunities, not only for FS, but also for other chronic inflammatory and fibrotic conditions. Addressing these interconnected mechanisms through precision medicine and personalized metabolic–immune interventions could transform FS management, offering long-term solutions that go beyond conventional orthopedic treatments.

Funding: This research received no external funding.

Acknowledgments: This publication is part of the project Ref. No.: MEL-02-UGR24, funded by the Autonomous City of Melilla as part of its commitment to research.

Conflicts of Interest: The author declares no conflict of interest.

References

1. Abrassart, S.; Kolo, F.; Piotton, S.; Chih-Hao Chiu, J.; Stirling, P.; Hoffmeyer, P.; Lädermann, A. 'Frozen shoulder' is ill-defined. How can it be described better? *EFORT Open Rev.* **2020**, *5*, 273–279. [CrossRef]
2. Brue, S.; Valentin, A.; Forssblad, M.; Werner, S.; Mikkelsen, C.; Cerulli, G. Idiopathic adhesive capsulitis of the shoulder: A review. *Knee Surg. Sports Traumatol. Arthrosc.* **2007**, *15*, 1048–1054. [CrossRef]
3. Date, A.; Rahman, L. Frozen Shoulder: Overview of Clinical Presentation and Review of the Current Evidence Base for Management Strategies. *Future Sci. OA* **2020**, *6*, FSO647. [CrossRef] [PubMed]
4. Mertens, M.G.; Struyf, F.; Verborgt, O.; Dueñas, L.; Balasch-Bernat, M.; Navarro-Ledesma, S.; Fernandez-Sanchez, M.; Luque-Suarez, A.; Lluch Girbes, E.; Meeus, M. Exploration of the clinical course and longitudinal correlations in frozen shoulder: The role of autonomic function, central pain processing, and psychological variables. A longitudinal multicenter prospective observational study. *Musculoskelet. Sci. Pract.* **2023**, *67*, 102857. [CrossRef]
5. Mertens, M.G.; Meeus, M.; Verborgt, O.; Girbes, E.L.; Horno, S.M.-D.; Aguilar-Rodriguez, M.; Dueñas, L.; Navarro-Ledesma, S.; Fernandez-Sanchez, M.; Luque-Suarez, A.; et al. Exploration of the clinical course of frozen shoulder: A longitudinal multicenter prospective study of functional impairments. *Braz. J. Phys. Ther.* **2023**, *27*, 100539. [CrossRef] [PubMed]
6. Lyne, S.A.; Goldblatt, F.M.; Shanahan, E.M. Living with a frozen shoulder—A phenomenological inquiry. *BMC Musculoskelet. Disord.* **2022**, *23*, 318. [CrossRef] [PubMed]
7. Struyf, F.; Mertens, M.; Navarro-Ledesma, S. Causes of Shoulder Dysfunction in Diabetic Patients: A Review of Literature. *Int. J. Environ. Res. Public Health* **2022**, *19*, 6228. [CrossRef]
8. De la Serna, D.; Navarro-Ledesma, S.; Alayón, F.; López, E.; Pruimboom, L. A Comprehensive View of Frozen Shoulder: A Mystery Syndrome. *Front. Med.* **2021**, *8*, 663703. [CrossRef]
9. Navarro-Ledesma, S.; Hamed-Hamed, D.; Pruimboom, L. A new perspective of frozen shoulder pathology; the interplay between the brain and the immune system. *Front. Physiol.* **2024**, *15*, 1248612. [CrossRef]
10. Pérez-Pérez, A.; Sánchez-Jiménez, F.; Vilariño-García, T.; Sánchez-Margalet, V. Role of Leptin in Inflammation and Vice Versa. *Int. J. Mol. Sci.* **2020**, *21*, 5887. [CrossRef]
11. Pérez-Pérez, A.; Vilariño-García, T.; Fernández-Riejos, P.; Martín-González, J.; Segura-Egea, J.J.; Sánchez-Margalet, V. Role of leptin as a link between metabolism and the immune system. *Cytokine Growth Factor Rev.* **2017**, *35*, 71–84. [CrossRef] [PubMed]
12. Nataf, S. Evolution, immunity and the emergence of brain superautoantigens. *F1000Research* **2017**, *6*, 171. [CrossRef]
13. Sohnlein, P.; Muller, M.; Syren, K.; Hartmann, U.; Bohm, B.O.; Meinck, H.M.; Knip, M.; Akerblom, H.K.; Richter, W. Epitope spreading and a varying but not disease-specific GAD65 antibody response in Type I diabetes. *Diabetologia* **2000**, *43*, 210–217. [CrossRef]
14. Kawahara, K.; Hohjoh, H.; Inazumi, T.; Tsuchiya, S.; Sugimoto, Y. Prostaglandin E2-induced inflammation: Relevance of prostaglandin E receptors. *Biochim. Biophys. Acta Mol. Cell Biol. Lipids* **2015**, *1851*, 414–421. [CrossRef] [PubMed]
15. Leonardini, A.; Laviola, L.; Perrini, S.; Natalicchio, A.; Giorgino, F. Cross-Talk between PPAR γ and Insulin Signaling and Modulation of Insulin Sensitivity. *PPAR Res.* **2009**, *2009*, 818945. [CrossRef] [PubMed]
16. Thon, M.; Hosoi, T.; Ozawa, K. Possible Integrative Actions of Leptin and Insulin Signaling in the Hypothalamus Targeting Energy Homeostasis. *Front. Endocrinol.* **2016**, *7*, 138. [CrossRef]
17. Huang, X.; Liu, G.; Guo, J.; Su, Z. The PI3K/AKT pathway in obesity and type 2 diabetes. *Int. J. Biol. Sci.* **2018**, *14*, 1483–1496. [CrossRef]
18. Roh, J.S.; Sohn, D.H. Damage-Associated Molecular Patterns in Inflammatory Diseases. *Immune Netw.* **2018**, *18*, e27. [CrossRef]
19. Khorshidian, N.; Khanniri, E.; Koushki, M.R.; Sohrabvandi, S.; Yousefi, M. An Overview of Antimicrobial Activity of Lysozyme and Its Functionality in Cheese. *Front. Nutr.* **2022**, *9*, 833618. [CrossRef]
20. Hand, G.C.R.; Athanasou, N.A.; Matthews, T.; Carr, A.J. The pathology of frozen shoulder. *J. Bone Jt. Surg. Br.* **2007**, *89-B*, 928–932. [CrossRef]
21. Ng, M.T.H.; Borst, R.; Gacaferi, H.; Davidson, S.; Ackerman, J.E.; Johnson, P.A.; Machado, C.C.; Reekie, I.; Attar, M.; Windell, D.; et al. A single cell atlas of frozen shoulder capsule identifies features associated with inflammatory fibrosis resolution. *Nat. Commun.* **2024**, *15*, 1394. [CrossRef] [PubMed]

22. Yao, J.; Wu, D.; Qiu, Y. Adipose tissue macrophage in obesity-associated metabolic diseases. *Front. Immunol.* **2022**, *13*, 977485. [CrossRef]
23. Pellegrinelli, V.; Rodriguez-Cuenca, S.; Rouault, C.; Figueroa-Juarez, E.; Schilbert, H.; Virtue, S.; Moreno-Navarrete, J.M.; Bidault, G.; Vázquez-Borrego, M.C.; Dias, A.R.; et al. Dysregulation of macrophage PEPD in obesity determines adipose tissue fibro-inflammation and insulin resistance. *Nat. Metab.* **2022**, *4*, 476–494. [CrossRef]
24. Pruimboom, L.; Rocio, F.A.; Navarro-Ledesma, S. Psychoneuroimmunology in the Daily Clinic is Only Possible Within a Contextual Frame. In *PsychoNeuroImmunology: Volume 1: Integration of Psychology, Neurology, and Immunology*; Springer Nature: Cham, Switzerland, 2024; pp. 515–563.
25. Sarapultsev, A.; Gusev, E.; Komelkova, M.; Utepova, I.; Luo, S.; Hu, D. JAK-STAT signaling in inflammation and stress-related diseases: Implications for therapeutic interventions. *Mol. Biomed.* **2023**, *4*, 40. [CrossRef]
26. Hu, X.; Li, J.; Fu, M.; Zhao, X.; Wang, W. The JAK/STAT signaling pathway: From bench to clinic. *Signal Transduct. Target. Ther.* **2021**, *6*, 402. [CrossRef] [PubMed]
27. Gurzov, E.N.; Stanley, W.J.; Pappas, E.G.; Thomas, H.E.; Gough, D.J. The JAK/STAT pathway in obesity and diabetes. *FEBS J.* **2016**, *283*, 3002–3015. [CrossRef]
28. Yang, R.; Barouch, L.A. Leptin Signaling and Obesity. *Circ. Res.* **2007**, *101*, 545–559. [CrossRef]
29. Paz-Filho, G.; Mastronardi, C.; Wong, M.-L.; Licinio, J. Leptin therapy, insulin sensitivity, and glucose homeostasis. *Indian J. Endocrinol. Metab.* **2012**, *16*, 549. [CrossRef] [PubMed]
30. Cui, J.; Zhang, T.; Xiong, J.; Lu, W.; Duan, L.; Zhu, W.; Wang, D. RNA-sequence analysis of samples from patients with idiopathic adhesive capsulitis. *Mol. Med. Rep.* **2017**, *16*, 7665–7672. [CrossRef]
31. Burja, B.; Mertelj, T.; Frank-Bertoncelj, M. Hi-JAKi-ng Synovial Fibroblasts in Inflammatory Arthritis With JAK Inhibitors. *Front. Med.* **2020**, *7*, 124. [CrossRef]
32. Hu, Q.; Bian, Q.; Rong, D.; Wang, L.; Song, J.; Huang, H.-S.; Zeng, J.; Mei, J.; Wang, P.-Y. JAK/STAT pathway: Extracellular signals, diseases, immunity, and therapeutic regimens. *Front. Bioeng. Biotechnol.* **2023**, *11*, 1110765. [CrossRef] [PubMed]
33. Papaioannou, I.; Xu, S.; Denton, C.P.; Abraham, D.J.; Ponticos, M. STAT3 controls COL1A2 enhancer activation cooperatively with JunB, regulates type I collagen synthesis posttranscriptionally, and is essential for lung myofibroblast differentiation. *Mol. Biol. Cell* **2018**, *29*, 84–95. [CrossRef] [PubMed]
34. Yan, Z.; Gibson, S.A.; Buckley, J.A.; Qin, H.; Benveniste, E.N. Role of the JAK/STAT signaling pathway in regulation of innate immunity in neuroinflammatory diseases. *Clin. Immunol.* **2018**, *189*, 4–13. [CrossRef]
35. Kamal, N.; McGee, S.L.; Eng, K.; Brown, G.; Beattie, S.; Collier, F.; Gill, S.; Page, R.S. Transcriptomic analysis of adhesive capsulitis of the shoulder. *J. Orthop. Res.* **2020**, *38*, 2280–2289. [CrossRef]
36. Chen, P.-Y.; Qin, L.; Simons, M. TGFβ signaling pathways in human health and disease. *Front. Mol. Biosci.* **2023**, *10*, 1113061. [CrossRef]
37. Giarratana, A.O.; Prendergast, C.M.; Salvatore, M.M.; Capaccione, K.M. TGF-β signaling: Critical nexus of fibrogenesis and cancer. *J. Transl. Med.* **2024**, *22*, 594. [CrossRef]
38. Liu, J.; Wang, F.; Luo, F. The Role of JAK/STAT Pathway in Fibrotic Diseases: Molecular and Cellular Mechanisms. *Biomolecules* **2023**, *13*, 119. [CrossRef] [PubMed]
39. Chakraborty, D.; Šumová, B.; Mallano, T.; Chen, C.-W.; Distler, A.; Bergmann, C.; Ludolph, I.; Horch, R.E.; Gelse, K.; Ramming, A.; et al. Activation of STAT3 integrates common profibrotic pathways to promote fibroblast activation and tissue fibrosis. *Nat. Commun.* **2017**, *8*, 1130. [CrossRef]
40. Casado, M.E.; Collado-Pérez, R.; Frago, L.M.; Barrios, V. Recent Advances in the Knowledge of the Mechanisms of Leptin Physiology and Actions in Neurological and Metabolic Pathologies. *Int. J. Mol. Sci.* **2023**, *24*, 1422. [CrossRef]
41. Jain, M.; Budinger, G.R.S.; Lo, A.; Urich, D.; Rivera, S.E.; Ghosh, A.K.; Gonzalez, A.; Chiarella, S.E.; Marks, K.; Donnelly, H.K.; et al. Leptin promotes fibroproliferative acute respiratory distress syndrome by inhibiting peroxisome proliferator-activated receptor-γ. *Am. J. Respir. Crit. Care Med.* **2011**, *183*, 1490–1498. [CrossRef]
42. Dees, C.; Pötter, S.; Zhang, Y.; Bergmann, C.; Zhou, X.; Luber, M.; Wohlfahrt, T.; Karouzakis, E.; Ramming, A.; Gelse, K.; et al. TGF-β-induced epigenetic deregulation of SOCS3 facilitates STAT3 signaling to promote fibrosis. *J. Clin. Investig.* **2020**, *130*, 2347–2363. [CrossRef] [PubMed]
43. Choi, S.S.; Syn, W.-K.; Karaca, G.F.; Omenetti, A.; Moylan, C.A.; Witek, R.P.; Agboola, K.M.; Jung, Y.; Michelotti, G.A.; Diehl, A.M. Leptin promotes the myofibroblastic phenotype in hepatic stellate cells by activating the hedgehog pathway. *J. Biol. Chem.* **2010**, *285*, 36551–36560. [CrossRef]
44. Jain, M.; Singh, M.K.; Shyam, H.; Mishra, A.; Kumar, S.; Kumar, A.; Kushwaha, J. Role of JAK/STAT in the Neuroinflammation and its Association with Neurological Disorders. *Ann. Neurosci.* **2021**, *28*, 191–200. [CrossRef]
45. Dragano, N.R.V.; Haddad-Tovolli, R.; Velloso, L.A. Leptin, Neuroinflammation and Obesity. *Front. Horm. Res.* **2017**, *48*, 84–96.
46. Jais, A.; Brüning, J.C. Hypothalamic inflammation in obesity and metabolic disease. *J. Clin. Investig.* **2017**, *127*, 24–32. [CrossRef]

47. Martin, S.S.; Qasim, A.; Reilly, M.P. Leptin Resistance: A possible interface of inflammation and metabolism in obesity-related cardiovascular disease. *J. Am. Coll. Cardiol.* **2008**, *52*, 1201–1210. [CrossRef] [PubMed]
48. Philips, R.L.; Wang, Y.; Cheon, H.; Kanno, Y.; Gadina, M.; Sartorelli, V.; Horvath, C.M.; Darnell, J.E.; Stark, G.R.; O'Shea, J.J. The JAK-STAT pathway at 30: Much learned, much more to do. *Cell* **2022**, *185*, 3857–3876. [CrossRef]
49. Yang, H.; Cheng, H.; Dai, R.; Shang, L.; Zhang, X.; Wen, H. Macrophage polarization in tissue fibrosis. *PeerJ* **2023**, *11*, e16092. [CrossRef] [PubMed]
50. Xue, C.; Yao, Q.; Gu, X.; Shi, Q.; Yuan, X.; Chu, Q.; Bao, Z.; Lu, J.; Li, L. Evolving cognition of the JAK-STAT signaling pathway: Autoimmune disorders and cancer. *Signal Transduct. Target. Ther.* **2023**, *8*, 204. [CrossRef]
51. Xia, T.; Zhang, M.; Lei, W.; Yang, R.; Fu, S.; Fan, Z.; Yang, Y.; Zhang, T. Advances in the role of STAT3 in macrophage polarization. *Front. Immunol.* **2023**, *14*, 1160719. [CrossRef]
52. Li, L.; Li, D.; Wang, Z.; Li, J.; Shahzad, K.A.; Wang, Y.; Tan, F. Signaling pathways activated and regulated by stem cell-derived exosome therapy. *Cell Biosci.* **2024**, *14*, 105. [CrossRef]
53. Bjørbæk, C.; Lavery, H.J.; Bates, S.H.; Olson, R.K.; Davis, S.M.; Flier, J.S.; Myers, M.G. SOCS3 Mediates Feedback Inhibition of the Leptin Receptor via Tyr985. *J. Biol. Chem.* **2000**, *275*, 40649–40657. [CrossRef] [PubMed]
54. Wunderlich, C.M.; Hövelmeyer, N.; Wunderlich, F.T. Mechanisms of chronic JAK-STAT3-SOCS3 signaling in obesity. *JAK-STAT* **2013**, *2*, e23878. [CrossRef]
55. Jorgensen, S.B.; O'Neill, H.M.; Sylow, L.; Honeyman, J.; Hewitt, K.A.; Palanivel, R.; Fullerton, M.D.; Öberg, L.; Balendran, A.; Galic, S.; et al. Deletion of Skeletal Muscle SOCS3 Prevents Insulin Resistance in Obesity. *Diabetes* **2013**, *62*, 56–64. [CrossRef] [PubMed]
56. Brindisino, F.; Minnucci, S.; Sergi, G.; Lorusso, M.; Struyf, F.; Innocenti, T. Does the psychological profile of a patient with frozen shoulder predict future outcome? A systematic review. *Physiother. Res. Int.* **2024**, *29*, e2056. [CrossRef]
57. Perry, R.J.; Shulman, G.I. The Role of Leptin in Maintaining Plasma Glucose During Starvation. *Postdoc J.* **2018**, *6*, 3–19. [CrossRef] [PubMed]
58. Maurya, R.; Bhattacharya, P.; Dey, R.; Nakhasi, H.L. Leptin Functions in Infectious Diseases. *Front. Immunol.* **2018**, *9*, 2741. [CrossRef] [PubMed]
59. Alti, D.; Sambamurthy, C.; Kalangi, S.K. Emergence of Leptin in Infection and Immunity: Scope and Challenges in Vaccines Formulation. *Front. Cell. Infect. Microbiol.* **2018**, *8*, 147. [CrossRef]
60. Faggioni, R.; Moser, A.; Feingold, K.R.; Grunfeld, C. Reduced Leptin Levels in Starvation Increase Susceptibility to Endotoxic Shock. *Am. J. Pathol.* **2000**, *156*, 1781–1787. [CrossRef]
61. Oishi, K.; Hashimoto, C. Short-term time-restricted feeding during the resting phase is sufficient to induce leptin resistance that contributes to development of obesity and metabolic disorders in mice. *Chronobiol. Int.* **2018**, *35*, 1576–1594. [CrossRef]
62. Sánchez-Muñoz, F.; García-Macedo, R.; Alarcón-Aguilar, F.; Cruz, M. Adipocitokines, adipose tissue and its relationship with immune system cells. *Gac. Med. Mex.* **2005**, *141*, 505–512. [PubMed]
63. Hirayama, D.; Iida, T.; Nakase, H. The Phagocytic Function of Macrophage-Enforcing Innate Immunity and Tissue Homeostasis. *Int. J. Mol. Sci.* **2017**, *19*, 92. [CrossRef]
64. Birlutiu, V.; Boicean, L.C. Serum leptin level as a diagnostic and prognostic marker in infectious diseases and sepsis. *Medicine* **2021**, *100*, e25720. [CrossRef]
65. Kiernan, K.; MacIver, N.J. The Role of the Adipokine Leptin in Immune Cell Function in Health and Disease. *Front. Immunol.* **2021**, *11*, 622468. [CrossRef]
66. Francisco, V.; Pino, J.; Campos-Cabaleiro, V.; Ruiz-Fernández, C.; Mera, A.; Gonzalez-Gay, M.A.; Gómez, R.; Gualillo, O. Obesity, Fat Mass and Immune System: Role for Leptin. *Front. Physiol.* **2018**, *9*, 640. [CrossRef]
67. Franco, J.-S.; Amaya-Amaya, J.; Anaya, J.-M. Thyroid disease and autoimmune diseases. In *Autoimmunity: From Bench to Bedside*; Anaya, J.-M., Shoenfeld, Y., Rojas-Villarraga, A., Levy, R.A., Cervera, R., Eds.; El Rosario University Press: Bogotá, Colombia, 2013.
68. Timper, K.; Brüning, J.C. Hypothalamic circuits regulating appetite and energy homeostasis: Pathways to obesity. *Dis. Model. Mech.* **2017**, *10*, 679–689. [CrossRef] [PubMed]
69. Liu, Z.; Xiao, T.; Liu, H. Leptin signaling and its central role in energy homeostasis. *Front. Neurosci.* **2023**, *17*, 1238528. [CrossRef] [PubMed]
70. Czaja-Stolc, S.; Potrykus, M.; Stankiewicz, M.; Kaska, Ł.; Małgorzewicz, S. Pro-Inflammatory Profile of Adipokines in Obesity Contributes to Pathogenesis, Nutritional Disorders, and Cardiovascular Risk in Chronic Kidney Disease. *Nutrients* **2022**, *14*, 1457. [CrossRef]
71. Kirichenko, T.V.; Markina, Y.V.; Bogatyreva, A.I.; Tolstik, T.V.; Varaeva, Y.R.; Starodubova, A. V The Role of Adipokines in Inflammatory Mechanisms of Obesity. *Int. J. Mol. Sci.* **2022**, *23*, 14982. [CrossRef]
72. Kwon, O.; Kim, K.W.; Kim, M.-S. Leptin signalling pathways in hypothalamic neurons. *Cell. Mol. Life Sci.* **2016**, *73*, 1457–1477. [CrossRef]

73. Morris, R.; Kershaw, N.J.; Babon, J.J. The molecular details of cytokine signaling via the JAK/STAT pathway. *Protein Sci.* **2018**, *27*, 1984–2009. [CrossRef]
74. Islam, M.R.; Arthur, S.; Haynes, J.; Butts, M.R.; Nepal, N.; Sundaram, U. The Role of Gut Microbiota and Metabolites in Obesity-Associated Chronic Gastrointestinal Disorders. *Nutrients* **2022**, *14*, 624. [CrossRef]
75. Vetrani, C.; Di Nisio, A.; Paschou, S.A.; Barrea, L.; Muscogiuri, G.; Graziadio, C.; Savastano, S.; Colao, A. From Gut Microbiota through Low-Grade Inflammation to Obesity: Key Players and Potential Targets. *Nutrients* **2022**, *14*, 2103. [CrossRef] [PubMed]
76. Scheithauer, T.P.M.; Rampanelli, E.; Nieuwdorp, M.; Vallance, B.A.; Verchere, C.B.; van Raalte, D.H.; Herrema, H. Gut Microbiota as a Trigger for Metabolic Inflammation in Obesity and Type 2 Diabetes. *Front. Immunol.* **2020**, *11*, 571731. [CrossRef] [PubMed]
77. Beam, A.; Clinger, E.; Hao, L. Effect of Diet and Dietary Components on the Composition of the Gut Microbiota. *Nutrients* **2021**, *13*, 2795. [CrossRef]
78. Singh, R.K.; Chang, H.-W.; Yan, D.; Lee, K.M.; Ucmak, D.; Wong, K.; Abrouk, M.; Farahnik, B.; Nakamura, M.; Zhu, T.H.; et al. Influence of diet on the gut microbiome and implications for human health. *J. Transl. Med.* **2017**, *15*, 73. [CrossRef] [PubMed]
79. Rinninella, E.; Tohumcu, E.; Raoul, P.; Fiorani, M.; Cintoni, M.; Mele, M.C.; Cammarota, G.; Gasbarrini, A.; Ianiro, G. The role of diet in shaping human gut microbiota. *Best Pract. Res. Clin. Gastroenterol.* **2023**, *62–63*, 101828. [CrossRef]
80. Li, D.; Wu, M. Pattern recognition receptors in health and diseases. *Signal Transduct. Target. Ther.* **2021**, *6*, 291. [CrossRef]
81. Valentini, M.; Piermattei, A.; Di Sante, G.; Migliara, G.; Delogu, G.; Ria, F. Immunomodulation by Gut Microbiota: Role of Toll-Like Receptor Expressed by T Cells. *J. Immunol. Res.* **2014**, *2014*, 586939. [CrossRef]
82. Frosali, S.; Pagliari, D.; Gambassi, G.; Landolfi, R.; Pandolfi, F.; Cianci, R. How the Intricate Interaction among Toll-Like Receptors, Microbiota, and Intestinal Immunity Can Influence Gastrointestinal Pathology. *J. Immunol. Res.* **2015**, *2015*, 489821. [CrossRef]
83. Fitzgerald, K.A.; Kagan, J.C. Toll-like Receptors and the Control of Immunity. *Cell* **2020**, *180*, 1044–1066. [CrossRef] [PubMed]
84. Everard, A.; Lazarevic, V.; Derrien, M.; Girard, M.; Muccioli, G.G.; Neyrinck, A.M.; Possemiers, S.; Van Holle, A.; François, P.; de Vos, W.M.; et al. Responses of Gut Microbiota and Glucose and Lipid Metabolism to Prebiotics in Genetic Obese and Diet-Induced Leptin-Resistant Mice. *Diabetes* **2011**, *60*, 2775–2786. [CrossRef]
85. Piggott, D.A.; Higgins, Y.M.; Melia, M.T.; Ellis, B.; Carroll, K.C.; McFarland, E.G.; Auwaerter, P.G. Characteristics and Treatment Outcomes of Propionibacterium acnes Prosthetic Shoulder Infections in Adults. *Open Forum Infect. Dis.* **2015**, *3*, ofv191. [CrossRef] [PubMed]
86. Bunker, T.D.; Boyd, M.; Gallacher, S.; Auckland, C.R.; Kitson, J.; Smith, C.D. Association between Propionibacterium acnes and frozen shoulder: A pilot study. *Shoulder Elb.* **2014**, *6*, 257–261. [CrossRef]
87. Booker, S.J.; Boyd, M.; Gallacher, S.; Evans, J.P.; Auckland, C.; Kitson, J.; Thomas, W.; Smith, C.D. The colonisation of the glenohumeral joint by Propionibacterium acnes is not associated with frozen shoulder but is more likely to occur after an injection into the joint. *Bone Jt. J.* **2017**, *99-B*, 1067–1072. [CrossRef]
88. Cher, J.Z.B.; Akbar, M.; Kitson, S.; Crowe, L.A.N.; Garcia-Melchor, E.; Hannah, S.C.; McLean, M.; Fazzi, U.G.; Kerr, S.C.; Murrell, G.A.C.; et al. Alarmins in Frozen Shoulder: A Molecular Association Between Inflammation and Pain. *Am. J. Sports Med.* **2018**, *46*, 671–678. [CrossRef] [PubMed]
89. Portillo, M.E.; Corvec, S.; Borens, O.; Trampuz, A. Propionibacterium acnes: An Underestimated Pathogen in Implant-Associated Infections. *BioMed Res. Int.* **2013**, *2013*, 804391. [CrossRef]
90. Corvec, S.; Portillo, M.E.; Pasticci, B.M.; Borens, O.; Trampuz, A. Epidemiology and New Developments in the Diagnosis of Prosthetic Joint Infection. *Int. J. Artif. Organs* **2012**, *35*, 923–934. [CrossRef]
91. Capoor, M.N.; Ruzicka, F.; Schmitz, J.E.; James, G.A.; Machackova, T.; Jancalek, R.; Smrcka, M.; Lipina, R.; Ahmed, F.S.; Alamin, T.F.; et al. Propionibacterium acnes biofilm is present in intervertebral discs of patients undergoing microdiscectomy. *PLoS ONE* **2017**, *12*, e0174518. [CrossRef]
92. Lavergne, V.; Malo, M.; Gaudelli, C.; Laprade, M.; Leduc, S.; Laflamme, P.; Rouleau, D.M. Clinical impact of positive Propionibacterium acnes cultures in orthopedic surgery. *Orthop. Traumatol. Surg. Res.* **2017**, *103*, 307–314. [CrossRef]
93. Lockhart, P.B.; Brennan, M.T.; Sasser, H.C.; Fox, P.C.; Paster, B.J.; Bahrani-Mougeot, F.K. Bacteremia Associated with Toothbrushing and Dental Extraction. *Circulation* **2008**, *117*, 3118–3125. [CrossRef]
94. Tang, G.; Wang, Z.; Chen, J.; Zhang, Z.; Qian, H.; Chen, Y. Latent infection of low-virulence anaerobic bacteria in degenerated lumbar intervertebral discs. *BMC Musculoskelet. Disord.* **2018**, *19*, 445. [CrossRef]
95. Potgieter, M.; Bester, J.; Kell, D.B.; Pretorius, E. The dormant blood microbiome in chronic, inflammatory diseases. *FEMS Microbiol. Rev.* **2015**, *39*, 567–591. [CrossRef]
96. Pérez, S.; Rius-Pérez, S. Macrophage Polarization and Reprogramming in Acute Inflammation: A Redox Perspective. *Antioxidants* **2022**, *11*, 1394. [CrossRef] [PubMed]
97. Lis-López, L.; Bauset, C.; Seco-Cervera, M.; Cosín-Roger, J. Is the Macrophage Phenotype Determinant for Fibrosis Development? *Biomedicines* **2021**, *9*, 1747. [CrossRef] [PubMed]

98. Monteiro, L.d.B.; Prodonoff, J.S.; de Aguiar, C.F.; Correa-Da-Silva, F.; Castoldi, A.; Bakker, N.v.T.; Davanzo, G.G.; Castelucci, B.; Pereira, J.A.d.S.; Curtis, J.; et al. Leptin Signaling Suppression in Macrophages Improves Immunometabolic Outcomes in Obesity. *Diabetes* **2022**, *71*, 1546–1561. [CrossRef] [PubMed]
99. Monteiro, L.; Pereira, J.A.d.S.; Palhinha, L.; Moraes-Vieira, P.M.M. Leptin in the regulation of the immunometabolism of adipose tissue-macrophages. *J. Leukoc. Biol.* **2019**, *106*, 703–716. [CrossRef]
100. Lumeng, C.N.; Bodzin, J.L.; Saltiel, A.R. Obesity induces a phenotypic switch in adipose tissue macrophage polarization. *J. Clin. Investig.* **2007**, *117*, 175–184. [CrossRef]
101. Pan, D.; Li, G.; Jiang, C.; Hu, J.; Hu, X. Regulatory mechanisms of macrophage polarization in adipose tissue. *Front. Immunol.* **2023**, *14*, 1149366. [CrossRef]
102. Sun, J.-X.; Xu, X.-H.; Jin, L. Effects of Metabolism on Macrophage Polarization Under Different Disease Backgrounds. *Front. Immunol.* **2022**, *13*, 880286. [CrossRef]
103. Matarese, G.; Moschos, S.; Mantzoros, C.S. Leptin in Immunology. *J. Immunol.* **2005**, *174*, 3137–3142. [CrossRef] [PubMed]
104. Challoumas, D.; Biddle, M.; McLean, M.; Millar, N.L. Comparison of Treatments for Frozen Shoulder: A Systematic Review and Meta-analysis. *JAMA Netw. Open* **2020**, *3*, e2029581. [CrossRef] [PubMed]
105. de Luxán-Delgado, B.; Potes, Y.; Rubio-González, A.; Solano, J.J.; Boga, J.A.; Antuña, E.; Cachán-Vega, C.; Bermejo-Millo, J.C.; Menéndez-Coto, N.; García-González, C.; et al. Melatonin Alleviates Liver Mitochondrial Dysfunction in Leptin-Deficient Mice. *Int. J. Mol. Sci.* **2024**, *25*, 8677. [CrossRef]
106. Wang, W.; Shi, M.; Zhou, C.; Shi, Z.; Cai, X.; Lin, T.; Yan, S. Effectiveness of corticosteroid injections in adhesive capsulitis of shoulder: A meta-analysis. *Medicine* **2017**, *96*, e7529. [CrossRef]
107. Gaujoux-Viala, C.; Dougados, M.; Gossec, L. Efficacy and safety of steroid injections for shoulder and elbow tendonitis: A meta-analysis of randomised controlled trials. *Ann. Rheum. Dis.* **2009**, *68*, 1843–1849. [CrossRef] [PubMed]
108. Dueñas, L.; Balasch-Bernat, M.; Aguilar-Rodríguez, M.; Struyf, F.; Meeus, M.; Lluch, E. A Manual Therapy and Home Stretching Program in Patients With Primary Frozen Shoulder Contracture Syndrome: A Case Series. *J. Orthop. Sport. Phys. Ther.* **2019**, *49*, 192–201. [CrossRef]
109. Page, M.J.; Green, S.; Kramer, S.; Johnston, R.V.; McBain, B.; Chau, M.; Buchbinder, R. Manual therapy and exercise for adhesive capsulitis (frozen shoulder). *Cochrane Database Syst. Rev.* **2014**, *2014*, CD011275. [CrossRef]
110. Çelik, D.; Kaya Mutlu, E. Does adding mobilization to stretching improve outcomes for people with frozen shoulder? A randomized controlled clinical trial. *Clin. Rehabil.* **2016**, *30*, 786–794. [CrossRef]
111. Wagner, E.R.; Farley, K.X.; Higgins, I.; Wilson, J.M.; Daly, C.A.; Gottschalk, M.B. The incidence of shoulder arthroplasty: Rise and future projections compared with hip and knee arthroplasty. *J. Shoulder Elb. Surg.* **2020**, *29*, 2601–2609. [CrossRef]
112. Kraal, T.; The, B.; Boer, R.; van den Borne, M.P.; Koenraadt, K.; Goossens, P.; Eygendaal, D. Manipulation under anesthesia versus physiotherapy treatment in stage two of a frozen shoulder: A study protocol for a randomized controlled trial. *BMC Musculoskelet. Disord.* **2017**, *18*, 412. [CrossRef]
113. Zabeau, L.; Lavens, D.; Peelman, F.; Eyckerman, S.; Vandekerckhove, J.; Tavernier, J. The ins and outs of leptin receptor activation. *FEBS Lett.* **2003**, *546*, 45–50. [CrossRef] [PubMed]
114. Banerjee, S.; Biehl, A.; Gadina, M.; Hasni, S.; Schwartz, D.M. JAK-STAT Signaling as a Target for Inflammatory and Autoimmune Diseases: Current and Future Prospects. *Drugs* **2017**, *77*, 521–546. [CrossRef] [PubMed]
115. Curtis, J.R.; Lee, E.B.; Kaplan, I.V.; Kwok, K.; Geier, J.; Benda, B.; Soma, K.; Wang, L.; Riese, R. Tofacitinib, an oral Janus kinase inhibitor: Analysis of malignancies across the rheumatoid arthritis clinical development programme. *Ann. Rheum. Dis.* **2016**, *75*, 831–841. [CrossRef]
116. Reyes Diaz, R.A.; Cruz Lara, N.M. Papel de la microbiota intestinal en el desarrollo del síndrome metabólico: Revisión narrativa. *Rev. Nutr. Clínica y Metab.* **2024**, *7*, 45–54. [CrossRef]
117. García-Ríos, A.; Camargo Garcia, A.; Perez-Jimenez, F.; Perez-Martinez, P. Microbiota intestinal: ¿un nuevo protagonista en el riesgo de enfermedad cardiovascular? *Clínica e Investig. en Arterioscler.* **2019**, *31*, 178–185. [CrossRef]
118. Mallappa, R.; Rokana, N.; Duary, R.; Panwar, H.; Batish, V.; Grover, S. Management of metabolic syndrome through probiotic and prebiotic interventions. *Indian J. Endocrinol. Metab.* **2012**, *16*, 20. [CrossRef]
119. Uchida, F.; Oh, S.; Shida, T.; Suzuki, H.; Yamagata, K.; Mizokami, Y.; Bukawa, H.; Tanaka, K.; Shoda, J. Effects of Exercise on the Oral Microbiota and Saliva of Patients with Non-Alcoholic Fatty Liver Disease. *Int. J. Environ. Res. Public Health* **2021**, *18*, 3470. [CrossRef]
120. Hamed Hamed, D.; Struyf, F.; Pruimboom, L.; Navarro-Ledesma, S. Efficacy of combined strategies of physical activity, diet and sleep disorders as treatment in patients with chronic shoulder pain. A systematic review. *Front. Physiol.* **2023**, *14*, 1221807. [CrossRef] [PubMed]
121. Navarro-Ledesma, S.; Hamed-Hamed, D.; González-Muñoz, A.; Pruimboom, L. Physical Activity, Insulin Resistance and Cancer: A Systematic Review. *Cancers* **2024**, *16*, 656. [CrossRef]

122. Navarro-Ledesma, S.; Hamed-Hamed, D.; Gonzalez-Muñoz, A.; Pruimboom, L. Impact of physical therapy techniques and common interventions on sleep quality in patients with chronic pain: A systematic review. *Sleep Med. Rev.* **2024**, *76*, 101937. [CrossRef]
123. Casanova, A.; Wevers, A.; Navarro-Ledesma, S.; Pruimboom, L. Mitochondria: It is all about energy. *Front. Physiol.* **2023**, *14*, 1114231. [CrossRef] [PubMed]
124. Ansarin, A.; Mahdavi, A.M.; Javadivala, Z.; Shanehbandi, D.; Zarredar, H.; Ansarin, K. The cross-talk between leptin and circadian rhythm signaling proteins in physiological processes: A systematic review. *Mol. Biol. Rep.* **2023**, *50*, 10427–10443. [CrossRef]
125. Maury, E. Off the Clock: From Circadian Disruption to Metabolic Disease. *Int. J. Mol. Sci.* **2019**, *20*, 1597. [CrossRef] [PubMed]
126. Park, H.-K.; Ahima, R.S. Physiology of leptin: Energy homeostasis, neuroendocrine function and metabolism. *Metabolism* **2015**, *64*, 24–34. [CrossRef] [PubMed]
127. Civelek, E.; Ozturk Civelek, D.; Akyel, Y.K.; Kaleli Durman, D.; Okyar, A. Circadian Dysfunction in Adipose Tissue: Chronotherapy in Metabolic Diseases. *Biology* **2023**, *12*, 1077. [CrossRef]
128. Dibner, C.; Gachon, F. Circadian Dysfunction and Obesity: Is Leptin the Missing Link? *Cell Metab.* **2015**, *22*, 359–360. [CrossRef]
129. Dessie, G.; Ayelign, B.; Akalu, Y.; Shibabaw, T.; Molla, M.D. Effect of Leptin on Chronic Inflammatory Disorders: Insights to Therapeutic Target to Prevent Further Cardiovascular Complication. *Diabetes. Metab. Syndr. Obes.* **2021**, *14*, 3307–3322. [CrossRef]

Journal of
Clinical Medicine

MDPI

Review

Physiotherapy in Text Neck Syndrome: A Scoping Review of Current Evidence and Future Directions

Joanna Piruta [1,*] and Wojciech Kułak [2]

[1] Doctoral School, Medical University of Bialystok, 15-089 Bialystok, Poland
[2] Department of Pediatric Neurology and Rehabilitation, Medical University of Bialystok, 15-274 Bialystok, Poland
* Correspondence: joannapiruta@wp.pl

Abstract: Background: Musculoskeletal disorders associated with excessive smartphone use represent a significant health issue. Text neck syndrome is one such disorder within that group, increasingly affecting individuals worldwide across various age groups. The phenomenon of text neck may occur in individuals who frequently and for prolonged periods adopt a forward-flexed neck and head position while looking at the screens of mobile electronic devices. Various therapeutic methods are used in the treatment of text neck syndrome. However, there is no consensus on text neck rehabilitation, which poses a challenge for physiotherapists. **Objective:** The aim of this study is to analyze the phenomenon of text neck, with a particular emphasis on current scientific reports regarding the rehabilitation of text neck syndrome. The scoping review was conducted to determine the physiotherapy methods currently used in the treatment of individuals with text neck, assess their impact on symptom reduction, and identify existing knowledge gaps and limitations in the current literature on the rehabilitation of text neck syndrome. **Design:** A scoping review was conducted on the treatment of text neck syndrome based on electronic databases: PubMed, ResearchGate, Physiotherapy Evidence Database (PEDro), and the Cochrane Library. The databases were searched up to 1 December 2024. The inclusion criteria comprised studies investigating physiotherapy interventions for individuals with text neck, published between 2018 and 2024 and written in English. **Results:** A total of fifteen papers were reviewed, focusing on various methods used in text neck rehabilitation, including postural correction exercises, stabilization exercises, strengthening and stretching exercises, Pilates, PNF (Proprioceptive Neuromuscular Facilitation), kinesiology taping, Bowen therapy, and manual therapy. Nearly all studies were conducted in the adult population (93%), with the majority of studies taking place in India (60%). **Conclusions:** In summary, all studies suggest that appropriate physiotherapeutic interventions can provide significant benefits, including pain reduction, posture correction, and improved range of motion in the cervical spine. The best outcomes appear to be achieved by combining various therapeutic techniques. However, further high-quality research is needed to strengthen the evidence and offer reliable recommendations for clinical practice. Additionally, there is limited research on physiotherapy for text neck in the pediatric population, presenting a potential area for future studies.

Keywords: text neck syndrome; physiotherapy; rehabilitation; smartphone overuse; musculoskeletal disorders; neck pain; mobile phone users

1. Introduction

The advancement of technology has made nearly everyone an owner of a device such as a mobile phone [1]. In 2022, approximately 83% of people worldwide were estimated to own a mobile phone [2]. In 2024, 7.21 billion people are indicated to be smartphone users, accounting for 90% of the global population [3]. In the United States, as many as 97% of residents aged 18–29 are smartphone owners [3]. According to statistics, approximately 79% of people aged 18–44 virtually never part with their mobile phones, and 3.5 billion smartphone owners exhibit signs of addiction to those devices [4–6].

Undoubtedly, smartphones offer many attractive features. Mobile phones are no longer used solely for communication. They have become devices that provide entertainment, enable photography, allow users to stay updated with the latest news, and serve as tools for work and learning [7–9]. Unfortunately, despite their many advantages, prolonged screen time on smartphones may lead to numerous adverse health consequences [10]. Excessive use of smartphones may negatively affect sleep quality, cause vision problems (e.g., eye strain, blurred vision), lead to symptoms related to the peripheral nervous system, contribute to psychosocial issues (e.g., addiction, social isolation, depression), and also adversely impact posture [11–16].

Almost every day, one can observe people who, while using electronic devices, thrust their heads forward or maintain their cervical spine in a flexed position, staring at a smartphone screen for many hours throughout the day. Unfortunately, such behavior may adversely impact human health, leading to adverse consequences, such as musculoskeletal strain and the onset of neck and cervical pain [17,18]. Neck pain radiating to the upper limbs and headaches constitute a significant problem that affects the quality of life and limits daily functioning [19]. Neck pain affects many people worldwide across various age groups [20]. That issue also affects increasingly younger individuals, partly due to the more frequent and prolonged use of smartphones [21]. The prevalence of spinal pain among young adults is on the rise [22]. That phenomenon is influenced by many factors, one of which is the excessive use of computers and smartphones during leisure time [22]. It is estimated that the prevalence of neck pain in groups aged 7–11 years who are spending around 5–8 h daily using electronic devices is around 70% [23].

According to statistical data, nearly half of the people in the USA in 2024 spent about 5–6 h daily using a smartphone, which translates to 1825–2190 h annually (2.5–3 months per year spent solely on smartphone usage) [3]. A reduction in the time dedicated to physical activity, a sedentary lifestyle, lack of movement, and prolonged maintenance of static positions contribute to the occurrence of musculoskeletal disorders and spinal pain [19,20]. It is estimated that the prevalence of musculoskeletal disorders among smartphone users ranges from 50% to 84%, particularly affecting areas such as the neck, shoulders, upper back, and upper body [19]. One such disorder is the so-called 'text neck syndrome' [24]. The prevalence of text neck syndrome ranges from 16.7% to 93.2% [20,23,25–33].

The findings highlight the urgent need to address the issue of text neck syndrome. Various therapeutic methods are used in the treatment of text neck syndrome. However, there is no consensus on text neck rehabilitation, which poses a challenge for physiotherapists. The aim of this study is to analyze the phenomenon of text neck, with a particular emphasis on current scientific reports regarding the rehabilitation of text neck syndrome. The scoping review was conducted to determine the physiotherapy methods currently used in the treatment of individuals with text neck, assess their impact on symptom reduction, and identify existing knowledge gaps and limitations in the current literature on the rehabilitation of text neck syndrome.

Conducting a scoping review allows for the collection and summary of available studies related to the rehabilitation of text neck syndrome, providing a better understanding of the current state of knowledge regarding physiotherapeutic methods for treating this condition. This review helps identify areas where research is lacking or requires further exploration. It can guide future studies towards the most important aspects of text neck syndrome treatment that have not yet been sufficiently examined.

2. Text Neck Syndrome

2.1. *Definition*

Staring at the screen of a mobile device, such as a smartphone, for many hours a day with a flexed head and neck position predisposes to the development of text neck syndrome [24]. The term 'text neck' was first used by chiropractor Dr. L. Fischman [24]. Dr. Fischman noted that the tension associated with prolonged, repetitive, and frequent maintenance of a flexed neck and head position while using electronic devices such as smartphones or tablets leads to strain, injuries, and stiffness in the cervical spine area [8,34,35]. Text neck syndrome may be referred to as: 'turtle neck posture', 'smartphone neck syndrome', 'tech neck', 'SMS neck', or 'iNeck' [8,36]. The text neck posture is characterized by an increased flexion of the cervical spine and is caused by activities that require looking down, below eye level, such as when typing text messages [12]. Depending on the degree of progression, the text neck syndrome may present with a varied clinical picture [37].

The diagnosis of text neck syndrome is based on subjective (interview) and objective examinations, which include, among others, assessment of posture, pain intensity (e.g., using the Numerical Pain Rating Scale—NPRS or Visual Analogue Scale—VAS), disability (e.g., using the Neck Disability Index), muscle tension, and joint range of motion [5,38]. In some cases, imaging studies are recommended to rule out the presence of other medical conditions [38]. When diagnosing text neck syndrome, it is important to exclude the following conditions and diseases as the cause of the symptoms: osteoporosis, stenosis, scoliosis, spondylolisthesis, torticollis, spinal infections or inflammatory disorders, malignancies, herniation, and trauma [19,39].

In order to diagnose text neck syndrome, the following criteria are taken into account:

- Using the phone for 3 h or more per day;
- The presence of 3 out of the following 6 symptoms: neck pain, upper back pain, shoulder pain, headache, insomnia, tingling and numbness in the upper limbs;
- Using the phone with a neck flexion of approximately 15 degrees or greater [6].

These diagnostic criteria are taken into account when diagnosing text neck syndrome. However, it should be noted that clear diagnostic criteria for text neck syndrome have not yet been established.

2.2. *Symptomatology*

Correct posture ensures proper balance and functioning of the body. However, when there is a disturbance in one segment, it may lead to abnormalities and disorders in other parts of the body. Frequent use of smartphones causes the head and neck to often tilt forward toward the screen of the mobile device. That frequent adoption of an incorrect and burdening position may contribute to an increased risk of musculoskeletal problems in the neck and upper torso [19,40]. The set of symptoms associated with smartphone use is referred to as text neck syndrome [41]. In that musculoskeletal disorder, a muscular imbalance occurs. A correlation has been observed between smartphone addiction and a decrease in muscle strength and endurance [19]. Particularly, the deep neck flexor muscles become weakened [19]. Such a static flexed position leads to the overloading of the suboccipital muscles, the erector spinae, the levator scapulae, the trapezius, and the semispinalis muscles [37]. Tension in the suboccipital muscles may result in the onset of tension-type headaches [37].

In individuals with text neck syndrome, changes in posture and structural overload may occur. However, these are usually functional changes rather than structural ones in the sense of permanent, irreversible deformities. Prolonged strain on the neck can lead to excessive muscle tension, changes in the natural curvature of the cervical spine (e.g., flattening of cervical lordosis), pain and discomfort, and, in the long run, possible damage to spinal structures [5,23,42]. With prolonged flexion, continuous stress may result in the loosening of the posterior ligaments, instability of the vertebral segments, and degenerative joint disease, potentially causing plastic changes within the nervous system and resulting in clinical symptoms [12]. Neurological symptoms are additional manifestations that can occur in text neck syndrome. These may include tingling, numbness, or weakness in the arms or hands, often due to nerve compression or irritation in the cervical spine. While these symptoms are less common, they may indicate that the condition has progressed to affect the nerves [12,43].

The reinforcement of poor movement habits and the lack of correction of incorrect posture over time may lead to limited mobility in the cervical spine and further segments, disturbances in spinal curvature, reduced lung capacity, as well as the onset of neck pain, radiating pain to the upper limbs, and even numbness in the hands [24,34,35,44,45]. An unnatural, forced position with a tilted head puts excessive strain on the spine structures, eventually leading to the development of a herniated disc and degenerative changes [19,46]. Untreated text neck syndrome may lead to inflammation in the ligaments, muscles, or nerves [8]. The consequence in the future may be permanent changes in the musculoskeletal system [7]. Table 1 presents the symptoms and consequences of text neck syndrome.

Table 1. Symptoms and consequences of text neck syndrome.

Typical Symptoms	Additional Symptoms	Health Consequences
- Muscular tension imbalance - Neck pain - Neck stiffness - Neck soreness - Flattening of the cervical lordosis	- Radiating pain in the upper limbs - Upper back pain - Shoulder girdle pain - Headaches - Tingling in the hands - Numbness in the hands - Muscle weakness - Sleeplessness - Impaired range of motion in the cervical spine.	- Pressure on spinal nerves - Nerve and muscle damage - Cervical proprioception disturbances - Impaired range of motion in the thoracic spine - Degenerative changes - Herniated discs - Disruption of the spine's physiological curves - Reduced lung capacity - Cervical-origin dizziness - Early-onset arthritis - Disorders in the temporomandibular joint.

Own elaboration based on [6,7,19,25,34,37,39,40,47–50].

2.3. Pathophysiology

Thanks to the specific structural formation of the spine, it is possible to perform the appropriate functions [7]. The intervertebral disc is thicker at the front than at the back [2,5]. That structure of the disc, combined with the shape of the cervical vertebral bodies, creates cervical lordosis [46]. Thanks to the intervertebral discs and cervical lordosis, a cushioning function and a greater range of backward flexion are possible [35]. In an adult person in a neutral anatomical position, the cervical spine supports the weight of the head, which is approximately 5 kg [11]. The greater the flexion in the cervical spine, the greater the load placed on the spine [11]. Figure 1 shows the distribution of the load exerted on the cervical spine depending on the angle of neck flexion.

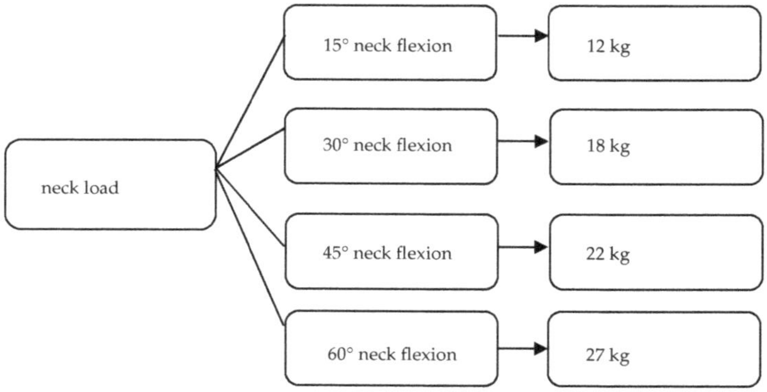

Figure 1. Distribution of the load exerted on the cervical spine depending on the angle of neck flexion. Own elaboration based on [4,11,40].

Prolonged, repetitive maintenance of a flexed position while using a mobile phone leads to the forward shift of the head's center of gravity [7,8]. Incorrect head positioning and prolonged positions with the head jutting forward, such as when using a mobile phone, increase the load on the spine joints and affect the length and endurance of the muscles [9]. Frequent, repetitive positioning of the neck in a flexed position with forward head protrusion may excessively stimulate the muscles, leading to muscular imbalance, functional changes, and overload [51]. Increased tension in specific muscles and a greater angle of neck flexion may lead to proprioceptive disturbances, limited mobility in the cervical spine, and referred pain to certain parts of the body, which may be caused, among other factors, by trigger points within the affected muscles [1]. In text neck syndrome, increased strain and stiffness are observed in the upper part of the trapezius muscle, the neck extensor muscles, and weakness of the deep neck flexor muscles [9,12,52]. Muscle imbalance and incorrect curvature of the cervical spine may lead to microdamage of soft tissues, overload of spinal structures, and the onset of pain [53,54].

2.4. Risk Factors

Risk factors that predispose to the onset and intensification of symptoms of text neck syndrome include the following:

- Frequency and duration of time spent in an improper position while using the phone;
- Position while using the smartphone;
- Height at which the mobile device is held;
- Lack of physical activity;
- Smartphone addiction;
- Female gender [12,39,55,56].

As reported by Elvan A. et al. [57], using a mobile phone for more than 3 h a day is a significant risk factor for the development of text neck syndrome. Studies conducted by Paek K.S. [58], Gong W. et al. [59], and Choi J.H. et al. [60] have indicated that a prolonged flexed position in the cervical spine negatively affects the endurance of the deep neck flexor muscles. Ayhualem S. et al. [1], in their publication, draw attention to the increased risk of neck pain in individuals who spend much time using smartphones. Shahzad Y. et al. [46] and Khan S. et al. [2] have demonstrated that neck pain occurs more frequently in individuals who spend more than 4 h a day using a mobile phone. De Vitta A. et al. [61], in a study conducted with a group of 1143 students, have also observed a correlation between the duration of smartphone use and the frequency of neck pain.

A study conducted by Sarraf F. and Varmazyar S. [18] confirms that the position adopted while looking at the screen of a mobile device affects the activity and degree of muscle strain. Researchers have shown that the best head and neck position is achieved when sitting with back support, while the worst position is sitting without back support [18]. The posture has an impact on the amount of strain placed on the cervical spine [18]. The lack of arm support while using a phone negatively affects the alignment of the cervical spine [62,63].

A study conducted by Raihan H.A. and Rahman F. [52] has demonstrated the relationship between the occurrence of text neck syndrome and the height at which the phone is held during use. According to Kokiwar P.R. et al. [34], neck pain symptoms are most commonly reported by individuals who hold their smartphones at the level of their abdomen. A similar correlation has been observed in studies conducted by Rashid M.K. et al. [26], where neck pain had been more commonly observed in individuals holding their smartphones with their necks bent at approximately 60 degrees. In turn, Correia I.M.T. et al. [64] have not confirmed any correlation between the body posture associated with text neck syndrome and the occurrence of neck pain in their study. Bertozzi L. et al. [65] also did not find a correlation between the angle of neck flexion while using a mobile phone and the occurrence of neck pain.

The differences in the above studies may stem from factors such as cultural or age-related differences among the participants. The studies by Raihan H.A. and Rahman F. [52] and Rashid M.K. et al. [26] were conducted in a population of adolescents and young adults attending Asian schools, while the studies by Correia I.M.T. et al. [64] and Bertozzi L. et al. [65] were conducted in a population of adult Europeans. Conducting research in a population that accounts for cultural differences could provide an interesting addition to the existing gap regarding the risk factors for the occurrence of text neck syndrome.

The relationship between smartphone addiction, the severity of neck pain, and the occurrence of text neck syndrome is confirmed by the study conducted by Mustafaoglu R. et al. [66]. A similar correlation has been found by Fatima S. et al. [67] and Shamsi R.F. et al. [17]. Gupta N. et al. [68], in a study of 957 students, have demonstrated that 22.4% of students have been found to be addicted to using electronic devices. In a study conducted by Paek K.S. [58] among 286 students, 15% were addicted to smartphones, and a trend was observed between addiction and the occurrence of neck pain. On the other hand, the study conducted by Alshahrani A. et al. [69] has demonstrated that as many as 60.3% of students at Qassim University were addicted to using smartphones, and a correlation has also been observed between addiction and the occurrence of cervical spine pain.

It is worth noting that neck pain affects women three times more often than men [61]. In turn, the analysis carried out by Chen Y.L. et al. [70] has proven that neck pain significantly more often affects women than men. Studies show that neck pain related to the text neck syndrome occurs more frequently in women [61,70]. An inverse relationship has been noted in the study by Kokiwar P.R. et al. [34] conducted among 306 students. Their study has shown a higher incidence of neck pain among men.

3. Occurrence of Text Neck

Approximately 30–50% of the adult population experiences neck pain [71]. The occurrence of neck pain has a tendency to increase [72]. However, those complaints are increasingly observed in adolescents and young adults. In the young adult population, the annual occurrence of neck pain ranges from 42% to 67% [72]. Epidemiological data indicate that pain syndromes in the cervical spine are one of the most common causes of disability and reduced quality of life in individuals aged 20–24 years [72]. Factors such as improper, forced body posture adopted while using electronic devices may contribute to an increased risk of neck pain [73].

Ayhualem S. et al. [1], in their publication, highlight that the risk of cervical spine pain is increased among students who spend much time using smartphones. They report that in a study conducted in Canada, 68% of students complained of musculoskeletal pain in the cervical spine related to smartphone use [1]. In a study conducted by Hassnain S. et al. [27] among 118 students in Lahore, the prevalence of text neck syndrome was very high, with 93.2% of the participants exhibiting symptoms of the syndrome. A high prevalence of text neck syndrome has also been noted in the research conducted by Javed A. et al. [28] and Khalid R. et al. [25].

Kumari S. et al. [20] have demonstrated the occurrence of text neck syndrome in 64.3% of the participants. A similar result has been obtained by Alsiwed K.T. et al. [29]—the text neck syndrome was present in 68.1% of the participants and in a study conducted by Rashid M.K. et al. [26]—64.5%. A low prevalence of text neck syndrome was observed in the study conducted by Kamaraj P.N. et al. [30] on a group of 354 individuals aged 18–22, where only 16.7% of the participants showed signs of smartphone-related neck syndrome. In turn, in a study conducted by Parmar N. et al. [31] among 428 individuals aged 17–24, 29.2% of them had text neck syndrome. A similar result was obtained in the study by Sathya P. and Tamboli S.A. [32], where among 100 physiotherapy students from Mumbai, aged 18–25, the occurrence of text neck syndrome was found in 32% of the students.

Atakla H.G. et al. [33] conducted a study in a significantly larger group than in the aforementioned studies. The researchers conducted a study among 1835 students at the University of Abomey Calavi in Benin. It has been found that 850 participants in the study exhibited symptoms of text neck syndrome. As shown by the cited studies, the prevalence of text neck syndrome in the adult population ranges from 16.7% to 93.2% [20,25–33].

4. Text Neck in Children

Due to the widespread availability of electronic devices, it is increasingly common for children to own mobile phones, giving them easier access to use those devices more frequently. According to Warda D.G. et al. [12], children aged 8–12 spend 41% of their time using electronic devices on smartphones, while adolescents aged 13–18 spend 46% of this time on smartphones.

Excessive smartphone use can be particularly harmful to children. While the young body is still developing, it receives inappropriate stimuli. Children may experience speech development issues, psychosocial disorders, vision problems, sensory integration disorders, or musculoskeletal disorders [11,12]. The last group includes, among others, text neck syndrome. The ratio of a child's head size to body size is greater than in adults, which means the load placed on the cervical spine is higher in children than in adults, increasing the risk of developing text neck syndrome in that age group [12].

The issue of text neck syndrome in children and adolescents is addressed by Warda D.G. et al. [12], David D. et al. [11], and Jyothsna G. [74]. Children and adolescents spend an average of 5–7 h using smartphones, which puts them at an increased risk of experiencing issues related to text neck syndrome in the future [11]. It is estimated that the prevalence of neck pain in groups aged 7–11 years who are spending around 5–8 h daily using electronic devices is around 70% [23].

Neck pain is the eighth leading cause of disability among individuals aged 15 to 19 [13]. Musculoskeletal pain in the pediatric population shows similar patterns: specific symptoms (such as headache and musculoskeletal pain) are more prevalent in females than in males, and these rates tend to be higher in adolescents compared to children [11].

The above statements are confirmed by the research conducted by Fares J. et al. [75]. A study conducted by Fares J. et al. [75] in Beirut, Lebanon, involving patients under 18 years of age presenting with nonspecific neck pain. The average age of the participants was 14 years. In total, 207 children and adolescents were identified, with 180 diagnosed with musculoskeletal neck pain and spasms. The majority of participants (57%) were female, and more adolescents (60%) were affected compared to children (40%). All 180 participants reported flawed neck and back flexion while studying or using electronic devices such as smartphones and tablets. The study found a significant association between poor posture during technology use and musculoskeletal neck pain in adolescents [75].

Song M.K. at al. [76] conducted a study among 308 school-age children. The researchers have found that children with poor posture and those dependent on smartphones more often experienced neck and shoulder pain.

There are fewer reports of text neck syndrome among children than among adults. However, there have been publications describing case studies of children with text neck syndrome [11,43,77]. David D. et al. [11] described the occurrence of text neck based on a case study of a 16-year-old girl. Chu E. et al. [43] also described the prevalence of text neck syndrome in a case study of a 6-year-old boy. The boy underwent 9 months of chiropractic treatment, resulting in improved cervical spine mobility, reduction of neurological symptoms, and decreased pain. The researcher emphasizes the importance of early therapeutic intervention and prevention.

Aziz A.N. et al. [78] conducted a cross-sectional study aimed at assessing the prevalence of text neck syndrome and its associated factors in children and adolescents attending primary health centers (PHCs) in Erbil, Iraqi Kurdistan, in 2022. The study included children aged 5–15 years attending primary and secondary schools in Erbil. A total of 352 participants were recruited. The study found a high prevalence of text neck syndrome, with 69.0% of children reporting neck pain. Adolescents who used smartphones for more than 3 h daily (83.56%), those studying at the secondary school level, and those with psychological, social, and physical dysfunctions were more likely to develop text neck syndrome. Additionally, children who slept less, played fewer sports, used computers more, watched more TV, and played video games for more than 3 h were also at higher risk for text neck. The study concluded that the high prevalence of text neck syndrome is associated with increased smartphone use, screen time, and psychological and physical dysfunctions. The findings suggest the need for interventions to reduce screen time and promote better physical health practices in this population [78].

The study conducted by Rathi P. et al. [13] aimed to assess adolescents' awareness, perceptions, and knowledge regarding the preventive measures, health hazards, and causes of text neck syndrome. The study included 302 adolescents from Pune city. The results revealed that 67.2% had heard of text neck syndrome, 47.7% were aware of its causes, and only 20.5% knew about holding smartphones at eye level. The study concluded that while awareness of text neck syndrome causes and health risks is good, knowledge of preventive measures remains limited, highlighting the need for enhanced educational efforts focused on prevention [13].

The authors emphasize that text neck syndrome is a serious problem that, if left untreated, may lead to significant health consequences for both children and adults. They highlight that prevention is the key, especially for children and adolescents [11,12,74].

Research on pain related to text neck syndrome in children is limited, with most existing studies focusing on young adults and college students. Therefore, additional research involving children and adolescents is necessary, particularly cross-cultural studies with large sample sizes.

5. Preventive Measures

Due to the increasing prevalence of text neck syndrome in the global population, the shifting age threshold, and the appearance of the condition in younger individuals, it is extremely important to raise awareness and knowledge about the consequences of improper excessive use of electronic devices.

The study conducted by Medani K.T. et al. [53] within a group of 229 students at Majmaah University has indicated that among the study participants, 71.2% have a low level of knowledge about text neck syndrome. On the other hand, the study conducted by Samani P.P. et al. [7] in a group of 311 people indicated that 35% of them had heard of text neck syndrome, but only 8% had knowledge about it. Accordingly, the study carried out by Rathi P. et al. [13] in a group of 302 teenagers has indicated that about 33% of the respondents have never heard of that term. The study conducted by Dolah J. et al. [79] has demonstrated that 39% of students are familiar with the term 'text neck', and the study conducted by Kumar S. et al. [22] among 200 respondents aged 18–25 has proven 50.3% of them to have no knowledge of text neck.

From a young age, children should be educated in schools about what text neck syndrome is, what the risk factors are, the health consequences of excessive and improper use of mobile devices, and what preventive and treatment methods are available [12]. A good solution could be the implementation of educational programs in schools or the use of smartphone applications that would inform users when they exceed the recommended screen time or adopt an incorrect head and neck posture during use [12,53].

Education is crucial both in prevention and in the therapeutic process. If a disorder has already occurred, the patient should be taught how to correct the posture, properly perform exercises, how to carry out self-therapy, modify movement habits, and adopt the correct posture when using electronic devices [5]. In addition, it is important to change harmful habits, adjust the workspace and study environment to individual needs, take regular breaks, and develop the awareness that the patient is responsible for the outcomes of their therapy and must follow recommendations if they wish to achieve results. Success requires perseverance, motivation, and commitment to the therapy.

The importance of education in the therapeutic process is emphasized by Farooq M. et al. [5]. Fouda K.Z. and Abdelsalam M.S. [80] also highlight that the combination of exercises to strengthen the deep flexor muscles of the neck with proper education and learning how to maintain a correct posture while using mobile devices significantly influences the achievement of positive treatment outcomes. A similar relationship between changing habits and therapy has been observed in the study by Shah J. and Soni K [54].

Regular physical activity is effective in preventing the occurrence of text neck syndrome [8,78]. Spinal stabilization exercises and exercises for maintaining a proper posture, when performed regularly, constitute an effective preventive measure [8,48].

Additionally, the position adopted while using a smartphone should be modified. Specifically, attention should be paid to holding the smartphone at eye level, thus preventing excessive neck flexion [12,40]. The study conducted by Namwongsa S. et al. [81] has evidenced that maintaining the neck at an angle of 0 to 15 degrees while using a smartphone significantly reduces neck muscle activity and the risk of developing neck pain.

In addition, activities that require frequent repetition of the same motion, such as texting or scrolling for extended periods, should be avoided [12,82]. It is also recommended to use both hands and index fingers when typing text messages, take frequent breaks every 20–30 min, frequently change positions, avoid using items that are too large and too heavy to hold in one hand for extended periods, and if necessary, use those items with arm support [12,40,82,83].

The study conducted by Vahedi Z. et al. [84] investigated the impact of smartphone use on musculoskeletal stress, specifically focusing on head forward flexion, lateral bending, and viewing distance during sitting/standing postures and one-handed/two-handed grips. The study monitored neck kinematics and evaluated performance in tasks such as typing, video watching, and reading. Results showed a significant increase in neck and upper limb pain after smartphone use. Sitting and standing postures were associated with greater head forward flexion and viewing distance during two-handed typing. One-handed tasks resulted in higher left lateral bending in standing posture. Overall, performance was better with two-handed grips [84]. These findings provide insights for recommending healthier smartphone usage practices.

It is also important to pay attention to reducing the amount of time spent using mobile phones. The Australian Department of Health guidelines from 2012 recommend that children under the age of 2 should not be exposed to mobile phones [12]. Children aged 2–5 years should not spend more than one hour per day using a mobile phone, while children and adolescents aged 5–17 years should limit their usage to 2 h per day during leisure time [12]. It is also worth mentioning that taking breaks and stretching during that time is an important preventive factor in the occurrence of unpleasant discomfort [48,74].

As reported by Elvan A. et al. [57], using a mobile phone for more than 3 h a day is a significant risk factor for the development of text neck syndrome. Shahzad Y. et al. [46] and Khan S. et al. [2] have demonstrated that neck pain occurs more frequently in individuals who spend more than 4 h a day using a mobile phone. De Vitta A. et al. [61], in a study conducted with a group of 1143 students, have also observed a correlation between the duration of smartphone use and the frequency of neck pain.

General recommendations suggest limiting non-essential screen time to 2–3 h per day for adults and less than 2 h for children and adolescents to reduce the risk of musculoskeletal issues. These recommendations are supported by the study by Aziz et al. [78]. Aziz et al. [78] conducted a cross-sectional study aimed at assessing the prevalence of text neck syndrome and its associated factors in children and adolescents in 2022. The study included children aged 5–15 years in Erbil. A total of 352 participants were recruited. Adolescents who used smartphones for more than 3 h daily were more likely to develop text neck syndrome. Additionally, children who slept less, played fewer sports, used computers more, watched more TV, and played video games for more than 3 h were also at higher risk for text neck. The findings suggest the need for interventions to reduce screen time and promote better physical health practices in this population [78].

The study conducted by Cevik S. et al. [85] aimed to explore the relationship between spinal degeneration parameters and increased smartphone usage time. Conducted as a cross-sectional study, it involved young adults aged 20–35 years. MRI was used to measure cervical disc degeneration, disc placement, Modic changes, and sagittal balance in 107 patients. Additionally, participants provided information about their daily smartphone usage through a questionnaire completed at the time of admission. Results suggested that smartphone use exceeding three hours daily had a greater impact on spinal degeneration parameters, including degenerative disc severity, disc placement, and Modic changes, compared to use for less than three hours [85].

The studies referenced in this chapter highlight the importance and relevance of the preventive guidelines for text neck syndrome. However, there is still a need for longitudinal cohort studies to assess the effectiveness of these preventive measures and validate their impact on reducing the risk of the condition.

6. Physical Therapy in Text Neck Syndrome—Literature Review

6.1. Literature Search

A scoping review was conducted on the treatment of text neck syndrome based on electronic databases: PubMed, ResearchGate, Physiotherapy Evidence Database (PEDro), and the Cochrane Library. The databases were searched up to 1 December 2024. The search phrases used were: "text neck syndrome", "text neck", "tech neck", "tech neck syndrome", "rehabilitation", "physiotherapy", and with the Boolean operator "and". The search strategy for the databases is presented in Table 2. Data were independently charted by one reviewer.

Table 2. The search strategy for the databases.

PEDro	Cochrane Library	PubMed	ResearchGate
- text neck and physiotherapy - text neck and rehabilitation - tech neck and physiotherapy - tech neck and rehabilitation - text neck syndrome - tech neck - text neck syndrome and rehabilitation - text neck syndrome and physiotherapy	- text neck and physiotherapy - text neck and rehabilitation - tech neck and physiotherapy - tech neck and rehabilitation - text neck syndrome - tech neck	- text neck syndrome and physiotherapy - text neck and rehabilitation - tech neck syndrome and physiotherapy - text neck syndrome - tech neck syndrome	- text neck and physiotherapy - text neck and rehabilitation - tech neck and physiotherapy - text neck syndrome - tech neck syndrome

The inclusion and exclusion criteria for the review are presented in Table 3. The review included clinical trials and experimental studies on rehabilitation methods used in patients with text neck syndrome, published between 2018 and 2024 and written in English and in full text. Papers were excluded if they did not align with the conceptual framework of the study.

Table 3. Inclusion and exclusion criteria for review.

Inclusion Criteria	Exclusion Criteria
- year of publication: 2018–2024 - language: publications written in English - type of study: clinical trial, experimental study - topic—rehabilitation in text neck syndrome - full text available	- year of publication: below 2018 - language: publications written in languages other than English - systematic review, case study - topics not of main interest - duplication of other publications already included in the review - full text not available

6.2. Included Studies

As a result of searching the literature, 811 records were found. After removing duplicates, 502 publications were eligible for screening. Following title and abstract screening, 39 articles were eligible for full-text assessment. After meeting the inclusion criteria, 15 articles qualified for the review. Figure 2 presents a flow diagram demonstrating the scoping review process.

The latest literature highlights the use of, among others, postural correction exercises, stabilization exercises, strengthening and stretching exercises, Pilates, PNF (Proprioceptive Neuromuscular Facilitation), Kinesiology Taping, Bowen therapy, and manual therapy in the rehabilitation of text neck syndrome [5,19,23,38,39,42,50,86–92]. The summary of the latest research on the use of rehabilitation methods in the treatment of text neck syndrome is presented in Table 4.

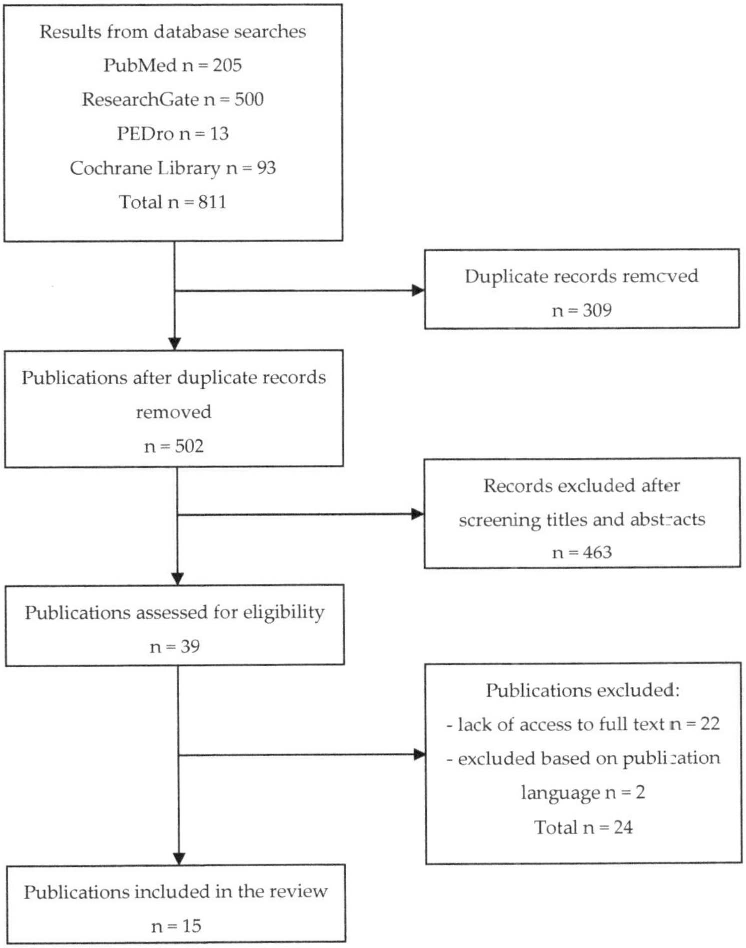

Figure 2. Flow diagram demonstrating the scoping review process.

Table 4. The summary of the latest research on the use of rehabilitation methods in the treatment of text neck syndrome.

Primary Author (Year of Publication)	Number of Study Participants	Intervention	Intervention Duration	Studied Parameters	Results
Kaya M. (2024) [19]	n = 38	G1—exercises to improve CROM, strengthen, and correct posture. G2—exercises to improve CROM, strengthen, and correct posture, as well as PNF (contract–relax technique, replication technique)	Exercises in both groups: 10 repetitions, once a day, 3 days a week; PNF: 3 days a week; Duration: 6 weeks	VAS, CROM, NFEMET, NYPRC, NDI	Improvement of the studied parameters in both groups, but greater improvement in G2. CROM improvement was observed in G2.

Table 4. *Cont.*

Primary Author (Year of Publication)	Number of Study Participants	Intervention	Intervention Duration	Studied Parameters	Results
Bhende R. (2024) [42]	n = 80	G1—conventional exercise program G2—integrated postural training	3 times a week; 6 weeks	VAS, NDI, CROM, TTW, CPJE Testing	Improvement of parameters in both groups, but CPJE testing was better in G2 than in G1.
Nathani H.R. (2024) [38]	n = 54	Individually tailored rehabilitation protocol	3 weeks	VAS, NDI, SAS, CHDQ, ROM	Improvement in VAS, NDI, and CHDQ after the treatments.
Rajopadhye S. (2023) [86]	n = 63	PNF (Dynamic Reversal Technique, Rhythmic Stabilization Technique)	4 times a week, 2 weeks	VAS, CROM (cervical spine extension)	Improvement in CROM and pain reduction.
Bharal S. (2023) [50]	n = 75	G1—isometric neck exercises G2—neck stabilization training G3—Contrology training	4 weeks	CVA, NPRS, NDI	Better results in G2 and G3 than in G1. CVA increased, and NPRS and NDI decreased. In G2, better results than in G3.
Bhanu Sri P.L. (2023) [23]	n = 60	G1—Pilates, G2—Gong's Mobilization	5 sessions a week; 6 weeks	VAS, NDI, CROM	Improvement of parameters in both groups, Better results in G1.
Sarraf F. (2023) [87]	n = 60	G1—corrective exercises G2—no therapy	1 daily, 5 times a week; 8 weeks	NDI, VAS, photogrammetry	Improvement in posture and VAS, NDI parameters in G1.
Afzal H. (2023) [88]	n = 24	G1—Kendall's intervention G2—Gong's mobilization	3 times a week; 6 weeks	NDI, NPRS, CROM, CVA, RSA, neck muscle strength	Greater improvement in parameters in G2.
Farooq M. (2023) [5]	n = 40	G1—10 min hot pack session, ELDOA, ergonomic recommendation, G2—10-minute hot pack session, post-facilitation stretching, ergonomic recommendation.	3 sessions weekly, 45 min each, 6 weeks	NPRS, NDI, SAS	Greater improvement in parameters in G1.
Seemal P. (2022) [39]	n = 22	G1—hot packs and METs G2—hot packs, METs, and Bowen therapy	3 sessions weekly; 6 weeks	CROM, CVA, NPRS, NDI, RSA	Improvement of the studied parameters in both groups, but better results in G2.
Shikha B. (2022) [35]	n = 30	G1—balloon blowing activity, G2—modified cervical exercise along with Swiss ball exercise.	4 weeks	FEV, FVC (spirometry)	Improvement in FEV and FVC in both groups, but better results in G1.

Table 4. *Cont.*

Primary Author (Year of Publication)	Number of Study Participants	Intervention	Intervention Duration	Studied Parameters	Results
Varyani S. (2022) [89]	n = 36	Traditional exercises (neck strengthening exercises, upper body stretching, side bends with chin tuck, chin tucks) and eye muscle exercises.	25–30 min daily, 5 times a week; 4 weeks	NDI, OSDI, NPRS	Reduction of neck pain, improvement in NDI and OSDI.
Shah J. (2019) [90]	n = 30	G1—conventional exercise program, ergonomic advice G2—the same as above, plus Pilates	6 weeks	NPRS, NDI, neck muscle strength and endurance	Improvement of the studied parameters in both groups.
Kothare H. (2019) [91]	n = 50	KT application on UT	3 days	NPRS, NDI	Improvement of the studied parameters.
Areeudomwong P. (2018) [92]	n = 25	Two conditions: - shoulder taping, - no taping	30 min	NPRS, muscle activity, and fatigue during smartphone writing were assessed using electromyography	Reduction of pain and discomfort with KT application. No effect of KT on muscle activity and fatigue.

Abbreviations: G1—group 1; G2—group 2; CROM—Cervical Range of Motion; PNF—Proprioceptive Neuromuscular Facilitation; VAS—Visual Analogue Scale; NFMET—Neck flexor-extensor muscle endurance test; NYPRC—New York Posture Rating Chart; NDI—Neck Disability Index; TTW—tragus to wall test; CPJE Testing—Vernier Caliper measurements for rounded shoulders and cervical joint position error testing; SAS—Smartphone Addiction Scale; CHDQ—Cornell Hand Discomfort Questionnaire; ROM—range of motion; G3—group 3; CVA—Craniovertebral angle; NPRS—Numerical Pain Rating Scale; RSA—Rounded Shoulder Angle; ELDOA—Elongation Longitudinaux Avec Decoapton Osteo-Articulaire; METs—Muscle energy technique; FEV—Forced Expiratory Volume; FVC—Forced Vital Capacity; OSDI—Ocular Surface Disease Index; KT—Kinesiology Taping; UT—upper trapezius.

All studies were published within the last seven years. Most studies focused on adult populations aged 18–35, with three studies including individuals aged 18–44 [19,42,50] and one study involving adolescents [92]. The majority of studies were conducted in Asia, including countries such as India, Thailand, Pakistan, Iran, and Turkey in Eurasia [5,19,35,38,39,42,50,86–92].

In most studies, no funding was received (80%) [19,35,38,39,86–92], with only three studies receiving funding [5,42,50].

The physiotherapy methods identified as useful and effective in reducing pain and correcting posture in individuals with text neck syndrome include PNF (Proprioceptive Neuromuscular Facilitation) [19,86], corrective exercises, strengthening the deep neck flexor muscles [87], dynamic correction exercises [49], Pilates [23,90], Gong's mobilization [88], ELDOA [5], and kinesiology taping (KT) [91,92].

Regarding the improvement of cervical range of motion (CROM), the most effective methods were PNF [19,86], Gong's mobilization [88], and Pilates [23,90].

6.3. Summary of Current Evidence

Due to the fact that text neck syndrome primarily affects young adults, i.e., the working population, the symptoms associated with that syndrome may significantly impact the deterioration of their functioning and quality of life [1,93–96]. Therefore, early implementation of treatment is crucial to prevent the progression of symptoms, avoid degenerative changes in the cervical spine, and further impairment of function. In order to minimize the negative effects and reverse the symptoms of that syndrome as much as possible, various physiotherapeutic methods are used.

Depending on the severity of symptoms, different forms of therapy can be applied. For acute symptoms of text neck syndrome, rest, hot or cold compresses, massage, stretching, exercises, postural correction, and lifestyle changes are recommended. For chronic symptoms of text neck syndrome, physical therapy treatments, painkillers, injections, and acupuncture are used [5].

The duration of physical therapy for text neck syndrome varies depending on the severity of the condition. On average, for mild cases, physical therapy may last for 2–4 weeks with exercises aimed at improving posture, strengthening muscles, and increasing flexibility. In more severe cases, physical therapy could be required for 6–8 weeks or longer, with ongoing exercises and possibly additional treatments like manual therapy. Early intervention often leads to quicker recovery, while chronic cases may require longer treatment [5,19,23,38,39,42,50,86–92].

The main goal of physiotherapy treatment is to eliminate the problem and, if that is not possible, to reduce the perceived discomfort and prevent the disorder from progressing [5,90,97]. That goal may be achieved through the normalization of muscle tension, improvement of mobility in the cervical spine joints, enhancement of tissue trophism, and biomechanics [5]. An individually tailored therapeutic program may bring numerous benefits.

The scoping review was aimed to determine the physiotherapy methods currently used in the treatment of individuals with text neck, assess their impact on symptom reduction, and identify existing knowledge gaps and limitations in the current literature on the rehabilitation of text neck syndrome.

This review analyzes studies from the last 7 years, written in English, where the full text was available and clearly stated that the participants had text neck syndrome. The reviewed studies examined the effectiveness of the following rehabilitation methods: postural correction exercises, stabilization exercises, strengthening and stretching exercises, Pilates, PNF (Proprioceptive Neuromuscular Facilitation), Kinesiology taping, Bowen therapy, and manual therapy in the rehabilitation of text neck syndrome [5,19,23,38,39,42,50,86–92].

Before any therapeutic intervention is applied, it is essential to conduct diagnostics to identify abnormalities and functional disorders, which will enable the creation of an appropriate rehabilitation plan [38]. Detailed diagnostics should facilitate the identification of 'red flags' that indicate serious dysfunctions, such as the presence of a tumor or atlanto-axial subluxations. After a thorough assessment, the physiotherapist sets rehabilitation goals and establishes a treatment plan that is modified according to the patient's progress and condition changes [74]. The selection of therapy forms, methods, and techniques depends on the patient's current health status, reported symptoms, and coexisting conditions.

6.3.1. Kinesiotherapy

In the therapy of text neck syndrome, exercises should be carefully selected to normalize muscle tension. The forward shift of the head's center of gravity in text neck syndrome places increased strain on the cervical spine joints and muscles, such as the cervical extensor muscle and the upper part of the trapezius muscle. At the same time, deep neck flexor muscles, such as the longus capitis, longus colli, and rectus capitis anterior, lose their strength and endurance. Such a muscle imbalance may contribute to pain and dysfunction, which is why targeted exercises aim to strengthen the weakened muscles while relieving the overburdened ones [18]. The rhomboid muscles, as well as the middle and lower portions of the trapezius muscle, also weaken [18]. The pectoralis minor muscles and muscles of the rotator cuff are subjected to tension [18]. Due to that, it is recommended to incorporate exercises into the therapy that strengthen weakened muscles, such as deep neck flexors and stretching exercises for the shortened muscles [80].

Based on the analysis of available studies, there is noticeable effectiveness of stabilizing, corrective, and strengthening exercises for deep neck flexors in the treatment of text neck syndrome [19,38,42,50,86,87,89,90]. It is important to emphasize that adopting the appropriate position, duration, intensity, frequency, and difficulty level, tailored to the individual needs of the patient as well as health conditions is crucial in these exercises [38,42].

Sarraf F. et al. [87] demonstrated the effectiveness of corrective exercises in reducing pain and the NDI (Neck Disability Index) score in their study. The researchers have been able to achieve that effect because the corrective exercises contributed to strengthening the deep neck flexor muscles and stretching the tense muscles in both the neck and shoulder girdle areas [87]. Stretching and strengthening exercises are effective in maintaining the correct position of the cervical spine and improving stability in individuals with text neck syndrome [19,38,50,87]. The research conducted by Kang D.Y. [98] and Agrawal Y.K. and Hande D. [99] confirms that exercises targeting the deep neck flexors are highly effective in restoring the muscle tension balance and, consequently, alleviating pain in that area.

Wissem D.W. and Saadc H.B. [49] emphasize the superiority of dynamic correction over static postural correction exercises. Traditional static postural correction exercises focus on restoring and maintaining the cervical spine in a neutral position and adhering to ergonomic principles [49]. On the other hand, dynamic correction is based on the joint-by-joint approach, which focuses on restoring mobility and stability throughout the entire kinetic chain, including the thoracic spine and shoulder girdle, rather than just focusing on the cervical spine [49]. That approach provides a long-term effect rather than temporary relief, as is the case with traditional static postural correction exercises [49]. According to the joint-by-joint approach, the therapeutic process for text neck should include mobilization of the thoracic spine, stabilization exercises, scapular control exercises, and exercises incorporating rotational movements in the thoracic spine [49].

In order to improve the patient's functionality, the proprioceptive neuromuscular facilitation (PNF) method is also used, which utilizes developed movement patterns [19]. PNF is based on neurophysiological principles, using tri-planar and diagonal movement [19,86]. In a study conducted by Kaya M. et al. [19] on a group of 38 individuals with text neck, comparing the use of exercises improving CROM, strengthening, and postural correction with the application of PNF techniques—contract–relax and replication—a statistically significant better improvement in the range of motion of the cervical spine was observed in the group using PNF. It may be due to the fact that PNF techniques improve the range of motion by activating both agonist and antagonist muscles, which helps lengthen muscles and tendons. PNF, particularly the contract–relax and hold–relax methods, is often more effective than static stretching due to mechanisms like reciprocal and autogenic inhibition. During PNF, when a muscle contracts against resistance, tension builds up, activating Golgi tendon organs, which then reduce muscle tension by inhibiting excessive contraction. This process helps improve flexibility and range of motion, as supported by this study [19].

Similar results were obtained in a study conducted by Rajopadhye S. and Honkalas P. [86], evaluating the effectiveness of the Dynamic Reversal technique for improving the range of motion of the cervical spine and the Rhythmic Stabilization technique for reducing neck pain in individuals with text neck syndrome. After eight therapeutic sessions conducted over 2 weeks, the researchers observed statistically significant improvements in the measured parameters [86].

The positive effects on pain reduction in the PNF group may be due to the activation of impaired proprioception centers through various PNF techniques. These techniques stimulate proprioceptive receptors in muscles and tendons, improving nerve control, muscle tone, and circulation. Additionally, the decrease in pain intensity could be linked to the local afferent input generated by PNF interventions, which help modulate pain perception [19,86].

It is important to note that the key to success is to perform exercises correctly and safely. The therapist should provide guidance on how to exercise. The duration, type, intensity, frequency, and level of difficulty of the exercises should be tailored individually to the patient, health status, functional abilities, and preferences. In order to achieve benefits such as an improved range of motion and tissue nourishment, increased functional capabilities, alleviation of pain, and improved posture, it is necessary to work with the entire body of the patient, eliminate coexisting dysfunctions rather than just working locally [83,97].

Shah J. and Soni K. [90] recommend incorporating Pilates into the therapy for text neck syndrome. The Pilates method positively influences psychophysical functioning, strengthens muscles, improves core stabilization, and enhances mobility, balance, flexibility, and endurance [23,90]. The effectiveness of using Pilates in therapy for text neck syndrome was evaluated by Bhanu Sri P.L. et al. [23]. The researchers evaluated the impact of the Gong mobilization technique and Pilates on pain intensity, range of motion, and function. It has been shown that after 6 weeks of therapy, a greater improvement in the studied parameters was observed in the Pilates group [23]. Pilates helps activate the deep neck flexor muscles—it strengthens and improves the endurance of the deep muscles, thereby relieving and reducing the activity and fatigue of the superficial muscles, which in turn leads to pain reduction and improvement of overall functioning [23,50,90].

Pilates promotes a neutral cervical spine position with slight flexion at the craniocervical junction, activating the deep neck flexor muscles. By combining breathing techniques with specific stretches, Pilates helps manage neck pain. Neck pain is often linked to weakness in the deep cervical flexors, and Pilates aids in re-educating the stabilizing muscles of the spine and shoulder girdle. This not only alleviates pain but also improves function by strengthening and increasing endurance in the cervical muscles [23,90].

In Pilates, it is important to combine exercises with proper breath control [90]. Shikha B. et al. [35] emphasize the importance of breath work in the treatment of text neck syndrome. The researchers compared the effectiveness of balloon-blowing exercises with modified neck exercises and exercises using a Swedish ball on lung capacity. After 4 weeks of therapy, improvement in the measured parameters (FEV, FVC) was observed in both groups, with a greater improvement in the group performing balloon-blowing exercises [35].

Bhende R. et al. [42] investigated whether integrated postural training, focusing on the involvement of three systems—visual, vestibular, and somatosensory—that coordinate postural control of the neck, would be effective in treating text neck syndrome. The training included neck proprioception exercises, deep neck muscle strengthening exercises, and strengthening exercises; the McKenzie program focused on postural correction, as well as oculomotor exercises and eye–head coordination exercises [42]. The authors have demonstrated that a holistic approach, rather than merely addressing symptomatic relief, offers numerous benefits. A six-week integrated postural training program for individuals with text neck syndrome resulted in improved posture, strengthened weakened muscles, restored joint mobility, reduced pain, and enhanced overall functional capacity [42].

In turn, Varyani S. et al. [89] focused on applying a conventional exercise program that included isometric neck exercises combined with eye muscle exercises for individuals with text neck syndrome. In the study group of 36 participants, the researchers observed improvements in neck flexor muscle endurance, pain reduction, alleviation of asthenopic symptoms, and enhanced functionality after four weeks of therapy [89].

Many authors emphasize that combining physiotherapeutic methods yields better results than using individual treatments alone [5,19,39,42]. Nakhate S. et al. [48] recommend implementing a 1–4-week rehabilitation program that should begin with soft tissue mobilization, followed by joint mobilization and both active and passive stretching of tense muscles. The next recommended steps include strengthening weakened muscles, correcting posture, changing habits, performing home exercises, and reducing time spent using a phone [48].

6.3.2. Manual Therapy

Manual therapy is used to increase the range of motion, restore proper joint mechanics, normalize the tension of paraspinal tissues, and reduce pain during movement [5,100]. Manual therapy not only addresses the cervical spine but also works on the thoracic spine and the cervicothoracic junction [49]. It may include manipulations, mobilizations, or Muscle Energy Techniques (MET) [5].

The muscle energy technique is a form of manual therapy aimed at improving joint mobility by lengthening tense muscles and strengthening weakened muscles through the use of isotonic or isometric contractions [39]. The Bowen therapy, on the other hand, employs gentle rolling movements applied to soft tissues in a specific manner and at designated points [39].

The effectiveness of the MET and Bowen therapy in the treatment of text neck syndrome was assessed by Seemal P. et al. [39]. The researchers observed that the combination of the Muscle Energy Technique and Bowen therapy yielded better results than using the MET alone in the treatment. The combination of both therapies resulted in a statistically significant reduction in perceived pain as well as improvements in the function and mobility of the cervical spine [39]. Afzal H. et al. [88] also demonstrated the effectiveness of manual therapy—Gong's mobilization in the reduction of neck pain, disability, and improvement of CROM and neck muscle strength in individuals with text neck syndrome.

The effectiveness of manual therapy has also been demonstrated in individual case reports of people with text neck syndrome [37,43]. One study focused on the use of manual therapy and instrument-assisted therapy in a 6-year-old boy with text neck syndrome [43]. The treatment applied resulted in a reduction of pain and neurological symptoms and an improvement in the Cervical Range of Motion (CROM) [43].

Farooq M. et al. [5] demonstrated the effectiveness of the ELDOA (Elongation Longitudinaux Avec Decoapton Osteo-Articulaire) method and post-facilitation stretching in a group of 40 participants with text neck syndrome, aged 18–35. The ELDOA group and the stretching group each consisted of 20 individuals. Each group received the assigned therapy three times a week for 6 weeks. Both groups showed a reduction in neck pain and NDI scores, but the ELDOA group showed a statistically significantly greater improvement than the post-facilitation stretching group.

Better results in the ELDOA group may be related to the fact that ELDOA focuses on maximizing spinal and fascial stretching by holding specific postures. This technique aims to strengthen and decompress the spine. Originating from various treatment methods, ELDOA has both local and overall effects. It helps decompress the zygapophyseal joints, enhances fluid absorption in the discs, improves circulation, and boosts muscle tone and range of motion. Additionally, it aids in correcting posture, improving breathing, and enhancing proprioception in the targeted segment [5].

6.3.3. Kinesiology Taping

In the rehabilitation of text neck syndrome, the Kinesiology Taping (KT) method is used. It involves applying an elastic tape with a specific structure to the skin surface using a technique appropriately selected for the therapeutic goal. The application of the tape is performed after properly preparing the patient's skin for the application. The pain-relieving effect is achieved by improving the microcirculation of blood and lymph, activating alpha and beta nerve fibers and their skin connections, and unloading the subcutaneous nociceptors [91,92]. In addition to its analgesic effect, Kinesiology Taping influences the normalization of muscle tone, improvement of posture, and stabilization of the achieved therapeutic effects—maintaining the corrected position [92]. For example, in individuals with head protrusion, excessive stretching of the extensors and neck pain may occur, so the use of KT will, in such a case, serve as a supportive function for the extensor muscles in maintaining the head in the correct position.

However, it should be noted that Kinesiology Taping is not used as a standalone method in the treatment of text neck syndrome. It serves as an attractive complement to other therapeutic methods; for example, it may be used to maintain the effects of manual therapy [91,92,101].

KT is a complementary form that supports proper treatment [91,92]. Kothare H. et al. [91] have noted that the appropriate application of KT may be effective in alleviating the symptoms of text neck syndrome as early as 3 days after application. The effectiveness of KT in reducing pain symptoms is supported by studies conducted by Areeudomwong P. et al. [92]. The authors of the study examined whether shoulder taping would affect the perceived discomfort in the neck area as well as the activity and endurance of the upper part of the trapezius muscle, neck extensors, and sternocleidomastoid muscles during 30 min of smartphone use. The results have demonstrated that KT reduced pain and discomfort but had no impact on muscle activity or fatigue [92]. Shoulder taping was found to reduce neck discomfort compared to no taping. While the exact mechanisms behind this effect are not fully understood, it is possible that the tension from the tape plays a role in alleviating discomfort. Participants who received shoulder taping reported only moderate skin tension, which may activate skin mechanoreceptors and reduce pain through the gate control theory, thus lessening their discomfort [92].

6.4. Limitations of the Included Studies

One of the primary limitations identified in the cited literature on physical therapy for text neck syndrome is the lack of blinding of both the researchers and the participants [5,19,35,38,42,50,86–92]. Additionally, most of the studies were conducted with a young adult population [5,35,38,86–91], which may not be representative of other age groups. The studies also utilized small sample sizes, limiting the generalizability of the results to a larger population. Furthermore, the studies were geographically restricted, which may reduce the applicability of the findings to other regions. The majority of studies were conducted in India [23,35,38,42,50,86,89–91]. Lastly, the studies were short-duration and lacked long-term follow-up, making it difficult to assess the sustained effects of the interventions.

6.5. Limitations of the Study

In a scoping review, the process of selecting, evaluating, and synthesizing the included studies may be less rigorous and potentially prone to bias, as it generally does not involve a formal quality assessment of the literature. Nevertheless, the strength of this type of review lies in its ability to provide a clear and accessible summary and critique of existing literature, providing valuable new insights. To enhance the methodological rigor of our review, we have clearly defined the eligibility criteria, search strategies, and databases used, as well as specified the number of records to be included, which helps to better outline the scope of the study.

This review has analyzed publications written in English for the last seven years regarding the use of physical therapy in text neck syndrome, which may lead to bias in study selection due to the lack of data on text neck syndrome described in languages other than English. Additionally, many articles are not publicly available. As a result, our findings can only be generalized to studies that are publicly available, which is a limitation of the study. Despite these limitations, this scoping review serves as a valuable resource for understanding the current state of research on the rehabilitation of text neck syndrome.

6.6. Future Research Objectives

This review highlights several key areas for future research on text neck syndrome. Most existing studies have focused on young adults and college students, leaving gaps in research regarding other age groups. Notably, there is a lack of studies on children and adolescents, an area that warrants further investigation. Research on pain related to text neck syndrome in children is limited, and establishing its prevalence along with clear diagnostic criteria using validated tools is a crucial step. Developing a standardized instrument for assessing text neck syndrome in the pediatric population would enable cross-cultural comparisons and facilitate the comparison of different sample sizes, accounting for cultural differences. As a result, cross-cultural studies involving large sample sizes are recommended to improve the generalizability and applicability across various populations.

Furthermore, long-term cohort studies are essential for evaluating the effectiveness of preventive measures and assessing the lasting impact of interventions. The need for longitudinal studies with long-term follow-up periods is critical to understanding the sustained effects of interventions over time.

Recommendations for future research on physical therapy in text neck syndrome include conducting longitudinal studies with extended follow-up periods to observe the long-term effects of interventions. Increasing sample sizes and conducting studies with diverse populations, including children, adolescents, and elderly individuals, is also essential. Expanding the geographical scope and incorporating cross-cultural studies to improve the generalizability of findings is crucial. Utilizing randomized controlled trials (RCTs) would be a good approach to strengthen the evidence base.

7. Conclusions

It is not possible to eliminate electronic devices from daily use, so it is important to maintain a proper posture while using them, reduce the time spent using smartphones, and ensure regular physical activity. When text neck syndrome does occur, it is crucial to start treatment promptly to prevent further functional decline and irreversible changes. The studies cited in this paper indicate the effectiveness of physiotherapy in treating text neck syndrome. All studies suggest that appropriate physiotherapeutic interventions can provide significant benefits, including pain reduction, posture correction, and improved range of motion in the cervical spine. The most effective therapeutic approach involves combining various rehabilitation methods, including postural correction exercises, stabilization exercises, strengthening and stretching exercises, Pilates, PNF (Proprioceptive Neuromuscular Facilitation), kinesiology taping, Bowen therapy, and manual therapy. The best treatment outcomes are achieved through a combination of strengthening and stretching exercises, manual therapy, and postural correction. In addition to physiotherapy, education is essential at every stage, both in prevention and treatment. However, further high-quality research is needed to strengthen the evidence and offer reliable recommendations for clinical practice. Additionally, there is limited research on physiotherapy for text neck in the pediatric population, presenting a potential area for future studies.

Author Contributions: Conceptualization, J.P. and W.K.; Investigation, J.P.; Resources, J.P.; Writing—Original Draft Preparation, J.P. and W.K.; Writing—Review and Editing, J.P. and W.K.; Visualization, J.P. and W.K.; Supervision, W.K.; Funding Acquisition, J.P. and W.K. All authors have read and agreed to the published version of the manuscript.

Funding: This research was funded by the Medical University of Bialystok, Bialystok, Poland under grants B.SUB.24.168 and B.SUB.25.181. The authors are grateful to the Medical University of Bialystok, Bialystok, Poland, for funding this study.

Institutional Review Board Statement: Not applicable.

Informed Consent Statement: Not applicable.

Conflicts of Interest: The authors declare no conflicts of interest.

References

1. Ayhualem, S.; Alamer, A.; Dabi, S.D.; Bogale, K.G.; Abebe, A.B.; Chala, M.B. Burden of neck pain and associated factors among smart phone user students in University of Gondar, Ethiopia. *PLoS ONE* **2021**, *16*, e0256794. [CrossRef]
2. Khan, S.; Kumari, B.; Kataria, S.; Sultan, R.; Hakim, A.; Quratulain; Faiz, A.; Mazhar, S.; Aslam, I. Impact of Smartphone Addiction on Neck Pain Among University Students. *J. Health Rehabil. Res.* **2024**, *4*, 1–5. [CrossRef]
3. Demandsage. Available online: https://www.demandsage.com/smartphone-usage-statistics/ (accessed on 17 November 2024).
4. Iqbal, K.; Hafeez, K.; Rashad, A.; Lodhi, A.A. Prevalence of Neck Pain and its Association with Smartphone Use Among University Students. *J. Health Rehabil. Res.* **2024**, *4*, 96–101. [CrossRef]
5. Farooq, M.; Bashir, M.S.; Arif, A.; Kashif, M.; Manzoor, N.; Abid, F. Effects of elongation longitudinaux avec decoaption osteo-articulaire and postfacilitation stretching technique on pain and functional disability in mobile users with text neck syndrome during COVID-19 pandemic: A randomized controlled trial. *Medicine* **2023**, *102*, e33073. [CrossRef] [PubMed]
6. Purushothaman, V.K.; Ramalingam, V.; Xian, R.W.Y.; Pillai, S.G.K.; Jabbar, M.A.; Muniandy, Y.; Subbarayalu, A.V.; Vasanthi, R.K. The Relationship Between Smartphone Usage Pattern and Cervical Proprioception in Adults with Text Neck Syndrome in Malaysia. *Natl. J. Community Med.* **2023**, *14*, 821–826. [CrossRef]
7. Samani, P.P.; Athavale, N.A.; Shyam, A.; Sancheti, P.K. Awareness of text neck syndrome in young-adult population. *Int. J. Community Med. Public Health* **2018**, *5*, 154–159. [CrossRef]
8. Kamalakannan, M.; Rakshana, R.; Padma, P.R. Estimation and prevention of text neck syndrome among smart phone users. *Biomedicine* **2020**, *40*, 372–376. [CrossRef]
9. Tsantili, A.R.; Chrysikos, D.; Troupis, T. Text Neck Syndrome: Disentangling a New Epidemic. *Acta Med. Acad.* **2022**, *51*, 123–127. [CrossRef]
10. Thorburn, E.; Pope, R.; Wang, S. Musculoskeletal symptoms among adult smartphone and tablet device users: A retrospective study. *Arch. Physiother.* **2021**, *11*, 1. [CrossRef]
11. David, D.; Giannini, C.; Chiarelli, F.; Mohn, A. Text Neck Syndrome in Children and Adolescents. *Int. J. Environ. Res. Public Health* **2021**, *18*, 1565. [CrossRef]
12. Warda, D.G.; Nwakibu, U.; Nourbakhsh, A. Neck and Upper Extremity Musculoskeletal Symptoms Secondary to Maladaptive Postures Caused by Cell Phones and Backpacks in School-Aged Children and Adolescents. *Healthcare* **2023**, *11*, 819. [CrossRef] [PubMed]
13. Rathi, P.; Talwar, J.K.; Athavale, N.; Dabadghav, R.; Shyam, A.; Sancheti, P. Awareness about text neck syndrome amongst adolescents. *Physiother. J. Indian Assoc. Physiother.* **2022**, *16*, 72–76. [CrossRef]
14. Pacheco Salles, F.L.; Feitanin Basso, M.; Leonel, A. Smartphone use: Implications for musculoskeletal symptoms and socio-demographic characteristics in students. *Interdiscip. Rehab.* **2024**, *4*, 1–9. [CrossRef]
15. Shetty, S.; Umesh, K.; Adersh, C.P.; Akshay, R.; Fathimath Sumayya, N.E.; Midhun, P.M.; Shehin, P.K.M.; Sadique Ali, K.T.; Shahul Hameed, A.M. Prevalence of text neck syndrome associated with smart phone addiction: A cross sectional study. *IJPESH* **2022**, *9*, 350–353.
16. Fiebert, I.; Kistner, F.; Gissendanner, C.; DaSilva, C. Text neck: An adverse postural phenomenon. *Work* **2021**, *69*, 1261–1270. [CrossRef]
17. Shamsi, R.F.; Sadeeqa, A.; Khan, A.A.; Khan, F.M.; Saeed, A.; Sheeraz, S.N. Correlation of smartphone addiction with text neck syndrome during COVID-19 pandemic. *Rehabil. J.* **2022**, *6*, 442–445. [CrossRef]
18. Sarraf, F.; Varmazyar, S. Comparing the effect of the posture of using smartphones on head and neck angles among college students. *Ergonomics* **2022**, *65*, 1631–1638. [CrossRef] [PubMed]
19. Kaya, M.; Ucgun, H.; Denizoglu Kulli, H. The effect of proprioceptive neuromuscular facilitation on individuals with text neck syndrome: A randomized controlled study. *Medicine* **2024**, *103*, e38716. [CrossRef] [PubMed]

20. Kumari, S.; Kumar, R.; Sharma, D. Text neck syndrome: The pain of modern era. *Int. J. Health Sci. Res.* **2021**, *11*, 161–165. [CrossRef]
21. Jahre, H.; Grotle, M.; Smedbraten, K.; Dunn, K.M.; Qiestad, B.E. Risk factors for non—Specific neck pain in young adults. A systematic review. *BMC Musculoskelet. Disord.* **2020**, *21*, 366. [CrossRef]
22. Kumar, S.; Khaleeluddin, K.B.; Jayakumar, S.; Vendhan, E. Prevalence and Awareness of Text Neck and Texting Thumb Syndrome in Young Adult Population. *J. Appl. Pharm. Res.* **2024**, *12*, 22–28. [CrossRef]
23. Bhanu Sri, P.L.; Pundarikaksha, P.; Apparao, P.; Swamy, C.G. Effectiveness of Pilates and gong's mobilization on pain, range of motion and function in text neck syndrome among young adults. *Int. J. Health Sci. Res.* **2023**, *13*, 138–154. [CrossRef]
24. Neupane, S.; Ifthikar, A.; Mathew, A. Text neck syndrome—Systematic review. *Imp. J. Interdiscip. Res.* **2017**, *3*, 141–148.
25. Khalid, R.; Amjad, F.; Hashim, A.; Ain, Q. Text neck syndrome, an emerging public health threat during COVID-19 situation. *Rawal. Med. J.* **2022**, *47*, 527–531.
26. Rashid, M.K.; Jadoo, S.A.A.; Al-Hussainy, A.H.; Latif, I.I. Prevalence of text neck syndrome among Iraqi medical students: A cross-sectional study. *J. Ideas Health* **2022**, *5*, 693–699. [CrossRef]
27. Hassnain, S.M.; Nouman Latif, M.; Hassan Arshad, M.; Aneeque, A.; Noor, S. Association of Text Neck Pain with Prolonged Studying and Excessive Smart Phone Usage Among Medical Students. *J. Bahria Uni Med. Dent. Coll.* **2023**, *13*, 29–33. [CrossRef]
28. Javed, A.; Andama, G.; Rehman, A.; Ahmed, M.W.; Ali, S.H.; Ahmed, M.A.; Bibi, M.; Khalid, A. Text Neck Syndrome and Associated Risk Factors: Prevalence in Medical Students: Text Neck Syndrome and Associated Risk Factors. *Ther. (J. Ther. Rehabil. Sci.)* **2023**, *4*, 38–42. [CrossRef]
29. Alsiwed, K.T.; Alsarwani, R.M.; Alshaikh, S.A.; Howaidi, R.A.; Aljahdali, A.J.; Bassi, M.M. The prevalence of text neck syndrome and its association with smartphone use among medical students in Jeddah, Saudi Arabia. *J. Musculoskelet. Surg. Res.* **2021**, 266–272. [CrossRef]
30. Kamaraj, P.N.; Rajasekar, V.D.; Rangasamy, S. A study on prevalence of text neck syndrome among under-graduate students of a medical college in Puducherry. *Int. J. Community Med. Public Health.* **2022**, *9*, 2919–2922. [CrossRef]
31. Parmar, N.; Agrawal, M.; Solanki, S.; Solanki, J. Impact of text neck symptoms on posture and mobili ty among college students: A study utilizing a self-designed questionnaire. *World J. Adv. Res. Rev.* **2024**, *21*, 363–375. [CrossRef]
32. Sathya, P.; Tamboli, S.A. Prevalence of Text Neck Nyndrome in young-adult population. *Ijmaes* **2020**, *6*, 749–759. [CrossRef]
33. Atakla, H.G.; Mbaye, M.; Dakurah, T.K.; Quenum, M.K.; Barry, L.F.; Wague, D.; Sossa, C.I.; Houinato, D.S.; Thiam, A.B.; Code Ba, M. Tech Neck Syndrome: A global epidemic of the modern era among students at the University of Abomey Calavi in Benin. *Interdiscip. Neurosurg.* **2023**, *34*, 101812. [CrossRef]
34. Kokiwar, P.R.; Shruthi, C.; Vaishnavi, I.; Kavya, S.; Manognya, K.; Ghouse, M.; Sajid, S.; Shravya, G.; Tejaswini, S.; Snigdha, P.; et al. Prevalence and risk factors of text neck syndrome among medical students. *MRIMS J. Health Sci.* **2020**, *8*, 10–13. [CrossRef]
35. Shikha, B.; Thapa, B.; Zafar, S. Effect of balloon blowing exercise vs modified cervical exercise along with Swiss ball exercise on the lung capacity of patient suffering from text neck syndrome due to improper posture. *Int. J. Health Sci.* **2022**, *6*, 7497–7507. [CrossRef]
36. Melhorn, J.M.; Goff, W.J. "Text neck pain" and Hand held devices. *Med. Res. Innov.* **2019**, *3*, 1–2. [CrossRef]
37. Chu, E. Preventing the progression of text neck in a young man: A case report. *Radiol. Case Rep.* **2022**, *17*, 978–982. [CrossRef]
38. Nathani, H.R.; Phansopkar, P. Effectiveness of Tailor-Made Physiotherapy Protocol in Smartphone-Addicted Individuals with Text Neck Syndrome and Short Message Service (SMS) Thumb. *Cureus* **2024**, *16*, e57453. [CrossRef]
39. Seemal, P.; Noor, R.; Riaz, S.; Afzal, H.; Anwar, S.; Niaz, M. Effects of Muscle Energy Technique with and Without Bowen Therapy in Text Neck Syndrome. *Pak. J. Med. Health Sci.* **2022**, *16*, 164–166. [CrossRef]
40. Bhattacharya, S.; Saleem, S.M.; Juyal, R.; Kaur, R.; Singh, A. "Texting neck" or "iNeck pain" syndrome—An emerging public health threat: In the era of NEW NORMAL. *J. Prim. Care Spec.* **2021**, *2*, 1–3. [CrossRef]
41. Kataria, J. Text neck—Its effects on posture. *IJCRT* **2018**, *6*, 817–819.
42. Bhende, R.; Shinde, S.; Jain, P. Effect of Integrated Postural Training in Individuals with TextNeck Syndrome. *J. Kinesiol. Exerc. Sci.* **2024**, *108*, 1–18. [CrossRef]
43. Chu, E.; Mok, T.; Ng, G.; Chu, E. Pediatric Text Neck Syndrome. *Cureus* **2023**, *15*, e38034. [CrossRef] [PubMed]
44. Hend, H.A.; Samah, A.A.; Haytham, M.E.; Al Shimaa, S.A. Effect of text-neck syndrome on scapular index and respiratory functions in different age groups. *Int. J. Recent Adv. Multidiscip. Res.* **2021**, *8*, 7115–7120.
45. Thiyagarajan, S.; Telegbal, S.V. Text Neck: Is it a new term for physiotherapist? *Indian J. Med. Health Sci.* **2015**, *2*, 119–121. [CrossRef]
46. Shahzad, Y.; Mehmood, F.; Sarwar, S.; Ramooz, K.; Akhtar, N.; Akram, A.; Yaqoob, E.; Javed, S. The Text Neck Epidemic: Unveiling the Hidden Burden of Neck Pain Among Medical Students. *Pak. J. Neurol. Surg.* **2023**, *27*, 174–181. [CrossRef]
47. Bashir, U.; Noor, R.; Shoukat, H.; Ali, M.L.; Javed, M.T.; Hassan, Z. Correlation of mobile phone usage on grip strength, disabilities and posture in young adults. *Rehabil. J.* **2022**, *7*, 495–498. [CrossRef]

48. Nakhate, S.; Asutkar, S.; Asutkar, V.; Yadav, Y.; Puri, G.; Paliwal, A. Text neck syndrome and its perspective through Ayurveda: A literary review. *Afr. J. Bio. Sc.* **2024**, *6*, 8658–8666.
49. Wissem, W.D.; Saadc, H.B. Revolutionizing "Text Neck Syndrome" Management: Paradigm Shifting from "Posture Correction" to "Posture Change". *Acta Kinesiol.* **2024**, *18*, 37–40. [CrossRef]
50. Bharal, S.; Rizvi, M.R.; Alqahtani, M.M.; Alajam, R.A.; Sharma, A.; Ahmad, I.; Al-Otaibi, M.L.; Alshehri, M.M.; Ahmad, M.M.; Shaphe, M.A.; et al. Effectiveness of neck stabilization and Contrology training in comparison to conventional therapy amongst individuals with Text Neck Syndrome. *Eur. Rev. Med. Pharmacol. Sci.* **2023**, *27*, 8340–8349. [CrossRef]
51. Hofstetter, L.; Häusler, M.; Schweinhardt, P.; Heggli, U.; Bron, D.; Swanenburg, J. Influence of Axial Load and a 45-Degree Flexion Head Position on Cervical Spinal Stiffness in Healthy Young Adults. *Front. Physiol.* **2021**, *12*, 786625. [CrossRef] [PubMed]
52. Raihan, H.A.; Rahman, F. Effect of Ergonomic Levels on Text Neck Syndrome Among Students: A Correlational Study. *J. Kesehat.* **2023**, *16*, 301–308. [CrossRef]
53. Medani, K.T.; Ahmad, M.S.; Sami, W.; Shaik, R.A.; Mohamed, E.; Alhammad, M.A.; Almutlaq, M.M.S.; Alodaini Alotiabi, Z.A.M.; Alshammary, F.H. Perspective, awareness and behaviour towards Text-Neck among medical students of Majmaah University—A cross sectional study. *J. Evol. Med. Dent. Sci.* **2021**, *10*, 294–298. [CrossRef]
54. Shah, P.P.; Sheth, M.S. Correlation of smartphone use addiction with text neck syndrome and SMS thumb in physiotherapy students. *Int. J. Community Med. Public Health* **2018**, *5*, 2512. [CrossRef]
55. Hakami, I.; Sherwani, A.; Hadadi, M.; Alzahrani, R.; Albukhari, A.; Omar, Y.; Alsaedi, K.; Aljadani, F.; Ali, N.; Khan, M.; et al. Assessing the Impact of Smartphone Use on Neck Pain and Related Symptoms Among Residents in Jeddah, Saudi Arabia: A Cross-Sectional Study. *Cureus* **2024**, *16*, e64299. [CrossRef] [PubMed]
56. Anand, B.; Thakur, S.; Sharma, P. Association between discomfort and fatigue around neck area due to portable electronic devices in college students. *J. Exerc. Sci. Physiother.* **2020**, *16*, 16–22. [CrossRef]
57. Elvan, A.; Cevik, S.; Vatansever, K.; Erak, I. The association between mobile phone usage duration, neck muscle endurance, and neck pain among university students. *Sci. Rep.* **2024**, *14*, 20116. [CrossRef]
58. Paek, K.S. A convergence study the association between addictive smartphone use, dry eye syndrome, upper extremity pain and depression among college students. *J. Korea Converg. Soc.* **2017**, *8*, 61–69. [CrossRef]
59. Gong, W.; Kim, C.; Lee, Y. Correlations between cervical lordosis, forward head posture, cervical ROM and the strength and endurance of the deep neck flexor muscles in college students. *J. Phys. Ther. Sci.* **2012**, *24*, 275–277. [CrossRef]
60. Choi, J.H.; Jung, M.H.; Yoo, K.T. An analysis of the activity and muscle fatigue of the muscles around the neck under the three most frequent postures while using a smartphone. *J. Phys. Ther. Sci.* **2016**, *28*, 1660–1664. [CrossRef]
61. De Vitta, A.; Candido, J.P.; Bento, T.; Cornelio, G.P.; Perrucini, P.O.; Fernandes, J.A.A.; Ramos, W. Neck pain and factors associated in university students: A cross sectional study. *CiênciaemMovimento-Reabil. Saúde* **2020**, *22*, 89–101. [CrossRef]
62. Cankurtaran, D.; Yigman, Z.A.; Yigman, F.; Celik, G. How does smartphone usage affect the severity of neck pain, neck-pain related disability, and cervical lordosis? A pilot study. *Med. Sci. Discov.* **2021**, *8*, 254–259. [CrossRef]
63. Maayah, M.F.; Nawasreh, Z.H.; Gaowgzeh, R.A.M.; Neamatallah, Z.; Alfawaz, S.S.; Alabasi, U.M. Neck pain associated with smartphone usage among university students. *PLoS ONE* **2023**, *18*, e0285451. [CrossRef]
64. Correia, I.M.T.; Sa' Ferreira, A.; Fernandez, J.; Reis, F.J.J.; Nogueira, L.A.C.; Meziat-Filho, N. Association Between Text Neck and Neck Pain in Adults. *Spine* **2021**, *46*, 571–578. [CrossRef]
65. Bertozzi, L.; Negrini, S.; Agosto, D.; Costi, S.; Guccione, A.A.; Lucarelli, P.; Villafañe, J.H.; Pillasrini, P. Posture and time spent using a smartphone are not correlated with neck pain and disability in young adults: A cross-sectional study. *J. Bodyw. Mov. Ther.* **2020**, *14*, 12994. [CrossRef]
66. Mustafaoglu, R.; Yasaci, Z.; Zirek, E.; Griffiths, M.D.; Ozdincler, A.R. The relationship between smartphone addiction and musculoskeletal pain prevalence among young population: A cross-sectional study. *Korean J. Pain.* **2021**, *34*, 72–81. [CrossRef]
67. Fatima, S.; Fatima, M.; Taufiq, A.; Fiaz, S.; Afzal, M. Association Between Nomophobia and Text Neck Syndrome in Students in Lahore: A Cross-Sectional Study. *J. Health Rehabil. Res.* **2024**, *4*, 1–4. [CrossRef]
68. Gupta, N.; Krishnamurthy, V.; Majhi, J.; Gupta, S. Gadget dependency among medical college students in Delhi. *Indian J. Community Health* **2013**, *25*, 362–366.
69. Alshahrani, A.; Samy Abdrabo, M.; Aly, S.M.; Alshahrani, M.S.; Alqhtani, R.S.; Asiri, F.; Ahmad, I. Effect of smartphone usage on neck muscle endurance, hand grip and pinch strength among healthy college students: A cross-sectional study. *Int. J. Environ. Res. Public Health* **2021**, *18*, 6290. [CrossRef] [PubMed]
70. Chen, Y.L.; Chan, Y.C.; Alexander, H. Gender differences in neck muscle activity during near-maximum forward head flexion while using smartphones with varied postures. *Sci. Rep.* **2024**, *14*, 12994. [CrossRef]
71. Sultan, N.; Khushnood, K.; Mehmood, R. Effects of sustained natural apophyseal glides with Muscle energy technique on mechanical neck pain. *Int. J. Allied Health Sci.* **2018**, *4*, 202–207.

72. Jahre, H.; Grotle, M.; Småstuen, M.; Guddal, M.H.; Smedbråten, K.; Richardsen, K.R.; Stensland, S.; Storheim, K.; Øiestad, B.E. Risk factors and risk profiles for neck pain in young adults: Prospective analyses from adolescence to young adulthood—The North-Trøndelag Health Study. *PLoS ONE* **2021**, *16*, e0256006. [CrossRef] [PubMed]
73. Kim, S.D. Fatigue and pain related to internet usage among university students. *J. Phys. Ther. Sci.* **2016**, *28*, 1233–1237.
74. Jyothsna, G. Text Neck Syndrome in Adolescents: How to Stem the Tide. *Int. J. Pediatr. Nurs. IJPEN* **2019**, *5*, 35–40.
75. Fares, J.; Fares, M.Y.; Fares, J. Musculoskeletal neck pain in children and adolescents: Risk factors and complications. *Surg. Neurol. Int.* **2017**, *10*, 72. [CrossRef]
76. Song, M.K.; Park, J.H.; Kong, J.Y.; Kang, H.S. The Relationships of Smartphone Usage with Spinal Curvature and Neck or Shoulder Pain in School Children. *Coll. Sport* **2020**, *29*, 394–401. [CrossRef]
77. George, S.A.; Rajashekhar, A.T.A. A case study on text neck syndrome and gamers' thumb in 10-year old nomophobic student with attention deficit hyperactivity disorder (ADHD). *IJSHR* **2022**, *7*, 354–357. [CrossRef]
78. Aziz, A.N.; Bakir, L.A. Prevalence of Text Neck Syndrome in Children and Adolescents Using Smartphones in Erbil City. *Med. J. Babylon* **2022**, *19*, 540–546. [CrossRef]
79. Dolah, J.; Yie, J.L.J.; Gee, L.L.S. Improving knowledge of text neck and neck pain using interactive smartphone application for undergraduate students in University Sains Malaysia. *Gendang Alam* **2020**, *10*, 143–158. [CrossRef]
80. Fouda, K.Z.; Abdelsalam, M.S. Effect of cervical exercises with corrective instructions on neck pain and disability in smartphone addicted users. *Physiother. Quart.* **2022**, *30*, 1–6. [CrossRef]
81. Namwongsa, S.; Puntumetakul, R.; Neubert, M.S.; Boucaut, R. Effect of neck flexion angles on neck muscle activity among smartphone users with and without neck pain. *Ergonomics* **2019**, *62*, 1524–1533. [CrossRef] [PubMed]
82. Anand, B.; Sharma, P. Association of Hand Performance with Neck Disability in Text Neck Syndrome Among College Students. *Indian J. Physiother. Occup. Ther.* **2020**, *14*, 13–19.
83. Soyer, O.; Akarırmak, Z.U. The Effect of Postural Correction and Exercise on Neck Pains in Cell Phone Users. *Turk. J. Osteoporos.* **2020**, *26*, 81–91. [CrossRef]
84. Vahedi, Z.; Mazloumi, A.; Sharifnezhad, A.; Kazemi, Z.; Garosi, E. Head forward flexion, lateral bending and viewing distance in smartphone users: A comparison between sitting and standing postures. *Work* **2020**, *67*, 837–846. [CrossRef]
85. Cevik, S.; Kaplan, A.; Katar, S. Correlation of Cervical Spinal Degeneration with Rise in Smartphone Usage Time in Young Adults. *Niger. J. Clin. Pr.* **2020**, *23*, 1748–1752. [CrossRef]
86. Rajopadhye, S.; Honkalas, P. Effectiveness of PNF Techniques on Neck Pain and Cervical ROM (Cervical Extension) in College with Text Neck Syndrome—An Experimental Study. *Int. J. Health Sci. Res.* **2023**, *13*, 152–157. [CrossRef]
87. Sarraf, F.; Abbasi, S.; Varmazyar, S. Self-Management Exercises Intervention on Text Neck Syndrome Among University Students Using Smartphones. *Pain Manag. Nurs.* **2023**, *24*, 595–602. [CrossRef]
88. Afzal, H.; Noor, R.; Mumtaz, N.; Bashir, M.S.; Saqulain, G. Effects of Kendall exercise versus Gong's mobilization on pain, range of motion, function, and strength in cases with text neck syndrome. *Iran. Rehabil. J.* **2023**, *21*, 411–419. [CrossRef]
89. Varyani, S.; Deshmukh, K.; Nagulkar, J.; Shinde, M.; Raghani, P. Effectiveness of conventional exercise program and ocular muscle retraining in UG medical students with text neck syndrome and asthenopic symptoms due to smartphone adversity. *IJCRT* **2022**, *10*, 47–59.
90. Shah, J.; Soni, K. Effectiveness of Pilates along with Conventional Exercise Program and Conventional Exercise Program Alone in Subjects with Text Neck Syndrome. *IJSR* **2021**, *10*, 1322–1326. [CrossRef]
91. Kothare, H.; Patil, C.; Muley, R. Immediate effects of kinesio taping on upper trapezius muscle on subjects having text neck. *Int. J. Physiol. Nutr. Phys. Educ.* **2019**, *4*, 131–133.
92. Areeudomwong, P.; Oapdunsalam, K.; Havicha, Y.; Tantai, S.; Buttagat, V. Effects of Shoulder Taping on Discomfort and Electromyographic Responses of the Neck While Texting on a Touchscreen Smartphone. *Saf. Health Work* **2018**, *9*, 319–325. [CrossRef] [PubMed]
93. Ahmed, A.U.; Media, S.Q. The Relationship of Neck pain and Smart Phones Usage among students: A Cross-Sectional Study in Erbil City. *Adv. Med. J.* **2024**, *9*, 27–36. [CrossRef]
94. Sirajudeen, M.S.; Alzhrani, M.; Alanazi, A.; Alqahtani, M.; Waly, M.; Unnikrishnan, R.; Muthusamy, H.; Alrubaia, W.; Alanazi, N.; Seyam, M.K.; et al. Prevalence of text neck posture, smartphone addiction, and its association with neck disorders among university students in the Kingdom of Saudi Arabia during the COVID-19 pandemic. *PeerJ* **2022**, *10*, e14443. [CrossRef] [PubMed]
95. Sirajudeen, M.S.; Alzhrani, M.; Alanazi, A.; Alqahtani, M.; Waly, M.; Manzar, M.D.; Hegazy, F.A.; Jamali, M.N.; Reddy, R.S.; Kakaraparthi, V.N.; et al. Prevalence of Upper Limb Musculoskeletal Disorders and Their Association with Smartphone Addiction and Smartphone Usage Among University Students in the Kingdom of Saudi Arabia During the COVID-19 Pandemic—A Cross-Sectional Study. *Healthcare* **2022**, *10*, 2373. [CrossRef]
96. Ahmed, S.; Akter, R.; Pokhrel, N.; Samuels, A.J. Prevalence of text neck syndrome and SMS thumb among smartphone users in college-going students: A cross-sectional survey study. *J. Public Health* **2019**, *29*, 411–416. [CrossRef]

97. Buttagat, V.; Kluayhomthong, S.; Areeudomwong, P. Effects of the combination of traditional Thai massage, scapular stabilization exercise, and chest mobilization in subjects with forward head posture: A single-blinded randomized clinical trial. *Chiropr. Man. Therap.* **2023**, *31*, 31. [CrossRef]
98. Kang, D.Y. Deep cervical flexor training with a pressure biofeedback unit is an effective method for maintaining neck mobility and muscular endurance in college students with forward head posture. *J. Phys. Ther. Sci.* **2015**, *27*, 3207–3210. [CrossRef]
99. Agrawal, Y.K.; Hande, D. Effect of activation of deep neck flexor muscle exercise on neck pain due to smart phone addiction. *Int. J. Multidiscip. Res. Dev.* **2017**, *4*, 489–492.
100. Kumar, R.; Sharma, S.; Setia, K. Effect of Cyriax Manipulation on Individuals with Text Neck Syndrome: A Research Protocol for Quasi-experimental Study. *J. Clin. Diagn. Res.* **2023**, *7*, YK01–YK04. [CrossRef]
101. Gałczyk, M.; Kułak, W.; Zalewska, A. Is the use of mobile phones good for your neck? Text neck syndrome as an awareness of the existing threat—Literature review. *Med. Ogólna Nauk. Zdrowiu* **2020**, *26*, 240–243. [CrossRef]

Journal of
Clinical Medicine

MDPI

Systematic Review

Effects of Resistance Training on Pain, Muscle Strength, and Function in Patients Undergoing Total Knee Arthroplasty: A Systematic Review and Meta-Analysis

Jaehyun Lim [1] and Byeonggeun Kim [2,*]

1 Department of Physical Therapy, Graduate School, Nambu University, Gwangju 62271, Republic of Korea
2 Regional Health & Medical Center for Persons with Disabilities, Chonnam National University Hospital, Gwangju 61469, Republic of Korea
* Correspondence: qudrms_92@naver.com

Abstract: Background/Objectives: The importance of resistance training for functional recovery in Total Knee Arthroplasty (TKA) patients has been emphasized. Therefore, this systematic review and meta-analysis was conducted to analyze its effects on pain, muscle strength, and function in patients with TKA. **Methods**: The following databases were used: PubMed, Web of Science, the Cochrane Library, and Embase. Randomized controlled trials that administered resistance training to patients undergoing TKA and measured pain, strength, and function were included. The risk of bias was assessed using the Cochrane Risk of Bias 2.0 tool. Effect sizes were calculated using Hedges' g and are presented as Standardized Mean Differences (SMDs) with 95% Confidence Intervals (CIs). Subgroup analyses were conducted to determine the effect size based on the type and duration of the intervention. **Results**: The study selection process resulted in the inclusion of seven studies comprising a total of 439 participants. The bias assessment found that three studies had a low risk of bias and four had some concerns. Resistance training was effective in improving pain (SMD: 0.84, 95% CI: 0.11; 1.57, I^2: 89.6%), muscle strength (SMD: 1.03, 95% CI: 0.29; 1.77, I^2: 83.1%), self-reported function (SMD: 1.58, 95% CI: 0.15; 3.01, I^2: 93.1%), and performance-based function (SMD: 0.74, 95% CI: 0.38; 1.11, I^2: 68.9%). Subgroup analysis revealed significant differences in pain, strength, and performance-based function by comparison group, performance-based function by intervention duration, and self-reported function by intervention type. **Conclusions**: Resistance training improves pain, muscle strength, and function in TKA patients. Additionally, resistance training appears particularly effective when implemented as a standalone intervention or for durations under 12 weeks. These findings suggest that the design of resistance training protocols should be considered in clinical practice.

Keywords: total knee arthroplasty; resistance training; pain; muscle strength; function

1. Introduction

Osteoarthritis (OA) is one of the most common musculoskeletal diseases. It causes severe disability, particularly in weight-bearing knee joints; surgical intervention is often required due to pain and stiffness [1]. Total Knee Arthroplasty (TKA) is a common surgery for patients with end-stage OA. Over 100,000 cases are performed each year in the UK and 700,000 cases are performed each year in the US. This number is expected to increase in the future [2]. TKA is the most clinically and cost-effective method for maintaining patients' long-term health and functional status [3]. However, complications such as instability, stiffness, and disruption of the extensor mechanism may occur after surgery, so postoperative management is important [4].

In particular, the strength of the quadriceps femoris muscle decreases over the course of several months following TKA surgery [5]. Quadriceps femoris strength after TKA surgery is a key factor that positively affects patient expectations, symptoms, satisfaction, and functional activities [6]. In particular, it is closely related to functional outcomes such as functional mobility, stair climbing, quality of life, and activities of daily living [7]. Therefore, interventions such as preserving motor control, improving nutrition, and strengthening muscles are necessary after TKA surgery [5]. Among these interventions, resistance training has been reported to effectively strengthen muscles [8,9]. The American Physical Therapy Association recommends that TKA patients begin resistance exercise within seven days of surgery, and that it be performed gradually to improve strength, function, and range of motion [10].

Accordingly, the importance of resistance training has been increasingly emphasized for patients who have undergone TKA, and meta-analyses are continuously being conducted to analyze its effects [11–13]. However, previous meta-analyses included studies that implemented interventions or measurements prior to TKA surgery. Moreover, there remains a lack of studies that compare the effects of different intervention durations, as well as the single and multicomponent effects of resistance training. Therefore, this systematic review and meta-analysis aimed to evaluate the effects of resistance training on pain, muscle strength, and function in patients after TKA surgery, and to explore differences according to intervention duration and type through subgroup analysis.

2. Materials and Methods

This systematic review and meta-analysis was conducted in accordance with the PRISMA 2020 guidelines and the Cochrane Handbook for Systematic Reviews of Interventions [14,15]. Additionally, the study was prospectively registered in PROSPERO prior to its commencement (CRD42025640995).

2.1. Eligibility Criteria and Exclusion Criteria

The study inclusion criteria were selected using the PICOS method. Patients: Patients who underwent TKA surgery; Intervention: Inclusion of resistance or strength training in the intervention protocol; Comparison: No-intervention, usual care, or comparator without resistance or strength training in the protocol; Outcome: Pain, muscle strength, performance-based function, and patient-reported function; Study: Randomized clinical trials (RCTs). Studies were excluded from the analysis if they met any of the following criteria: Presence of other diseases after TKA, lack of information on resistance or strength training in the intervention protocol, absence of the full text, or non-English language version.

2.2. Search Strategy

The data search was conducted on 22 January 2025. The databases used were PubMed, Web of Science, the Cochrane Library, and Embase. The search included studies from database inception to 22 January 2025. The search terms were "Total knee arthroplasty", "Resistance training", and "Strength training". The Supplementary Material includes detailed search strategies (Table S1). In addition, the reference lists of the included studies were reviewed to identify further relevant studies. Two independent reviewers (J.-H.L. and B.-G.K.) conducted the study selection. Any disagreements were resolved through discussion and consensus.

2.3. Data Collection

The retrieved studies were managed using EndNote 2018, and the collected data were organized using Excel 2022. The collected data items were the study title, year of publication, number of participants, sex, age, Body Mass Index (BMI), the intervention method of the experimental and comparison groups, the number of sessions, exercise intensity, outcome, and the pre- and post-intervention mean and standard deviation values.

To prevent overestimating the effect size when outcomes of the same category exist, we collected them in a prioritized manner. For pain, we prioritized structured tools such as the Western Ontario and MacMaster Universities Osteoarthritis Index (WOMAC) and the Knee Injury and Osteoarthritis Outcome Score (KOOS) over simple measures such as Visual Analogue Scale (VAS). For strength, we prioritized the strength of the quadriceps femoris muscle. Function collected self-reported and performance-based outcomes. The self-reported function included tools to assess Activities of Daily Living (ADL), such as the WOMAC function, the KOOS ADL, and the Hospital for Special Surgery (HSS) knee score. Two independent reviewers (J.-H.L. and B.-G.K) conducted the study selection and data extraction. Any discrepancies were resolved through discussion and consensus.

2.4. Assessment of Risk of Bias and Certainty of Evidence

The risk of bias in the included studies was assessed using the Cochrane Risk of Bias 2 (ROB 2) tool. The ROB 2 tool assesses five domains: The randomization process, deviations from intended interventions, missing outcome data, measurement of the outcome, and selection of the reported result. In addition, the certainty of evidence for the overall pooled results was evaluated using the GRADE (Grading of Recommendations, Assessment, Development and Evaluations) approach, which considers five factors: Risk of bias, inconsistency, indirectness, imprecision, and publication bias. Based on these domains, the overall certainty of evidence was rated as high, moderate, low, or very low [16]. Based on these domains, the overall certainty of evidence was rated as high, moderate, low, or very low. Two independent reviewers (J.-H.L. and B.-G.K) conducted the risk of bias and certainty of evidence assessments and compared the results. Any discrepancies were resolved through discussion and consensus.

2.5. Statistical Analysis

A meta-analysis was conducted using R Studio 4.3.1 software. Since all collected outcomes were continuous and the characteristics of the participants and intervention methods were diverse, a random-effects model with restricted maximum likelihood (REML) estimation was selected. The mean difference was calculated using the pre- and post-intervention means and standard deviations of the experimental and comparison groups. Since the same outcome was assessed using different instruments across studies, the effect sizes were expressed as Standardized Mean Differences (SMDs). The effect size was calculated using Hedges' g. A small effect size is 0.3, a medium effect size is 0.5, and a large effect size is 0.8 [17]. The results are presented as SMDs and 95% Confidence Intervals (CIs) via forest plots for visual analysis. Heterogeneity between studies was assessed using both the I^2 statistic and Cochran's Q test. I^2 values of 25%, 50%, and 75% were interpreted as indicating low, moderate, and high heterogeneity [18], respectively, and a p-value less than 0.05 was considered statistically significant.

Subgroup analyses were conducted based on comparison group, intervention duration, and type. The comparison group was categorized as either no-intervention or other intervention to examine whether the type of control condition influenced the treatment effects. The duration was categorized as less than 12 weeks or 12 weeks or more to examine whether the duration of the intervention influenced the effect size. The intervention type was classified as either resistance training alone or multicomponent training to compare the effects of resistance training alone versus in combination with other components. These subgroupings were used to further explore the differential effects of intervention characteristics. Egger's regression analysis and funnel plots were not used to assess publication bias, as fewer than 10 studies were included. A sensitivity analysis was performed to assess whether exclusion of a study with an outlying effect size would substantially affect the overall results.

3. Results

3.1. Research Selection Process

A total of 942 studies were retrieved, including 165 from the PubMed database, 351 from the Web of Science database, 208 from the Cochrane Library database, and 198 from the Embase database. After removing 321 duplicates from the initial 621 records, 598 studies were excluded during title and abstract screening, and one study was excluded because the full-text report was not retrievable. As a result, 22 studies were selected for full-text review. After reading the original texts, 15 studies were excluded because they did not meet this study's selection criteria. As a result, seven studies were included in the final analysis [19–25] (Figure 1).

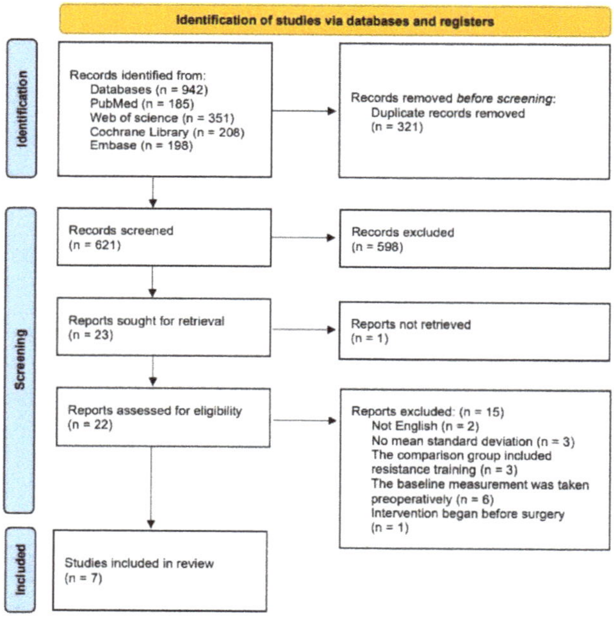

Figure 1. Research selection process.

The reasons for exclusion included not being written in English, lack of standard deviation data, inclusion of resistance training in the comparison group, baseline measurements taken preoperatively, and interventions applied before surgery [26–40]. The Jiao et al. study [40], which investigated high-intensity progressive training in TKA patients, was excluded because the strength training was conducted preoperatively. The reasons for excluding other papers are provided in Supplementary Table S2.

3.2. General Characteristics of Included Studies

A total of 439 participants were included across seven studies. The interventions applied included elastic band exercises, machine-based resistance training, aquatic resistance training, and isometric strength training. The intervention duration ranged from four weeks to one year. Various intensities were applied, including moderate intensity, One Repetition Maximum (1RM), and repetitions per set. The collected outcomes included pain, which was assessed using the WOMAC, the KOOS, VAS, and activity-specific pain. Muscle strength assessment focused on knee extensor strength. Self-reported function was assessed using the WOMAC Function, KOOS ADL, and the HSS knee score. Performance-based function was measured using the 40 m brisk walking test, the 8 ft up-and-go test, gait speed, maximal walking speed, and maximal velocity (Table S3).

3.3. Risk of Bias in Studies

Seven studies were assessed for bias using ROB 2. The randomization process was assessed as low risk in five studies and as having some concerns in two studies. The effect of intervention assignment was assessed as low risk in three studies and as having some concerns in four studies. Missing outcome data was assessed as low risk in four studies and as having some concerns in three studies. The measurement of the outcome was assessed as low risk in seven studies. The reported results were assessed as low risk in six studies and as having some concerns in one study. Overall, three studies were assessed as low risk, and four studies were assessed as having some concerns (Figure S1).

3.4. Meta-Analysis Results

3.4.1. Pain

Pain data were available from seven studies. A large effect size was observed for pain improvement through resistance training (SMD: 0.84, 95% CI: 0.11; 1.57). Heterogeneity was high ($I^2 = 89.6\%$) and statistically significant ($p < 0.05$) (Figure 2).

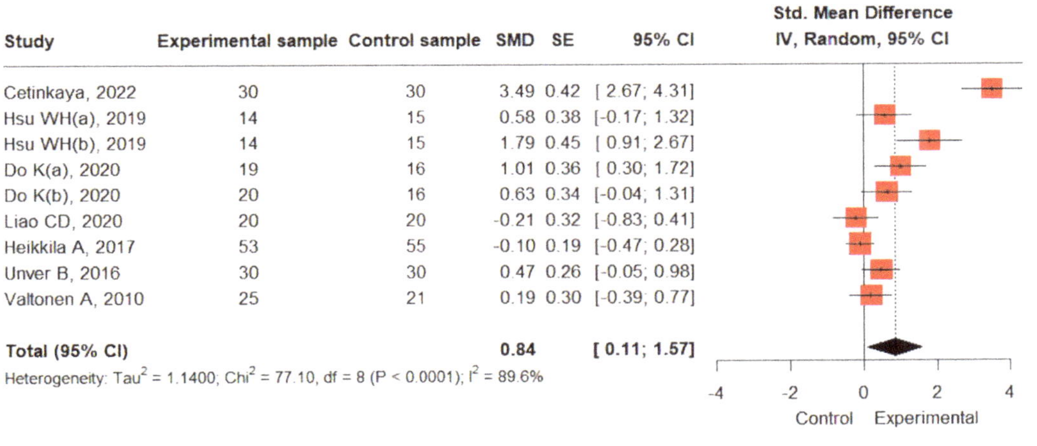

Figure 2. The effects of resistance training on pain [19–25].

3.4.2. Muscle Strength

Muscle strength data were available from four studies. A large effect size was observed for strength improvement through resistance training (SMD: 1.03, 95% CI: 0.29; 1.77). Heterogeneity was high ($I^2 = 83.1\%$) and statistically significant ($p < 0.05$) (Figure 3).

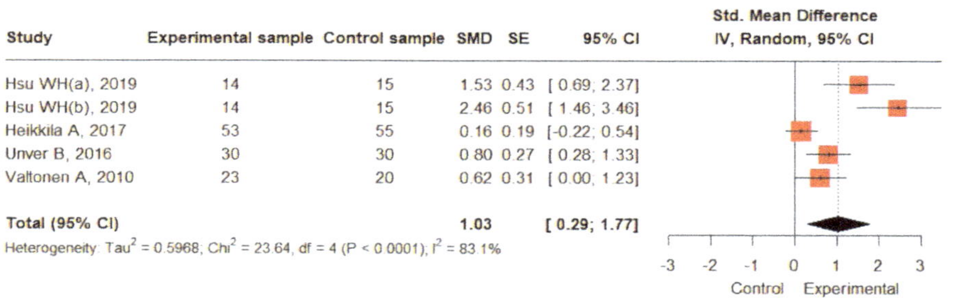

Figure 3. The effects of resistance training on muscle strength [20,23–25].

3.4.3. Self-Reported Function

Self-reported function data were available from six studies. A large effect size was observed for self-reported functional improvement through resistance training (SMD: 1.58, 95% CI: 0.15; 3.01). Heterogeneity was high ($I^2 = 93.1\%$) and statistically significant ($p < 0.05$) (Figure 4).

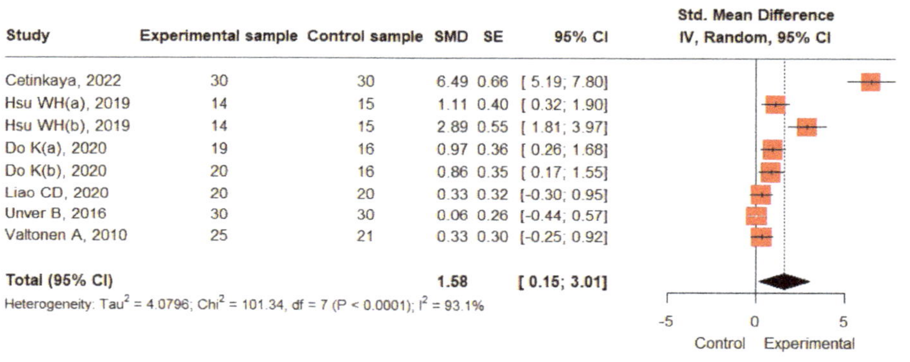

Figure 4. The effects of resistance training on self-reported function [19–22,24,25].

3.4.4. Performance-Based Function

Performance-based function data were available from seven studies. A moderate effect size was observed for performance-based functional improvement through resistance training (SMD: 0.74, 95% CI: 0.38; 1.11). Heterogeneity was moderate ($I^2 = 68.9\%$) and statistically significant ($p < 0.05$) (Figure 5).

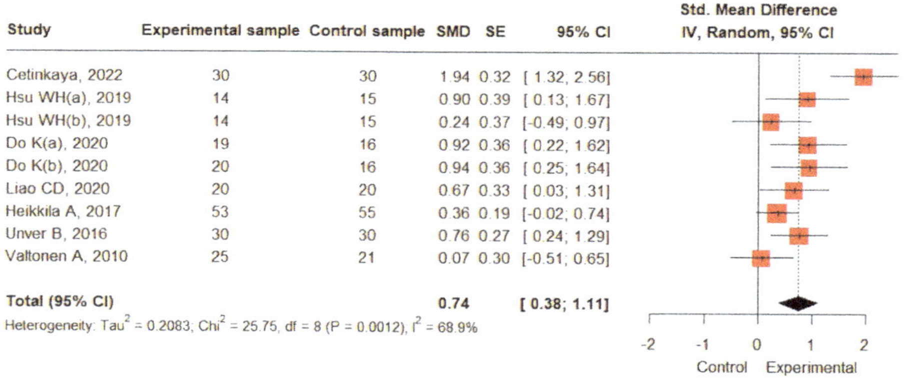

Figure 5. The effects of resistance training on performance-based function [19–25].

3.5. Subgroup Analysis

Subgroup analysis was conducted based on comparison group, intervention duration, and intervention type. Significant effects were observed in the other intervention group for all outcomes, whereas no significant effects were found in the no-intervention group. Subgroup differences were statistically significant for pain, strength, and performance-based function ($p < 0.05$), but not for self-reported function ($p > 0.05$). For intervention duration, pain showed a significant effect when the duration was less than 12 weeks, while strength and performance-based function showed significant effects regardless of duration. A significant subgroup difference was found only for performance-based function ($p < 0.05$). Subgroup differences for pain, strength, and self-reported function were not statistically significant ($p > 0.05$). Regarding intervention type, resistance training alone showed significant effects for strength and self-reported function, whereas multicomponent interventions did not. A significant subgroup difference was observed only for self-reported function ($p < 0.05$). Detailed results are shown in Table 2.

Table 1. Subgroup analysis of the effects of intervention duration and type.

Outcome	Subgroup	Study		Effect Size (SMD [95% CI])	I^2	Test for Subgroup Difference
Pain	Comparison group	[19–22,24]	Other intervention	1.08 [0.20; 1.97]	89.8%	$p = 0.023$
		[23,25]	No intervention	−0.01 [−0.33; 0.31]	0%	
	Intervention Duration	[19,21,24]	~11 weeks	1.38 [0.02; 2.74]	92.6%	$p = 0.199$
		[20,22,23,25]	12 weeks~	0.39 [−0.26; 1.04]	77.2%	
	Intervention type	[19–22,25]	Resistance only	1.05 [0.14; 1.96]	90.2%	$p = 0.101$
		[23,24]	Multicomponent	0.16 [−0.39; 0.71]	66.8%	
Muscle strength	Comparison group	[20,24]	Other intervention	1.52 [0.59; 2.46]	77.4%	$p = 0.022$
		[23,25]	No intervention	0.32 [−0.10; 0.75]	34.4%	
	Intervention Duration	[20,23,25]	~11 weeks	1.12 [0.14; 2.10]	87.1%	$p = 0.580$
		[24]	12 weeks~	0.80 [0.28; 1.33]	-	
	Intervention type	[20,25]	Resistance only	1.48 [0.43; 2.52]	80.4%	$p = 0.101$
		[23,24]	Multicomponent	0.46 [−0.17; 1.08]	73.5%	
Self-reported function	Comparison group	[19–22,24]	Other intervention	1.77 [0.15; 3.38]	93.9%	$p = 0.102$
		[25]	No intervention	0.33 [−0.25; 0.92]	-	
	Intervention Duration	[19,21,24]	~11 weeks	2.05 [−0.79; 4.90]	96.3%	$p = 0.542$
		[20,22,25]	12 weeks~	1.10 [−0.02; 2.22]	84.7%	

Table 2. Subgroup analysis of the effects of intervention duration and type.

Outcome	Subgroup	Study		Effect Size (SMD [95% CI])	I^2	Test for Subgroup Difference
	Intervention type	[19–22,25]	Resistance only	1.80 [0.22; 3.39]	93.3%	$p = 0.041$
		[24]	Multicomponent	0.06 [−0.44; 0.57]	-	
Performance-based function	Comparison group	[19–22,24]	Other intervention	0.92 [0.53; 1.31]	59.2%	$p = 0.011$
		[23,25]	No intervention	0.27 [−0.05; 0.59]	0%	
	Intervention Duration	[19,21,24]	~11 weeks	1.14 [0.60; 1.68]	66.9%	$p = 0.014$
		[20,22,23,25]	12 weeks~	0.39 [0.14; 0.65]	0%	
	Intervention type	[19–22,25]	Resistance only	0.81 [0.34; 1.28]	72.6%	$p = 0.345$
		[23,24]	Multicomponent	0.52 [0.13; 0.91]	34.4%	

SMD: Standardized mean difference; CI: Confidence interval.

3.6. Sensitivity Analysis

Due to the high heterogeneity of the study results, a sensitivity analysis was conducted. Additional analyses were conducted after excluding the study by Çetinkaya [17], due to its high heterogeneity in effect sizes. As a result, significant effects were found on pain (SMD: 0.48, 95% CI: 0.07; 0.89, I^2: 79.2%), self-reported function (SMD: 0.86, 95% CI: 0.24; 1.47, I^2: 77.2%), and performance-based function (SMD: 0.56, 95% CI: 0.33; 0.79, I^2: 14.5%).

3.7. Certainty of Evidence

The certainty of the evidence was assessed using the GRADE approach. The certainty was rated as moderate for pain, strength, and performance-based function due to serious risk of bias and inconsistency, but with no serious concerns about indirectness or imprecision. For self-reported function, the certainty was rated as low because of very serious inconsistency, serious imprecision, and serious risk of bias (Table S4).

4. Discussion

This systematic review and meta-analysis suggests that resistance training may lead to improvements in pain, muscle strength, and functional outcomes (WOMAC, KOOS, HSS knee score, and gait speed) among patients undergoing TKA. Additionally, subgroup analyses revealed that the effects were more pronounced when the interventions lasted fewer than 12 weeks and when resistance training was the only type of exercise performed. However, heterogeneity was high, and the risk of bias assessment showed that three studies were at low risk and four had some concerns, indicating that the overall findings were favorable but should be interpreted with caution.

A previous meta-analysis reported that active resistance exercise of the lower limbs was positively associated with pain relief, recovery of muscle strength, improved mobility, and enhanced physical function in patients who underwent TKA [11]. Another meta-analysis reported that strength training improved the distance covered in the six-minute walking test in patients with TKA [12]. In contrast, a meta-analysis with conflicting findings reported that, compared to standard rehabilitation, progressive resistance training did not significantly change functional capacity or muscle strength in patients with TKA or total hip arthroplasty [13]. The observed variations in outcomes are hypothesized to be attributable to disparities in the characteristics of the subjects included in the study and the outcomes collected. Only TKA patients were included in this meta-analysis. To ensure consistency in effect size calculation when multiple outcomes were available, subitems of the WOMAC and KOOS and walking speed were prioritized for inclusion. This may explain why the results differed from those of previous studies.

Resistance training contributes to pain relief through physiological mechanisms, including protein remodeling, reduced relative load, and decreased pain sensitivity via central inhibitory mechanisms [41–43]. Additionally, weakness in the quadriceps femoris negatively affects the long-term prognosis and functional recovery of TKA patients. Incorporating resistance training into the intervention program effectively improves physical function [44]. Following TKA surgery, lower extremity muscles such as the quadriceps femoris and biceps femoris lose 50–60% of their preoperative strength. This loss results in a decline in patients' functional mobility and ability to perform activities of daily living, such as rising from a chair, stair climbing, and walking at an adequate speed [45]. Walking speed is a critical outcome for TKA patients, strongly influenced by quadriceps femoris strength [46].

Between comparison groups, statistically significant subgroup differences were observed for pain, strength, and performance-based function, with the other intervention group showing more effective outcomes compared to the no-intervention group. For self-reported function, the effect size was also somewhat larger in the other intervention group, although this difference was not statistically significant. When analyzing studies in this review that compared resistance training to no intervention, Heikkilä et al. [23] reported that it was difficult to control the exercise load in a home-based program, and participant compliance declined during the final month. Valtonen et al. [25] reported that the participants' favorable baseline condition may have limited the potential for additional improvements, and that the training intensity was difficult to define because it was unclear whether the participants had actually reached fatigue, despite being instructed to exercise at maximum effort. These results suggest that the intensity and control of resistance training could potentially affect the effectiveness of the intervention. A study analyzing the dose–response relationship of resistance training in adults found that setting the intensity at 50–69% of 1RM produced the greatest improvement in symptoms, function, and lower extremity muscle strength [47]. In contrast, some studies found no significant difference between high- and low-intensity training. [48]. To improve strength, it is necessary to consider various training variables such as intensity, number of sets, and training frequency, as their combination can influence the effectiveness of the intervention [49]. Therefore, more high-quality studies are needed to clarify the causes of these conflicting results and understand the effects of resistance training.

A statistically significant subgroup difference by intervention duration was found for performance-based function, with greater effects seen in interventions lasting less than 12 weeks. Similar trends were noted for the other outcomes, although these differences did not reach statistical significance. These findings regarding intervention duration in the current meta-analysis differ from those of a previous meta-analysis [12], which reported that increasing the duration and frequency of resistance training improved gait and functional outcomes in patients with TKA. This discrepancy may be attributed to differences in participant characteristics or intervention protocols. To clarify this issue, a future meta-analysis incorporating additional studies is warranted. Regarding the optimal duration of resistance training, Monsegue et al. [44] reported that high-intensity resistance training performed three times per week for at least eight weeks was most effective in improving muscle strength and function during recovery after TKA.

In terms of intervention type, a statistically significant subgroup difference was found for self-reported outcomes, with resistance training alone being more effective than when it was included as part of a multicomponent intervention. A similar tendency was observed for pain, strength, and performance-based function, although these differences did not reach statistical significance. A previous meta-analysis showed that, compared to resistance training alone, concurrent resistance and aerobic training was equally effective in increasing muscle mass in middle-aged and older adults [50]. Additionally, a meta-analysis targeting patients with knee osteoarthritis found that a single type of exercise was more effective than a combined exercise program that included resistance, aerobic, and functional training [51]. This may be due to training time and effort being divided among multiple components, potentially diluting the neuromuscular stimulus of resistance training. Another possible explanation is the interference effect. In this study, the multicomponent interventions included flexibility training and functional tasks such as toe raises and step exercises. Although these components do not constitute endurance training per se, their repetitive and low-intensity nature may resemble endurance-type activity. Prior research suggests that combining endurance and resistance training can attenuate muscular adaptations compared to resistance training alone, indicating the possibility that similar interference effects may have occurred in the multicomponent groups [52]. Wilson et al. [53] reported that performing endurance and strength training simultaneously may inhibit maximum power and rate of force development due to interference effects. These findings align with the trends observed in the present study and suggest that the proportion of resistance training within multicomponent protocols could potentially influence the outcomes. However, given the largely exploratory nature of these subgroup findings, cautious interpretation is warranted, and further studies are required to confirm these outcomes.

This meta-analysis has several limitations. First, the number of studies included was relatively small compared to previous meta-analyses. This was primarily due to the exclusion of studies that initiated interventions or measured baseline outcomes prior to surgery, as the present analysis focused exclusively on the effects of resistance training after TKA. These criteria allowed for the analysis of the isolated effects of resistance training following TKA surgery. However, preoperative age and WOMAC pain and function scores should be considered collectively due to their impact on postoperative prognosis [54]. Second, as reported in previous meta-analyses [11–13], overall heterogeneity was high. This likely stems from differences in subject characteristics, intervention methods, and training intensity. Future studies should be conducted to clearly evaluate the effectiveness of resistance training after TKA surgery. These studies should be high-quality RCTs that standardize the components of the interventions and minimize dropout rates and missing data. Third, this review did not include a search of grey literature, which may have resulted in the omission of unpublished studies. Furthermore, data collection may have been incomplete, as no attempts were made to contact study authors when full texts were unavailable.

5. Conclusions

This meta-analysis suggests that resistance training may contribute to improvements in pain, muscle strength, and function among patients with TKA. Furthermore, it was observed that the intervention tended to be more effective when the duration was less than 12 weeks and when resistance training was applied alone. These findings may help inform the design of resistance training protocols in clinical settings. Future studies should be high-quality RCTs with standardized intervention timing, intensity, and composition.

Supplementary Materials: The following supporting information can be downloaded at: https://www.mdpi.com/article/10.3390/jcm14144979/s1, Table S1: Search strategy; Table S2: List of excluded studies; Table S3: Characteristics of studies included in the systematic review; Table S4: Certainty of evidence; Figure S1: Risk of bias in studies.

Author Contributions: Author Contributions: Conceptualization, J.L. and B.K.; methodology, J.L. and B.K.; software, J.L.; validation, J.L. and B.K.; formal analysis, J.L. and B.K.; investigation, J.L. and B.K.; resources, J.L.; data curation, J.L.; writing—original draft preparation, J.L. and B.K.; writing—review and editing, J.L. and B.K.; visualization, J.L.; supervision, B.K.; project administration, B.K. All authors have read and agreed to the published version of the manuscript.

Funding: This research received no external funding.

Institutional Review Board Statement: Not applicable.

Informed Consent Statement: Not applicable.

Data Availability Statement: Data can be requested from the corresponding author and will be released on reasonable request.

Conflicts of Interest: The authors declare no conflicts of interest.

Abbreviations

The following abbreviations are used in this manuscript:

OA	Osteoarthritis
TKA	Total Knee Arthroplasty
RCTs	Randomized Clinical Trials
BMI	Body Mass Index
WOMAC	Western Ontario and MacMaster Universities Osteoarthritis Index
KOOS	Knee Injury and Osteoarthritis Outcome Score
VAS	Visual Analogue Scale
ADL	Activities of Daily Living
HSS	Hospital for Special Surgery
ROB 2	Risk of Bias 2
SMD	Standardized Mean Difference
CIs	Confidence Intervals
1RM	One Repetition Maximum

References

1. Neuprez, A.; Neuprez, A.H.; Kurth, W.; Gillet, P.; Bruyère, O.; Reginster, J.Y. Profile of osteoarthritic patients undergoing hip or knee arthroplasty, a step toward a definition of the "need for surgery". *Aging Clin. Exp. Res.* **2018**, *30*, 315–321. [CrossRef] [PubMed]
2. Hamilton, D.F.; Beard, D.J.; Barker, K.L.; Macfarlane, G.J.; Tuck, C.E.; Stoddart, A.; Wilton, T.; Hutchinson, J.D.; Murray, G.D.; Simpson, A.H.R.W.; et al. Targeting rehabilitation to improve outcomes after total knee arthroplasty in patients at risk of poor outcomes: Randomised controlled trial. *BMJ* **2020**, *371*, m3576. [CrossRef]
3. Ho, D.M.; Huo, M.H. Are critical pathways and implant standardization programs effective in reducing costs in total knee replacement operations? *J. Am. Coll. Surg.* **2007**, *205*, 97–100. [CrossRef] [PubMed]
4. Healy, W.L.; Della Valle, C.J.; Iorio, R.; Berend, K.R.; Cushner, F.D.; Dalury, D.F.; Lonner, J.H. Complications of total knee arthroplasty: Standardized list and definitions of the Knee Society. *Clin. Orthop. Relat. Res.* **2013**, *471*, 215–220. [CrossRef]
5. Paravlic, A.H.; Meulenberg, C.J.; Drole, K. The Time Course of Quadriceps Strength Recovery After Total Knee Arthroplasty Is Influenced by Body Mass Index, Sex, and Age of Patients: Systematic Review and Meta-Analysis. *Front. Med.* **2022**, *9*, 865412. [CrossRef] [PubMed]
6. Furu, M.; Ito, H.; Nishikawa, T.; Nankaku, M.; Kuriyama, S.; Ishikawa, M.; Nakamura, S.; Azukizawa, M.; Hamamoto, Y.; Matsuda, S. Quadriceps strength affects patient satisfaction after total knee arthroplasty. *J. Orthop. Sci.* **2016**, *21*, 38–43. [CrossRef]
7. Mizner, R.L.; Petterson, S.C.; Snyder-Mackler, L. Quadriceps strength and the time course of functional recovery after total knee arthroplasty. *J. Orthop. Sports Phys. Ther.* **2005**, *35*, 424–436. [CrossRef]

8. Currier, B.S.; Mcleod, J.C.; Banfield, L.; Beyene, J.; Welton, N.J.; D'Souza, A.C.; Keogh, J.A.J.; Lin, L.; Coletta, G.; Yang, A.; et al. Resistance training prescription for muscle strength and hypertrophy in healthy adults: A systematic review and Bayesian network meta-analysis. *Br. J. Sports Med.* **2023**, *57*, 1211–1220. [CrossRef]
9. Lim, J.H.; Choi, A.Y.; Kim, B.G. The Effects of Resistance Training on Pain, Strength, and Function in Osteoarthritis: Systematic Review and Meta-Analysis. *J. Pers. Med.* **2024**, *14*, 1130. [CrossRef]
10. Jette, D.U.; Hunter, S.J.; Burkett, L.; Langham, B.; Logerstedt, D.S.; Piuzzi, N.S.; Poirier, N.M.; Radach, L.J.L.; Ritter, J.E.; Scalzitti, D.A.; et al. Physical Therapist Management of Total Knee Arthroplasty. *Phys. Ther.* **2020**, *100*, 1603–1631. [CrossRef]
11. Wei, G.; Shang, Z.; Li, Y.; Wu, Y.; Zhang, L. Effects of lower-limb active resistance exercise on mobility, physical function, knee strength and pain intensity in patients with total knee arthroplasty: A systematic review and meta-analysis. *BMC Musculoskelet. Disord.* **2024**, *25*, 730. [CrossRef] [PubMed]
12. Wang, J.; Zhu, R.; Xu, X.T.; Liu, S.; Li, Z.; Guo, C.; Tao, X.; Qian, L.; Charles, R.; Fang, L. Effects of strength training on functional ambulation following knee replacement: A systematic review, meta-analysis, and meta-regression. *Sci. Rep.* **2023**, *13*, 10728. [CrossRef]
13. Chen, X.; Li, X.; Zhu, Z.; Wang, H.; Yu, Z.; Bai, X. Effects of progressive resistance training for early postoperative fast-track total hip or knee arthroplasty: A systematic review and meta-analysis. *Asian J. Surg.* **2021**, *44*, 1245–1253. [CrossRef]
14. Page, M.J.; McKenzie, J.E.; Bossuyt, P.M.; Boutron, I.; Hoffmann, T.C.; Mulrow, C.D.; Shamseer, L.; Tetzlaff, J.M.; Akl, E.A.; Brennan, S.E.; et al. The PRISMA 2020 statement: An updated guideline for reporting systematic reviews. *BMJ* **2021**, *372*, n71. [CrossRef]
15. Chandler, J.; Cumpston, M.; Li, T.; Page, M.J.; Welch, V.J.H.W. *Cochrane Handbook for Systematic Reviews of Interventions*; Wiley: Hoboken, NJ, USA, 2019.
16. Guyatt, G.; Oxman, A.D.; Akl, E.A.; Kunz, R.; Vist, G.; Brozek, J.; Norris, S.; Falck-Ytter, Y.; Glasziou, P.; DeBeer, H.; et al. GRADE guidelines: 1. Introduction-GRADE evidence profiles and summary of findings tables. *J. Clin. Epidemiol.* **2011**, *64*, 383–394. [CrossRef] [PubMed]
17. Cohen, J. *Statistical Power Analysis for the Behavioral Sciences*, 2nd ed.; Routledge: New York, NY, USA, 1988.
18. Higgins, J.P.; Thompson, S.G.; Deeks, J.J.; Altman, D.G. Measuring inconsistency in meta-analyses. *BMJ* **2003**, *327*, 557–560. [CrossRef]
19. Çetinkaya, F.; Karakoyun, A. The effects of elastic band exercise on the pain, kinesiophobia, functional, and psychological status after total knee arthroplasty: A randomized controlled trial. *Clin. Rheumatol.* **2022**, *41*, 3179–3188. [CrossRef] [PubMed]
20. Hsu, W.H.; Hsu, W.B.; Shen, W.J.; Lin, Z.R.; Chang, S.H.; Hsu, R.W. Twenty-four-week hospital-based progressive resistance training on functional recovery in female patients post total knee arthroplasty. *Knee* **2019**, *26*, 729–736. [CrossRef]
21. Do, K.; Yim, J. Effects of Muscle Strengthening around the Hip on Pain, Physical Function, and Gait in Elderly Patients with Total Knee Arthroplasty: A Randomized Controlled Trial. *Healthcare* **2020**, *8*, 489. [CrossRef]
22. Liao, C.D.; Chiu, Y.S.; Ku, J.W.; Huang, S.W.; Liou, T.H. Effects of Elastic Resistance Exercise on Postoperative Outcomes Linked to the ICF Core Sets for Osteoarthritis after Total Knee Replacement in Overweight and Obese Older Women with Sarcopenia Risk: A Randomized Controlled Trial. *J. Clin. Med.* **2020**, *9*, 2194. [CrossRef]
23. Heikkilä, A.; Sevander-Kreus, N.; Häkkinen, A.; Vuorenmaa, M.; Salo, P.; Konsta, P.; Ylinen, J. Effect of total knee replacement surgery and postoperative 12 month home exercise program on gait parameters. *Gait. Posture* **2017**, *53*, 92–97. [CrossRef] [PubMed]
24. Unver, B.; Bakirhan, S.; Karatosun, V. Does a weight-training exercise programme given to patients four or more years after total knee arthroplasty improve mobility: A randomized controlled trial. *Arch. Gerontol. Geriatr.* **2016**, *64*, 45–50. [CrossRef]
25. Valtonen, A.; Pöyhönen, T.; Sipilä, S.; Heinonen, A. Effects of aquatic resistance training on mobility limitation and lower-limb impairments after knee replacement. *Arch. Phys. Med. Rehabil.* **2010**, *91*, 833–839. [CrossRef]
26. Hold, M. Strength and balance training before implantation of a total knee replacement. *Z. Orthop. Unfallchir.* **2024**, *162*, 12.
27. Chen, H.; Du Shan-shan, F.L.J.; Jiang, J.; Liang, X.Y.; Zhen, P.; Li, X.S.; Liu, J. Effects of combination therapy on the movement function of lower extremity after total knee arthroplasty in the elderly. *Chin. J. Tissue Eng. Res.* **2017**, *21*, 4939.
28. Vuorenmaa, M.; Ylinen, J.; Piitulainen, K.; Salo, P.; Kautiainen, H.; Pesola, M.; Häkkinen, A. Efficacy of a 12-month, monitored home exercise programme compared with normal care commencing 2 months after total knee arthroplasty: A randomized controlled trial. *J. Rehabil. Med.* **2014**, *46*, 166–172. [CrossRef] [PubMed]
29. Trudelle-Jackson, E.; Hines, E.; Medley, A.; Thompson, M. Exploration of Habitual Walking Behavior and Home-Based Muscle Power Training in Individuals with Total Knee Arthroplasty. *J. Phys. Act. Health* **2020**, *17*, 331–338. [CrossRef]
30. Husby, V.S.; Foss, O.A.; Husby, O.S.; Winther, S.B. Randomized controlled trial of maximal strength training vs. standard rehabilitation following total knee arthroplasty. *Eur. J. Phys. Rehabil. Med.* **2018**, *54*, 371–379. [CrossRef]
31. Shabbir, M.; Umar, B.; Ehsan, S.; Munir, S.; Bunin, U.; Sarfraz, K. Comparison of functional training and strength training in improving knee extension lag after first four weeks of total knee replacement. *Biomed. Res.* **2017**, *28*, 5623–5627.
32. Fung, V.; Ho, A.; Shaffer, J.; Chung, E.; Gomez, M. Use of Nintendo Wii Fit™ in the rehabilitation of outpatients following total knee replacement: A preliminary randomised controlled trial. *Physiotherapy* **2012**, *98*, 183–188. [CrossRef]
33. Codine, P.H.; Dellemme, Y.; Denis-Laroque, F.; Herisson, C.H. The use of low velocity submaximal eccentric contractions of the hamstring for recovery of full extension after total knee replacement: A randomized controlled study. *Isokinet. Exerc. Sci.* **2004**, *12*, 215–218. [CrossRef]

34. Tanaka, R.; Hayashizaki, T.; Taniguchi, R.; Kobayashi, J.; Umehara, T. Effect of an intensive functional rehabilitation program on the recovery of activities of daily living after total knee arthroplasty: A multicenter, randomized, controlled trial. *J. Orthop. Sci.* **2020**, *25*, 285–290. [CrossRef] [PubMed]
35. Risso, A.M.; van der Linden, M.L.; Bailey, A.; Gallacher, P.; Gleeson, N. Exploratory insights into novel prehabilitative neuromuscular exercise-conditioning in total knee arthroplasty. *BMC Musculoskelet. Disord.* **2022**, *23*, 547. [CrossRef]
36. Mau-Moeller, A.; Behrens, M.; Finze, S.; Bruhn, S.; Bader, R.; Mittelmeier, W. The effect of continuous passive motion and sling exercise training on clinical and functional outcomes following total knee arthroplasty: A randomized active-controlled clinical study. *Health Qual. Life Outcomes* **2014**, *12*, 68. [CrossRef]
37. Li, Z.; Li, B.; Wang, G.; Wang, K.; Chen, J.; Liang, Y.; Tang, X.; Yang, Y. Impact of enhanced recovery nursing combined with limb training on knee joint function and neurological function after total knee arthroplasty in patients with knee osteoarthritis. *Am. J. Transl. Res.* **2021**, *13*, 6864–6872.
38. Jakobsen, T.L.; Kehlet, H.; Husted, H.; Petersen, J.; Bandholm, T. Early progressive strength training to enhance recovery after fast-track total knee arthroplasty: A randomized controlled trial. *Arthritis Care. Res.* **2014**, *66*, 1856–1866. [CrossRef] [PubMed]
39. Jacksteit, R.; Stöckel, T.; Behrens, M.; Feldhege, F.; Bergschmidt, P.; Bader, R.; Mittelmeier, W.; Skripitz, R.; Mau-Moeller, A. Low-Load Unilateral and Bilateral Resistance Training to Restore Lower Limb Function in the Early Rehabilitation After Total Knee Arthroplasty: A Randomized Active-Controlled Clinical Trial. *Front. Med.* **2021**, *8*, 628021. [CrossRef]
40. Jiao, S.; Feng, Z.; Dai, T.; Huang, J.; Liu, R.; Meng, Q. High-Intensity Progressive Rehabilitation Versus Routine Rehabilitation After Total Knee Arthroplasty: A Randomized Controlled Trial. *J. Arthroplast.* **2024**, *39*, 665–671. [CrossRef]
41. Hägg, G.M. Human muscle fibre abnormalities related to occupational load. *Eur. J. Appl. Physiol.* **2000**, *83*, 159–165. [CrossRef]
42. Belavy, D.L.; Van Oosterwijck, J.; Clarkson, M.; Dhondt, E.; Mundell, N.L.; Miller, C.T.; Owen, P.J. Pain sensitivity is reduced by exercise training: Evidence from a systematic review and meta-analysis. *Neurosci. Biobehav. Rev.* **2021**, *120*, 100–108. [CrossRef]
43. Coury, H.J.; Moreira, R.F.; Dias, N.B. Evaluation of the effectiveness of workplace exercise in controlling neck, shoulder and low back pain: A systematic review. *Braz. J. Phys. Ther.* **2009**, *13*, 461–479. [CrossRef]
44. Monsegue, A.P.; Emans, P.; van Loon, L.J.C.; Verdijk, L.B. Resistance exercise training to improve post-operative rehabilitation in knee arthroplasty patients: A narrative review. *Eur. J. Sport Sci.* **2024**, *24*, 938–949. [CrossRef] [PubMed]
45. Judd, D.L.; Eckhoff, D.G.; Stevens-Lapsley, J.E. Muscle strength loss in the lower limb after total knee arthroplasty. *Am. J. Phys. Med. Rehabil.* **2012**, *91*, 220–226. [CrossRef] [PubMed]
46. Pua, Y.H.; Seah, F.J.T.; Clark, R.A.; Poon, C.L.L.; Tan, J.W.M.; Chong, H.C. Factors associated with gait speed recovery after total knee arthroplasty: A longitudinal study. *Semin. Arthritis Rheum.* **2017**, *46*, 544–551. [CrossRef]
47. Wang, H.; Ma, B.; Wang, G.; Wang, P.; Long, H.; Niu, S.; Dong, C.; Zhang, H.; Zhao, Z.; Ma, Q.; et al. Dose-Response Relationships of Resistance Training in Adults with Knee Osteoarthritis: A Systematic Review and Meta-analysis. *J. Geriatr. Phys. Ther.* **2024**, *47*, 97–109. [CrossRef]
48. Messier, S.P.; Mihalko, S.L.; Beavers, D.P.; Nicklas, B.J.; DeVita, P.; Carr, J.J.; Hunter, D.J.; Lyles, M.; Guermazi, A.; Bennell, K.L.; et al. Effect of High-Intensity Strength Training on Knee Pain and Knee Joint Compressive Forces Among Adults with Knee Osteoarthritis: The START Randomized Clinical Trial. *JAMA* **2021**, *325*, 646–657. [CrossRef]
49. Silva, N.L.; Oliveira, R.B.; Fleck, S.J.; Leon, A.C.; Farinatti, P. Influence of strength training variables on strength gains in adults over 55 years-old: A meta-analysis of dose-response relationships. *J. Sci. Med. Sport* **2014**, *17*, 337–344. [CrossRef]
50. Khalafi, M.; Kheradmand, S.; Habibi Maleki, A.; Symonds, M.E.; Rosenkranz, S.K.; Batrakoulis, A. The Effects of Concurrent Training Versus Aerobic or Resistance Training Alone on Body Composition in Middle-Aged and Older Adults: A Systematic Review and Meta-Analysis. *Healthcare* **2025**, *13*, 776. [CrossRef]
51. Juhl, C.; Christensen, R.; Roos, E.M.; Zhang, W.; Lund, H. Impact of exercise type and dose on pain and disability in knee osteoarthritis: A systematic review and meta-regression analysis of randomized controlled trials. *Arthritis. Rheumatol.* **2014**, *66*, 622–636. [CrossRef]
52. Leveritt, M.; Abernethy, P.J.; Barry, B.K.; Logan, P.A. Concurrent strength and endurance training. A review. *Sports Med.* **1999**, *28*, 413–427. [CrossRef]
53. Wilson, J.M.; Marin, P.J.; Rhea, M.R.; Wilson, S.M.; Loenneke, J.P.; Anderson, J.C. Concurrent training: A meta-analysis examining interference of aerobic and resistance exercises. *J. Strength Cond. Res.* **2012**, *26*, 2293–2307. [CrossRef] [PubMed]
54. Chang, C.B.; Yoo, J.H.; Koh, I.J.; Kang, Y.G.; Seong, S.C.; Kim, T.K. Key factors in determining surgical timing of total knee arthroplasty in osteoarthritic patients: Age, radiographic severity, and symptomatic severity. *J. Orthop. Traumatol.* **2010**, *11*, 21–27. [CrossRef] [PubMed]

MDPI AG
Grosspeteranlage 5
4052 Basel
Switzerland
Tel.: +41 61 683 77 34

Journal of Clinical Medicine Editorial Office
E-mail: jcm@mdpi.com
www.mdpi.com/journal/jcm

www.ingramcontent.com/pod-product-compliance
Lightning Source LLC
Chambersburg PA
CBHW061447210926
51850CB00008B/1638